MRI of the Newborn, Part 1

Guest Editors

THIERRY A.G.M. HUISMAN, MD
CLAUDIA M. HILLENBRAND, PhD

MAGNETIC RESONANCE IMAGING CLINICS OF NORTH AMERICA

www.mri.theclinics.com

Consulting Editors
VIVIAN S. LEE, MD, PhD, MBA
LYNNE STEINBACH, MD
SURESH MUKHERJI, MD

November 2011 • Volume 19 • Number 4

SAUNDERS an imprint of ELSEVIER, Inc.

W.B. SAUNDERS COMPANY
A Division of Elsevier Inc.

1600 John F. Kennedy Boulevard • Suite 1800 • Philadelphia, Pennsylvania 19103-2899

http://www.theclinics.com

MRI CLINICS OF NORTH AMERICA Volume 19, Number 4
November 2011 ISSN 1064-9689, ISBN 13: 978-1-4377-2692-3

Editor: Barton Dudlick
Developmental Editor: Donald Mumford

Magnetic Resonance Imaging Clinics of North America (ISSN 1064-9689) is published quarterly by Elsevier Inc., 360 Park Avenue South, New York, NY 10010-1710. Months of issue are February, May, August, and November. Business and Editorial Offices: 1600 John F. Kennedy Blvd., Ste. 1800, Philadelphia, PA 19103-2899. Customer Service Office: 3251 Riverport Lane, Maryland Heights, MO 63043. Periodicals postage paid at New York, NY and additional mailing offices. Subscription prices are $337.00 per year (domestic individuals), $541.00 per year (domestic institutions), $172.00 per year (domestic students/residents), $376.00 per year (Canadian individuals), $678.00 per year (Canadian institutions), $488.00 per year (international individuals), $678.00 per year (international institutions), and $249.00 per year (international and Canadian students/residents). International air speed delivery is included in all *Clinics* subscription prices. All prices are subject to change without notice. **POSTMASTER:** Send address changes to *Magnetic Resonance Imaging Clinics*, Elsevier Health Sciences Division, Subscription Customer Service, 3251 Riverport Lane, Maryland Heights, MO 63043. Customer Service (orders, claims, online, change of address): Elsevier Health Sciences Division, Subscription Customer Service, 3251 Riverport Lane, Maryland Heights, MO 63043. Tel:1-800-654-2452 (U.S. and Canada); 314-447-8871 (outside U.S. and Canada). Fax: 314-447-8029. E-mail: journalscustomerservice-usa@elsevier.com (for print support); journalsonlinesupport-usa@elsevier.com (for online support).

Reprints. For copies of 100 or more of articles in this publication, please contact the Commercial Reprints Department, Elsevier Inc., 360 Park Avenue South, New York, NY 10010-1710. Tel.: 212-633-3812; Fax: 212-462-1935; E-mail: reprints@elsevier.com.

Magnetic Resonance Imaging Clinics of North America is covered in the *RSNA Index of Imaging Literature, MEDLINE/PubMed (Index Medicus),* and *EMBASE/Excerpta Medica.*

Printed in the United States of America.

GOAL STATEMENT

The goal of *Magnetic Resonance Imaging Clinics of North America* is to keep practicing physicians up to date with current clinical practice by providing timely articles reviewing the state of the art in patient care.

ACCREDITATION

The *Magnetic Resonance Imaging Clinics of North America* is planned and implemented in accordance with the Essential Areas and Policies of the Accreditation Council for Continuing Medical Education (ACCME) through the joint sponsorship of the University of Virginia School of Medicine and Elsevier. The University of Virginia School of Medicine is accredited by the ACCME to provide continuing medical education for physicians.

The University of Virginia School of Medicine designates this enduring material activity for a maximum of 15 *AMA PRA Category 1 Credit*(s)™ for each issue, 60 credits per year. Physicians should claim only the credit commensurate with the extent of their participation in the activity.

The American Medical Association has determined that physicians not licensed in the US who participate in this CME enduring material activity are eligible for a maximum of **15** *AMA PRA Category 1 Credit*(s)™ for each issue, 60 credits per year.

Credit can be earned by reading the text material, taking the CME examination online at http://www.theclinics.com/home/cme, and completing the evaluation. After taking the test, you will be required to review any and all incorrect answers. Following completion of the test and evaluation, your credit will be awarded and you may print your certificate.

FACULTY DISCLOSURE/CONFLICT OF INTEREST

The University of Virginia School of Medicine, as an ACCME accredited provider, endorses and strives to comply with the Accreditation Council for Continuing Medical Education (ACCME) Standards of Commercial Support, Commonwealth of Virginia statutes, University of Virginia policies and procedures, and associated federal and private regulations and guidelines on the need for disclosure and monitoring of proprietary and financial interests that may affect the scientific integrity and balance of content delivered in continuing medical education activities under our auspices.

The University of Virginia School of Medicine requires that all CME activities accredited through this institution be developed independently and be scientifically rigorous, balanced and objective in the presentation/discussion of its content, theories and practices.

All authors/editors participating in an accredited CME activity are expected to disclose to the readers relevant financial relationships with commercial entities occurring within the past 12 months (such as grants or research support, employee, consultant, stock holder, member of speakers bureau, etc.). The University of Virginia School of Medicine will employ appropriate mechanisms to resolve potential conflicts of interest to maintain the standards of fair and balanced education to the reader. Questions about specific strategies can be directed to the Office of Continuing Medical Education, University of Virginia School of Medicine, Charlottesville, Virginia.

The faculty and staff of the University of Virginia Office of Continuing Medical Education have no financial affiliations to disclose.

The authors/editors listed below have identified no professional or financial affiliations for themselves or their spouse/partner:
Paul Babyn, MDCM, FRCP(C); Sarah Barth, (Acquisition Editor); Eduard de Lange, MD (Test Author); Charlotte Gilbert, MBChB, RANZCR; Nadine Girard, MD; P. Ellen Grant, MD; Sylviane Hanquinet, MD; Claudia M. Hillenbrand, PhD (Guest Editor); Thierry A.G.M. Huisman, MD, EQNR, FICIS (Guest Editor); Izlem Izbudak, MD; Vivian S. Lee, MD, PhD, MBA(Consulting Editor); Edward Lee, MD, MPH; Zoltán Patay, MD, PhD; Pedro S. Pinto, MD; Charles Raybaud, MD, FRCPC; Andrea Rossi, MD; Jacques F. Schneider, MD; Mariasavina Severino, MD; Melissa R. Spevak, MD; Aylin Tekes, MD; Emanuela R. Valsangiacomo Buechel, MD; and Rick R. van Rijn, MD, PhD.

The authors/editors listed below identified the following professional or financial affiliations for themselves or their spouse/partner:
Mark A. Fogel, MD receives grant support from Siemens Medical Solutions and Edwards Life Sciences, and receives support from Kereos and NIH.
Rajesh Krishnamurthy, MD receives research support from Philips MRI, and is on the Advisory Board for Toshiba/Vital Images.
Suresh K. Mukheri, MD (Consulting Editor) is a consultant for Philips.
Lynne Steinbach, MD (Consulting Editor) is a consultant for Synarc and Pfizer, Inc.

Disclosure of Discussion of non-FDA approved uses for pharmaceutical products and/or medical devices:
The University of Virginia School of Medicine, as an ACCME provider, requires that all faculty presenters identify and disclose any "off label" uses for pharmaceutical and medical device products. The University of Virginia School of Medicine recommends that each physician fully review all the available data on new products or procedures prior to instituting them with patients.

TO ENROLL

To enroll in the Magnetic Resonance Imaging Clinics of North America Continuing Medical Education program, call customer service at 1-800-654-2452 or visit us online at www.theclinics.com/home/cme. The CME program is available to subscribers for an additional fee of $196.00.

Contributors

CONSULTING EDITORS

VIVIAN S. LEE, MD, PhD, MBA
Professor of Radiology, Physiology, and
Neurosciences; Vice-Dean for Science; Senior
Vice-President and Chief Scientific Officer at
New York University Langone Medical Center,
New York, New York

LYNNE STEINBACH, MD
Professor of Clinical Radiology and
Orthopaedic Surgery at the University of
California San Francisco, San Francisco,
California

SURESH MUKHERJI, MD
Professor and Chief of Neuroradiology and
Head and Neck Radiology; Professor of
Radiology, Otolaryngology Head and Neck
Surgery, Radiation Oncology, Periodontics
and Oral Medicine, University of Michigan
Health System, Ann Arbor, Michigan

GUEST EDITORS

**THIERRY A.G.M. HUISMAN, MD,
EQNR, FICIS**
Professor, Division of Pediatric Radiology,
Department of Radiology and Radiological
Science, Johns Hopkins Hospital, Baltimore,
Maryland

CLAUDIA M. HILLENBRAND, PhD
Division of Translational Imaging Research,
Department of Radiological Sciences,
St. Jude Children's Research Hospital,
Memphis, Tennessee

AUTHORS

PAUL BABYN, MDCM, FRCP(C)
Head, Department of Medical Imaging,
University of Saskatchewan and Saskatoon
Health Region, Royal University Hospital,
Saskatoon, Saskatchewan

**EMANUELA R. VALSANGIACOMO
BUECHEL, MD**
Associate Professor of Cardiology, Division
of Cardiology, Department of Pediatrics,
University Children's Hospital Zurich, Zurich,
Switzerland

MARK A. FOGEL, MD
Professor of Cardiology and Radiology,
Division of Cardiology, Departments of
Pediatrics and Radiology, The Children's
Hospital of Philadelphia, Philadelphia,
Pennsylvania

CHARLOTTE GILBERT, MBChB, RANZCR
Auckland, New Zealand

NADINE GIRARD, MD
Department of Neuroradiology, Hopital
Timone; CRMBM, UMR CNRS 6612, Faculté
de Médecine, Université de la Méditerranée,
Marseille, France

P. ELLEN GRANT, MD
Associate Professor, Division of Newborn
Medicine, Department of Medicine; Associate
Professor, Division of Neuroradiology,
Department of Radiology, Harvard Medical
School, Center for Fetal Neonatal
Neuroimaging & Developmental Science,
Children's Hospital Boston, Boston,
Massachusetts

SYLVIANE HANQUINET, MD
Head, Department of Pediatric Radiology,
University Children's Hospital Geneva,
Geneva, Switzerland

THIERRY A.G.M. HUISMAN, MD, EQNR, FICIS
Professor, Division of Pediatric Radiology,
Department of Radiology and Radiological
Science, Johns Hopkins Hospital, Baltimore,
Maryland

IZLEM IZBUDAK, MD
Assistant Professor, Neuroradiology Division,
Department of Radiology and Radiological
Science, Johns Hopkins University, Baltimore,
Maryland

RAJESH KRISHNAMURTHY, MD
Clinical Professor of Radiology and
Pediatrics, Director of Research, Edward B.
Singleton Department of Pediatric Radiology,
Texas Children's Hospital, Baylor College of
Medicine, Houston, Texas

EDWARD LEE, MD, MPH
Assistant Professor of Radiology,
Director, Pulmonary Imaging, Department
of Radiology; Pulmonary Division, Department
of Medicine, Children's Hospital Boston and
Harvard Medical School, Boston,
Massachusetts

ZOLTÁN PATAY, MD, PhD
Chief, Section of Neuroimaging,
Department of Radiological Sciences, St. Jude
Children's Research Hospital; Professor of
Radiology, College of Medicine, University of
Tennessee Health Science Center, Memphis,
Tennessee

PEDRO S. PINTO, MD
Visiting Fellow, Division of Pediatric Radiology,
Department of Radiology and Radiological
Science, Johns Hopkins Hospital, Baltimore,
Maryland

CHARLES RAYBAUD, MD, FRCPC
Division of Neuroradiology, Hospital for Sick
Children, Toronto, Ontario, Canada

ANDREA ROSSI, MD
Head, Department of Pediatric Neuroradiology,
G. Gaslini Children's Hospital, Genoa, Italy

JACQUES F. SCHNEIDER, MD
Head, Department of Pediatric Radiology,
University Children's Hospital Basel, UKBB,
Basel, Switzerland

MARIASAVINA SEVERINO, MD
Consultant, Department of Pediatric
Neuroradiology, G. Gaslini Children's Hospital,
Genoa, Italy

MELISSA R. SPEVAK, MD
Division of Pediatric Radiology, The Russell
H. Morgan Department of Radiology and
Radiological Science, Johns Hopkins
University, Baltimore, Maryland

AYLIN TEKES, MD
Assistant Professor, Division of Pediatric
Radiology, Department of Radiology and
Radiological Science, Johns Hopkins Hospital,
Baltimore, Maryland

RICK R. VAN RIJN, MD, PhD
Department of Radiology, Academic Medical
Centre/Emma Children's Hospital Amsterdam,
Amsterdam Zuid-Oost; Section of Pediatric
Forensics, Department of Forensic Medicine,
Netherlands Forensic Institute, The Hague,
The Netherlands

Contents

Neonates with Seizures: What to Consider, How to Image 685

Nadine Girard and Charles Raybaud

The immature brain is more prone to seize than the mature brain. Causes of seizure are multiple and affect different neuroimaging modalities. The most common associated diseases are hypoxia-ischemia, intracranial hemorrhage and cerebral infarction, central nervous system infections, and acute metabolic disturbances. Ultrasound (US) is not specific. Computed tomography (CT) carries the risk of irradiation and is not as productive as magnetic resonance (MR) imaging. MR imaging is the modality of choice; it is difficult to perform in a neonate, but it is more sensitive and versatile than US or CT, and is now widely used in specialized centers.

MR Imaging of the Term and Preterm Neonate with Diffuse Brain Injury 709

Izlem Izbudak and P. Ellen Grant

Both term and preterm neonates suffer from diffuse brain injury. Global hypoxic-ischemic injury (HII) describes the diffuse brain injury most common in term neonates. HII is thought to result from decreases in blood flow and oxygen supply. Diffuse white matter injury of prematurity describes the most common diffuse brain injury in preterm neonates. The cause is likely multifactorial. Magnetic resonance (MR) imaging is the most sensitive imaging technique for early diagnosis of brain injury in neonates. This article discusses neonatal diffuse brain injury, the role of MR imaging in predicting neurodevelopmental outcome, and research results using MR imaging techniques.

MR Imaging Workup of Inborn Errors of Metabolism of Early Postnatal Onset 733

Zoltán Patay

Immediate or early postnatal onset forms of neurometabolic disorders represent a clinically important subgroup because these often present as a life-threatening episode of metabolic decompensation shortly after birth. This article focuses on this group of diseases, often referred to as "devastating neurometabolic diseases" of the newborn. Awareness of the most common entities and their clinical, biochemical, and diagnostic imaging manifestations is important because if undiagnosed and untreated, the diseases may have catastrophic consequences. Although formal diagnosis relies on laboratory tests, diagnostic imaging is often pivotal in both reaching the correct diagnosis and/or orienting further targeted investigative efforts.

MR Imaging of Neonatal Brain Infections 761

Jacques F. Schneider, Sylviane Hanquinet, Mariasavina Severino, and Andrea Rossi

Infections of the brain in the postnatal period differ from those in older children as a result of a combination of distinct epidemiologic factors in general, and immaturity of neonatal brain and immunologic host response in particular. It has been recognized that clinical and neurologic signs are often nonspecific, sometimes scarce, and seldom correlate with the extent of neuroimaging findings, thus warranting an early MR imaging examination in the course of the disease, enabling rapid therapy institution and better clinical outcome. This article reviews most of postnatal pathogen agents involved in neonatal brain infections, related physiopathology, and neuroimaging findings.

Aylin Tekes, Pedro S. Pinto, and Thierry A.G.M. Huisman

Birth-related injury is defined as any traumatic or ischemic event sustained during the process of delivery. Perinatally acquired disease processes secondary to birth-related injury can be traumatic or ischemic in nature. In this article, the authors focus on traumatic/mechanical injuries. Other diseases of the perinatal time period, including germinal matrix hemorrhages and hypoxic-ischemic encephalopathy, are beyond the objective of this review.

Rick R. van Rijn and Melissa R. Spevak

Child abuse and neglect is a serious clinical and socioeconomic problem that is sometimes underestimated. One of the most devastating forms is abusive head trauma. This review addresses the radiological workup in cases of suspected child abuse. The use of all modalities, and their advantages and disadvantages, is discussed. A special section is devoted to the radiological report in cases of child abuse, as a clinical record and a legal document.

Rajesh Krishnamurthy and Edward Lee

Owing largely to advances in fetal echocardiography, in most developed countries the diagnosis of severe congenital heart disease (CHD) is now made during gestation, and delivery is electively planned in hospitals that have the facilities and expertise to manage these patients, with magnetic resonance (MR) imaging performing an important complementary role. MR imaging as a sole imaging modality for comprehensive presurgical evaluation is also increasingly being explored. This article focuses on the imaging of neonatal CHD by MR, followed by a brief discussion of the safety of gadolinium-based contrast agents in this age group.

Emanuela R. Valsangiacomo Buechel and Mark A. Fogel

In neonates and infants with congenital heart disease (CHD), cardiovascular magnetic resonance (CMR) is an established imaging modality in all patients in whom echocardiography does not provide sufficient information and definitive diagnosis. CMR is noninvasive, and does not involve vascular catheterization or ionizing radiation. Therefore the use of CMR obviates the potential risks of cardiac catheterization in critically ill infants. This article discusses the use of CMR in newborns with CHD before cardiac surgery, focusing on conotruncal anomalies, pulmonary venous anomalies, complex CHD in visceroatrial heterotaxy, borderline hypoplastic left heart syndrome, and the use of contrast medium in newborns.

Charlotte Gilbert and Paul Babyn

Experience in magnetic resonance (MR) imaging of the neonatal musculoskeletal system is rapidly increasing. The exquisite ability of MR to image the soft tissues, especially cartilage, without radiation is its key strength. Although it is not practical or sensible to undertake MR imaging in conditions in which radiography and ultrasound provide adequate information, MR is proving to be a useful adjunct and problem-solving tool in many neonatal musculoskeletal conditions.

Magnetic Resonance Imaging Clinics of North America

THE CLINICS ARE NOW AVAILABLE ONLINE!

Access your subscription at:
www.theclinics.com

Preface
MR Imaging of the Newborn

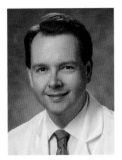 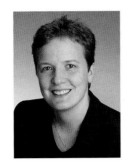

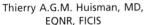

Thierry A.G.M. Huisman, MD,   Claudia M. Hillenbrand, PhD
EQNR, FICIS

Guest Editors

This issue of *Magnetic Resonance Imaging Clinics of North America* is dedicated to MRI of the Newborn Infant. Vast experience has been gained over the past decade in safely transporting, monitoring, and imaging this highly vulnerable patient group. Technological advances in MRI hardware such as higher field strength systems, multichannel coils, higher gradient performance, and MR-compatible incubators with integrated antennae laid the ground for more detailed, higher resolution anatomical MR imaging. In addition, the ongoing development of advanced functional MR imaging techniques (ie, diffusion-weighted/tensor imaging, perfusion-weighted imaging, susceptibility-weighted imaging, MR angiography and venography, dynamic contrast-enhanced MRI, and ^{1}H MR spectroscopy) rendered MRI the most versatile noninvasive diagnostic modality and an indispensable tool to investigate qualitatively and quantitatively neonatal injuries, malformations, congenital disorders, and tumors. Furthermore, the advanced MRI techniques allow collecting multiple "biomarkers" of injury that may monitor disease course or treatment results quantitatively. Today, neonate MRI is successfully performed in preterm newborns as young as 24 weeks of gestation and sequential imaging is carried out to assess development or response to injury and/or therapy.

The articles in this first issue—all written by international experts in the field—focus on topics directly relevant to patient care, thereby emphasizing once again the rapidly growing clinical importance of neonatal MRI. This issue is divided into three logical sections that cover all relevant anatomical and functional regions of the neonate. The first part covers, in accord with clinical appearance, the majority of MRI exams indicated for injuries and disorders of the brain and spine: hypoxic ischemic brain injury in preterm and term infants is discussed, as well as seizures, birth-related and inflicted head injuries, head trauma, and metabolic diseases. The second part focuses on congenital cardiac defects and cardiovascular malformations, and the third is dedicated to musculoskeletal indications of MRI. A second issue will be published shortly after the first issue, which will focus more on technical aspects of neonatal MR imaging.

We would like to express our sincere gratitude to the contributing authors for sharing their expertise and providing us with such exceptional material. We would also like to thank Barton Dudlick, Joanne Husovski, and the remainder of the staff at Elsevier for their assistance in preparing this issue. We hope

Magn Reson Imaging Clin N Am 19 (2011) xi–xii
doi:10.1016/j.mric.2011.10.003

you find the issue informative and educational. Enjoy this comprehensive update of neonate MR imaging!

Thierry A.G.M. Huisman, MD, EQNR, FICIS
Division of Pediatric Radiology
Department of Radiology and Radiological Science
Johns Hopkins Hospital
600 North Wolfe Street
Nelson, B-173
Baltimore, MD 21287–0842, USA

Claudia M. Hillenbrand, PhD
Division of Translational Imaging Research
Department of Radiological Sciences
St Jude Children's Research Hospital
262 Danny Thomas Place
Memphis, TN 38105, USA

E-mail addresses:
thuisma1@jhmi.edu (T.A.G.M. Huisman)
claudia.hillenbrand@stjude.org (C.M. Hillenbrand)

Neonates with Seizures: What to Consider, How to Image

Nadine Girard, MD[a,b],*, Charles Raybaud, MD, FRCPC[c]

KEYWORDS
- Seizures • Neonatal • Epilepsy • MR imaging

Seizures represent the most common clinical symptom of neurologic disorder in the neonatal period. The incidence is 1.3 to 3.5/1000 in term newborns, and as high as 10 to 130/1000 in preterm neonates.[1] Recognizing the seizure, a well-defined epileptic syndrome, and the many possible causes is important because some symptoms may mimic normal clinical manifestations, and causes of seizure may affect the choice of neuroimaging modality. However, there are no established evidence-based guidelines for management of neonatal seizures[2] and for the appropriate use of brain imaging. Ultrasonography (US), computed tomography (CT), and magnetic resonance (MR) imaging are widely used to image the neonatal brain, but MR (using diffusion-weighted imaging [DWI], diffusion tensor imaging [DTI], and MR spectroscopy) is likely to provide the most complete and useful information.

WHAT TO CONSIDER?
Identifying the Seizures

The immature brain is prone to seize. Neonatal seizures are defined clinically as abnormal, stereotyped, paroxysmal alterations in neurologic function occurring in the first 28 days after birth of a term neonate or before 44 weeks of gestational age in a preterm infant. This abnormal function may involve abnormal motor, sensory, or automatic activity, with or without a change in level of consciousness. Not all clinical seizures correlate with electroencephalograph (EEG) changes and not all seizures shown on

EEG recordings are clinically apparent.[1] Neonatal seizures may be epileptic or nonepileptic and are classified according to their characterization.[3,4] Electroclinical findings distinguish (1) clinical seizures with consistent electrocortical signature that are considered epileptic, (2) clinical seizures without consistent electrocortical signature that are presumed nonepileptic, and (3) electrical seizures without clinical manifestation. The first group may consist of focal clonic seizures (unifocal, multifocal, hemiconvulsive, axial), focal tonic seizures (asymmetrical truncal posturing, limb posturing, sustained eye deviation), myoclonic seizures (generalized or focal), and spasms (flexor, extensor, mixed extensor and flexor). The second group includes myoclonic seizures (generalized, focal, fragmentary), generalized tonic (flexor, extensor, mixed flexor and extensor), and motor automatisms (oral-buccal-lingual movements, ocular movements, movements of progression such as swimming and bicycling, complex purposeless movements).

It may be difficult to distinguish subtle neonatal seizures from other paroxysmal neurologic manifestations of the newborn. Apnea can express a subtle seizure. Most apneic episodes in preterm infants do not represent seizure activity but are associated with a bradycardia. In contrast, convulsive apnea is not accompanied by bradycardia but by other subtle phenomena such as eye opening, staring, and eye deviation. Jitteriness is a common benign neonatal movement disorder characterized by symmetric tremors of the extremities. It is

[a] Department of Neuroradiology, Hopital Timone, 264 Rue Saint Pierre, 13385 Marseille CEDEX 5, France
[b] CRMBM, UMR CNRS 6612, Faculté de Médecine, Université de la Méditerranée, 27 bd Jean Moulin, 13385 Marseille CEDEX 5, France
[c] Division of Neuroradiology, Hospital for Sick Children, 555 University Avenue, Toronto, Ontario M5G1X8, Canada
* Corresponding author. Department of Neuroradiology, Hopital Timone, 264 Rue Saint Pierre, 13385 Marseille CEDEX 5, France.
E-mail address: nadine.girard@ap-hm.fr

Magn Reson Imaging Clin N Am 19 (2011) 685–708
doi:10.1016/j.mric.2011.08.003
1064-9689/11/$ – see front matter © 2011 Published by Elsevier Inc.

generally induced by an external stimulus and ceases with gentle restraint or passive flexion. It occurs in infants without neurologic impairment and is not necessarily an abnormal feature. It is mainly encountered in hypoxic-ischemic encephalopathy (HIE), hypoglycemia, hypocalcemia, and drug withdrawal.

Epileptic Syndromes Occurring During the Neonatal Period

Idiopathic, symptomatic or cryptogenic, neonatal seizures often are part of specific epileptic syndromes. Idiopathic epilepsies include benign familial neonatal convulsions, benign neonatal convulsions, and benign familial neonatal-infantile seizures.[5,6]

Benign familial neonatal convulsions are a potassium voltage-gated channelopathy with an autosomal dominant inheritance and incomplete penetrance. This rare familial syndrome is characterized by unilateral or bilateral clonic, tonic-clonic, and apneic or tonic seizures on the second or third day of life, with normal interictal EEG. The outcome is generally favorable with seizures stopping early in life and normal psychomotor development. Some patients may develop febrile seizures or epilepsy later in life. It is genetically related to mutations of potassium channel genes KCNG2 and KCNQ3 on chromosomes 20q and 8q respectively.

Benign idiopathic neonatal seizures (also described as fifth day fits) differ from the familial syndrome: seizures occur later (fifth day of life), tonic seizures are never observed, and the interictal EEG commonly shows the θ pointu alternant.[5]

Benign familial neonatal-infantile seizures are characterized by tonic or clonic seizures that occur between 2 days and 3 to 5 months, later than benign familial neonatal convulsions but earlier than benign familial infantile convulsions. This epileptic syndrome has been related to chromosomes 19q, 16p, and 2q in which mutations of SCN2A (sodium channel) are found. Symptomatic epileptic syndromes include early myoclonic encephalopathy (EME) and early infantile epileptic encephalopathy (EIEE; also known as Otahara syndrome), which are often associated with structural abnormalities.[7] In both, the background EEG shows a suppression-burst pattern.

EIEE is characterized by a very early onset, often within the first 10 days of life. The main type of seizure is tonic spasms. Partial seizures and hemiconvulsions are also seen, whereas myoclonic seizures are rare. Seizures are accompanied by severe progressive encephalopathy that evolves to infantile spasms and Lennox-Gastaut syndrome.

Most cases are associated with structural brain damage, especially hemimegalencephaly. Metabolic disorders are also reported.

EME is also characterized by a very early onset. Partial to massive myoclonus as well as partial motor seizures are the main ictal phenomena, followed by infantile spasms. The clinical course is severe with, in half of the cases, death in the first year of life. Anatomic brain abnormalities are uncommon. The most common cause is nonketotic hyperglycinemia. It is also described in sulfite oxidase deficiency. Mutations of the glutamate carrier are also a cause of EME.[8] A high proportion of cryptogenic cases is described, and familial cases have also been reported.

Pyridoxine-dependent seizure is an autosomal recessive disorder with seizure onset between birth and age 3 months. The EEG abnormalities are nonspecific. The intravenous pyridoxine test is usually positive with cessation of seizures.[4]

Causes

Most cases of neonatal seizures are symptomatic with associated causal and risk factors, and few neonatal seizures are idiopathic (2%–5%).[1] The major categories of causal factors are (in decreasing order of frequency): HIE, acquired metabolic disorders (hypoglycemia, hypomagnesemia, hypocalcemia, hypernatremia, or hyponatremia), infections (meningitis, encephalitis, TORCH [toxoplasmosis, other, rubella, cytomegalovirus, and herpes]), acquired or developmental brain lesions (hemorrhage, infarction, malformations), inherited disorders, inborn error of metabolism (aminoacidurias, urea cycle defects, organic acidurias, mitochondrial disorders, peroxysomal disorders, metabolic substrate deficiencies), and maternal drug intoxication or neonatal drug withdrawal (eg, cocaine, heroin). The most common are hypoxia-ischemia, infections, hemorrhage and infarction, and acute metabolic disturbances. Infants prone to epilepsy of neonatal onset are most likely to have inborn errors of metabolism and cortical malformations.[3]

In general, the more acute the neurologic insult, the sooner the onset of neonatal seizures. For example HIE, hemorrhages, severe metabolic disturbances, maternal drug abuse, and some cases of sepsis present seizures in the first 24 hours after birth, whereas stroke, cerebral venous thrombosis, drug withdrawal, and metabolic defects in energy production and use, such as urea cycle defects, present seizures between 24 and 72 hours after birth. Other inborn errors of metabolism, such as aminoacidopathies and organic acidopathies, cerebral malformations, or congenital lesions, tend to present seizures after 72 hours to 1 week after birth.

Do Neonatal Seizures Damage the Brain?

In animal models, neonatal seizures impair cognition and learning ability, alter behavior and memory, increase anxiety, and are associated with later epileptogenesis. Despite this strong evidence from experimental studies, the issue remains largely unanswered in humans. However, significant changes are shown with MR spectroscopy in term neonates with perinatal asphyxia, which increase along with the severity of clinical seizures.[9] A recent clinical study suggests that clinical neonatal seizures and their treatment are associated with adverse long-term cognitive and neuromotor outcomes in perinatal asphyxia that are independent of the hypoxic-ischemic injury measured by MR imaging.[10] Moreover, high levels of excitatory amino acids pervade the epileptic brain during the interictal state, making it particularly vulnerable to seizure-induced damage.

Brain Maturation

The neonatal brain is immature at birth and this affects neuroimaging. Brain maturation, especially brain myelination, begins before birth and continues until adulthood. Brain maturation includes changes in morphology and in composition. Changes in brain morphology consist of increase in brain volume and weight, developing sulcation, changes in ventricular shape, and decrease in volume of the subarachnoid spaces. These changes are well depicted with fetal imaging. From midgestation to infancy, brain growth reflects synaptogenesis, dendritic arborization and spine formation, axonal elongation and collateral formation, myelination, gliogenesis, neurotransmitter development, and vascular development. The most rapid changes occur between midgestation and the end of the second postnatal year, with 2 partially overlapping stages: the first is a period of oligodendrocytic proliferation and differentiation, whereas the second is a period of rapid myelin synthesis and deposition. Myelination progresses in a caudorostral way, at different times and speeds depending on specific fiber tracts, and at variable speeds within a given functional unit. Because the rate of myelination in a particular pathway may change with time, the onset of myelination before or at birth is not necessarily associated with early myelin maturation. Motor and sensory tracts mature early compared with association fibers. As a consequence in the forebrain, myelination progresses from the somatosensory central sulcus toward all poles but also from the visual occipital lobe and the auditory Heschl gyrus: the occipital pole myelinates before the frontal pole, which in turn myelinates before the temporal pole. This progression implies that lesions that affect the processes of myelination have a different distribution from diseases that affect the already formed myelin.

The immature brain is more prone to seize than the mature brain. The immature neurons and networks generate periodic discharges. In addition, gamma aminobutyric acid (GABA) exerts a paradoxic excitatory action in the immature brain that increases excitability.[11] Maturational changes in excitatory amino acid (EAA) neurotransmission occur during the early postnatal period with consequent susceptibility to hypoxic seizures.[12] Excessive release of EAA neurotransmitters, especially glutamate, mediates seizure activity and hypoxoischemic neuronal damage.[13]

HOW TO IMAGE

US, cranial CT, and MR imaging are used extensively for the diagnosis of neonatal brain disorders.[14] In contrast, positron emission tomography (PET) is not commonly used in the neonatal period.

US

Cerebral US, whether in combination with Doppler technique or not, is an easily available modality that involves minimal or no disturbance to the neonate, even those who are sick and asphyxiated. However, cranial US has a low sensitivity, especially in term babies with hypoxic-ischemic injury. The signs for early detection of hypoxic-ischemic insult are small ventricles and subarachnoid spaces and increased echogenicity. However, it is not possible to determine whether an increased echogenicity reflects edema that may be transient, or permanent cell injury that will turn into a cystic lesion. Moreover, deep structures (brainstem, cerebellum) as well as superficial structures (cortical ribbon) are not easily imaged by cranial US (**Fig. 1**). US is reported to be normal in as many as 50% of neonates with hypoxic-ischemic injury.[15] It is also sometimes difficult to differentiate an ischemic stroke from a hemorrhagic infarction in the early stage because the echogenicity is similar. However, cranial US has improved significantly and is still the primary imaging modality in neonates for detecting intraventricular hemorrhages (IVH), hydrocephalus, and white matter changes. Periventricular leukomalacia (PVL) is suspected in cases of periventricular hyperechogenicity, but this may be confused with edema that can resolve without leaving residual damage. Normal sonograms have been

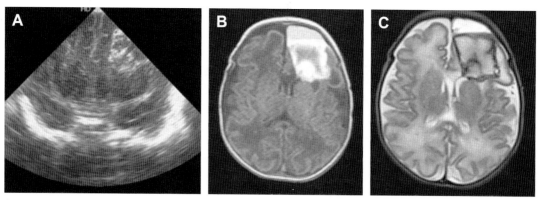

Fig. 1. US (*A*), axial T1-weighted image (T1WI) (*B*) and T1-weighted image (T2WI) (*C*). Well-limited hyperechoic lesion is seen on US, suggesting hemorrhage. MR imaging shows parenchymal hematoma associated with subdural frontal hematoma.

reported in children proved to have PVL at autopsy.[16] In very small premature babies (from 24 to 32 weeks), the white matter displays a diffuse hyperechogenicity, probably because of the interfaces that result from the multilayered pattern of the cerebral parenchyma (from outside to inside: the cortical ribbon, the subcortical white matter, the layers of migrant cell, the subventricular zone, and the germinal matrix; **Fig. 2**).[17–19] Although nodules of leukomalacia can be identified easily on US, persistent hyperechogenicities or asymmetry of echogenicity suggest white matter damage without being specific.[14] MR imaging is therefore the next step to consider

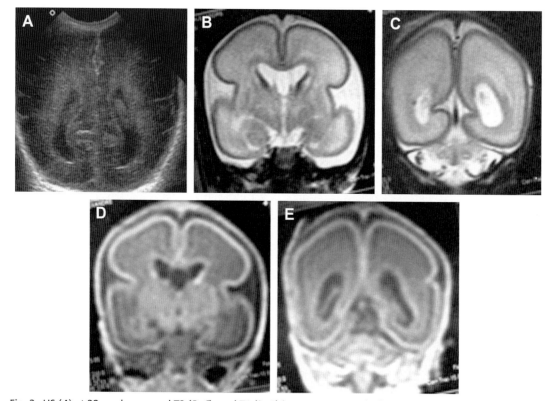

Fig. 2. US (*A*) at 28 weeks, coronal T2 (*B*, *C*), and T1 (*D*, *E*) images at 26 weeks from 2 different preterm neonates. Hyperechoic appearance of the periventricular white matter on US. This feature is related to the migrating cells seen on MR imaging as layers of low signal on T2 and bright signal on T1.

because it is more sensitive and has a prognostic value in severe cases (neonates without respiratory autonomy, maternofetal infection). This step helps therapeutic decision making because 30% to 50% of premature infants with normal US present with white matter abnormalities on MR imaging.[20,21] MR imaging is also the next step when cranial US does not explain the clinical state of a compromised neonate.

Midline malformations are easily depicted by US (Fig. 3), but with less precise information compared with MR imaging.

Cranial CT

Modern CT is fast and versatile, and easily available. However, it uses X-rays, and radiation is deemed to be harmful, especially in young children. CT is usually performed without iodine injection, except in cases of neonatal meningitis, to look for complications such as empyema and thrombophlebitis. CT vascular imaging can also be performed, when necessary, because it is considered the standard for venography.

The normal neonatal brain is characterized by a low attenuation of the white matter compared with the cortex and basal ganglia (Fig. 4). It is sensitive for detecting hemorrhage, HIE, and stroke (Fig. 5), as well as the complications of birth trauma. In contrast, white matter damage and

neuronal necrosis are more difficult to identify on CT, although the loss of gray-white contrast and the so-called laminar necrosis in the cortex show up well. Because of the low density of the white matter, it is difficult to detect nonhemorrhagic leukomalacia. Although CT is able to show cytotoxic edema by showing the effacement of the gray-white contrast (see Fig. 5B), it still lacks the sensitivity of MR in cases of HIE in term newborns. Midline malformations such as complete agenesis of commissures and posterior fossa cyst are easily identified. CT also efficiently depicts brain swelling, particularly the swelling seen in aminoacidopathies such as leucine toxicity (Fig. 6). However, MR imaging is better for optimally assessing malformations and inborn metabolic disorders. Epileptogenic tumors are not commonly detected in the neonatal period (Fig. 7).

MR Imaging

MR is the most sensitive and, with the use of DWI, DTI, susceptibility imaging (SWI), MR spectroscopy, MRA, and MR venography, the most versatile modality to investigate the neonatal brain.

- Conventional MR imaging is still extremely helpful. Given the brain immaturity, optimal MR imaging parameters have to be chosen: gradient echo and inversion

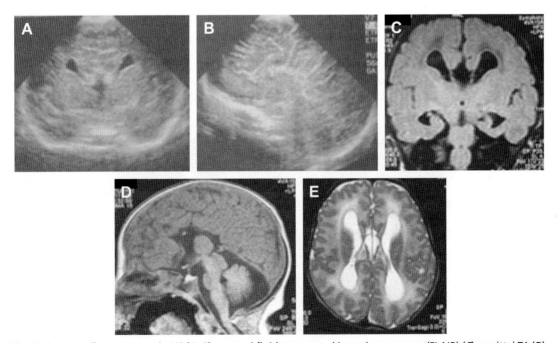

Fig. 3. Corpus callosum agenesis, US (*A, B*), coronal fluid attenuated inversion recovery (FLAIR) (*C*), sagittal T1 (*D*), axial T2 (*E*). Corpus callosum is not seen on US. Anterior commissure is not identified on the midline on MR imaging (*D*). Also note the disorganized gyration of the left parietal area.

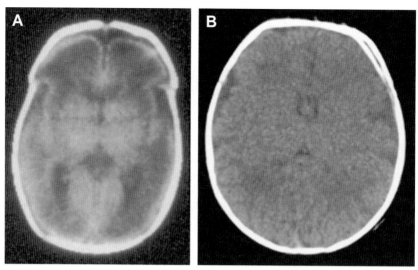

Fig. 4. CT of a preterm (*A*) and term (*B*) infant. Note the low attenuation of the white matter compared with cortex and basal ganglia, especially in preterm.

recovery T1-weighted images (T1WI) give excellent contrast between gray and white matter, and are highly sensitive to hemorrhage, calcifications, and neuronal necrosis. The recovery time (TR) and echo time (TE) of T2-weighted images (T2WI) have to be long enough in the neonate to adapt to the prolonged gray and white matter T1 and T2 relaxation times.[22] Single-shot T2WI (ie, HASTE) is not efficient enough in evaluating neonatal tissular changes: it may provide anatomic information, but brain maturation and brain damage are not well depicted. Fluid attenuated inversion recovery (FLAIR) images are usually not used in neonates except to identify cysts. Gadolinium is not

commonly given in neonates except in cases of meningitis, tumor, or vascular malformation.

The normal appearance of the neonatal brain is different (**Fig. 8**) from the mature brain. Water content is high, especially within the white matter, and is responsible for the low signal on T1WI and bright signal on T2WI compared with gray matter. In contrast, basal ganglia show low signal on T2 and bright signal on T1 because of the high cell density. Areas that are already even partially myelinated show low signal on T2 and bright signal on T1: areas of primary cortex (central sulcus, hippocampus, Heschl gyrus, calcarine sulcus), posterior brainstem, optic tracts, and white matter

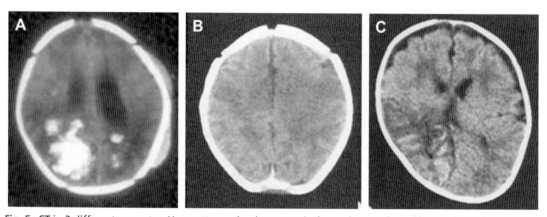

Fig. 5. CT in 3 different neonates. Hyperattenuating intraventricular and parenchymal hemorrhage (*A*). Bilateral cytotoxic edema with low attenuation of the cortex in right frontal and left frontoparietal areas in a neonate with hypoxic-ischemic injury (*B*). Right-sided stroke in the parietal area (*C*).

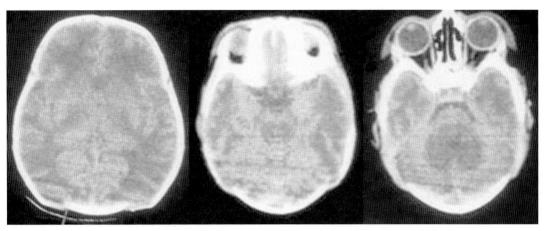

Fig. 6. CT of maple syrup disease. Note edematous appearance of the white matter and brainstem.

underlying the central area. Posterior limbs of internal capsules (PLICs) display bright signal on T1 but are not yet fully myelinated. This latter appearance is present from 33 weeks on. In premature babies of less than 30 weeks, the brain tissular layering is apparent: migrating cells form waves within the white matter and the germinal matrix is thick, giving a multilayered pattern of the cerebral mantle. In high premature neonates, gyration has not yet developed, resulting in a lissencephalic appearance, although with a normal cortical thickness (see **Fig. 2**).

- DWI seems to be more sensitive than standard MR imaging in the detection of acute brain damage related to hypoxic-ischemic

injury in the first day after the hypoxic event[23–26] and in excitotoxic damage seen in some inborn errors of metabolism. Echo planar (EP) diffusion images are routinely and easily performed in the neonate, with an acquisition time of 1.0 to 1.30 minutes. Sensitization gradients are applied following the 3 axes (x, y, z). Generated images consist of trace images and maps of apparent diffusion coefficient (ADC). DWI is also sensitive to changes in cell density and myelination and shows signal changes before T1 and T2 sequences. In the neonate (**Fig. 9**), ADC is lower in the hindbrain compared with the forebrain. The process of myelination is identified in the corticospinal

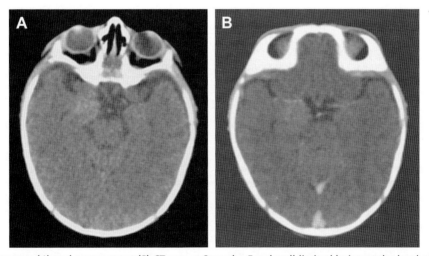

Fig. 7. Precontrast (*A*) and postcontrast (*B*) CT scan at 3 weeks. Focal well-limited lesion at the level of the amygdala shows slightly high attenuation compatible with focal cortical dysplasia. However, histology concluded glial tumor.

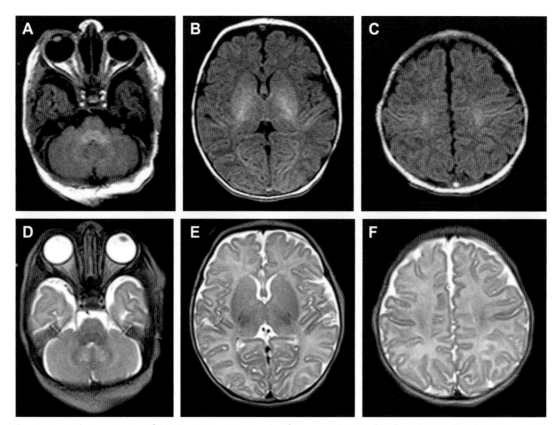

Fig. 8. Normal appearance of MR imaging at 1 month of age; axial T1WI (*A–C*) and T2WI (*D–F*). White matter displays low signal on T1WI and bright signal on T2WI compared with gray matter. In contrast, basal ganglia show a low signal on T2 and a bright signal on T1. Note areas already myelinated, although partially: central sulcus, posterior brainstem, and white matter underlying the central area with low signal on T2 and bright signal on T1. Posterior limbs of internal capsules display bright signal on T1 but are not yet fully myelinated on T2.

tracts as a bright signal on DWI and low signal on ADC within the pons, the central area, and the posterior limb of the internal capsules. This pattern is also seen in the optic radiations and the splenium of the corpus callosum. Unmyelinated white matter shows low signal on DWI and high signal on ADC. Pathologic restriction of diffusion is seen in anoxic-ischemic ischemic disease with cytotoxic edema (stroke, HIE, mitochondrial disorders), in metabolic disease with vacuolating myelinopathy, or in conditions in which an increased cellular density occurs, such as inflammation or pus collection. In contrast, lesions with increased diffusivity, such as vasogenic edema, display normal or low signal on diffusion images and high signal on ADC maps.

- DTI evaluates the changing microstructure of the developing brain.[27] Diffusion of water in the white matter becomes more restricted and gains anisotropy, which depends on the structural fascicular organization. Data are obtained from acquisitions made after applying diffusion gradients in multiple directions (at least 6 noncollinear). Acquisition time of this type of sequence is from 3 to 4 minutes with 6 directions, 5 to 6 minutes with 12 directions, and even longer with 20 directions when the pixels are isotropic. Shorter acquisition time is obtained with nonisotropic pixels. The images generated include trace images, ADC maps, fractional anisotropy (FA) maps, and color-coded orientation tractography maps (**Fig. 10**). Color-coded orientation tractography maps are useful in the assessment of focal cortical dysplasia (FCD; **Fig. 11**) or tumor (**Fig. 12**) in neonates by showing the disorganized tissue compared with conventional T1 and T2 images. White matter parcellation allows the assessment of FA ADC in a specific tract. However because of low FA in neonates, the

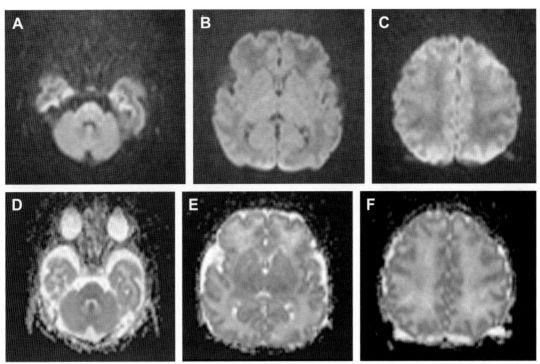

Fig. 9. Normal appearance of term infant with DWI (*A–C*) and ADC maps (*D–F*). ADC is lower in the posterior fossa compared with cerebral hemispheres. Note process of myelination within the corticospinal tracts as bright signal on DWI and low signal on ADC within the pons, the central area, and the posterior part of the internal capsules. Unmyelinated white matter shows increased diffusivity.

tractography postprocessing tool needs be modified from what is used in the mature brain. Tractography is also used to investigate brain connectivity such as parahippocampal connectivity,[28] corticothalamic connectivity,[29] and motor connectivity.[30] DTI studies in epileptic patients have shown increased diffusivity and decreased FA within and beyond the epileptic zone.[31–34] However, no study is available in the neonate.

- Proton MR spectroscopy can also be used to obtain complementary information on the brain status, especially in neonatal

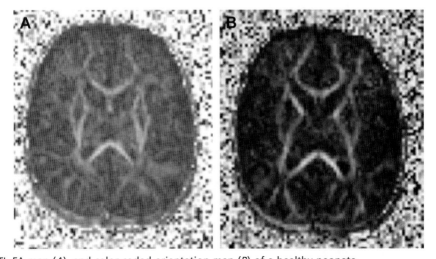

Fig. 10. DTI, FA map (*A*), and color-coded orientation map (*B*) of a healthy neonate.

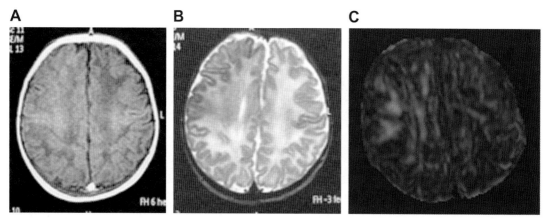

Fig. 11. FCD, axial T1 (*A*) and T2 (*B*) images, and FA color map (*C*). Note the poor differentiation between cortex and white matter within the right frontal area (*A*) with low signal on T2 (*B*). FA color map shows the disorganized tissue compared with T1 and T2 images.

encephalopathies.[23,35,36] Spectra may be acquired with the single-voxel technique or with chemical shift imaging (CSI) from 1 slab (two-dimensional CSI) or from multiple slices (three-dimensional CSI). Because of its robustness, position resolved spectroscopy sequence is commonly used, with short (30–35milliseconds) and long echo time (145 milliseconds). The neonatal brain is characterized by high concentration of choline (Cho), myo-inositol-glycine (mI), and glutamine plus glutamate (Glx) in relation to creatine (Cr) and *N*-acetylaspartate (NAA). Brain maturation is characterized by an increase of NAA and Cr, and a concomitant decrease of Cho, mI, and lipids.[37]

Inositol is a precursor molecule for inositol-lipid synthesis and is considered as an osmolyte and an astrocyte marker. Myo-inositol is the predominant peak from 22 to 28 weeks, and probably reflects the high density of glial cells that multiply and differentiate before myelinogenesis starts. The choline peak represents high levels of substrate needed for the formation of cell membranes, with gradual reduction as soon as incorporation of lipids has developed. NAA is considered a neuronal marker but is also expressed in oligo-type 2 astrocyte progenitors, immature oligodendrocytes, and mature oligodendrocytes. Therefore, NAA also reflects oligodendrocyte

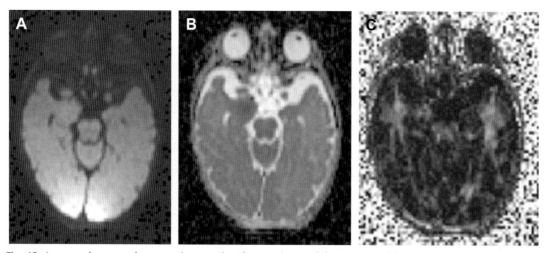

Fig. 12. Low-grade tumor (same patient as **Fig. 7**), trace image (*A*), ADC map (*B*), and FA color map (*C*). Focal lesion of the right amygdala shows slightly restricted diffusion. Note the disorganized tissues on the FA color map.

proliferation and differentiation.[38] As the neuronal cell density decreases with dendritic maturation in the cortex, the increase in NAA with age may reflect a contribution of nonneuronal origin. Creatine reflects energy metabolism and has been shown to increase before and around term, and postnatally.[37]

Regional variations are pronounced at all ages between gray and white matter, and also within different areas of gray and white matter. The highest choline, creatine, and NAA peak intensities are found in the thalami, followed by basal ganglia, and then other regions in preterm and term infants.[23] This probably reflects the high cellular density in these structures and their more advanced maturation compared with white matter. Concentration of NAA and creatine is higher in gray matter than in white matter ,whereas choline is slightly lower. The reason for this is unclear, but it may be that gray matter contains fewer myelin membrane. For white matter, NAA and choline peak intensities are higher in the parietooccipital area than in the frontal white matter[39] (the parietal area is myelinated before the frontal area, so the adult pattern is reached first in the parietooccipital region). The hindbrain has a peculiar metabolic pattern. The developing cerebellum shows a rapid NAA increase from infancy to childhood, and a rapid increase in creatine and Glx from fetal age, infancy, and childhood.[40] The cerebellum has the highest concentration of Cr and is also characterized by high contents of Glx, choline, and myo-inositol-glycine compared with the cerebral hemisphere. Regional variations are also observed: the lowest concentrations are in the vermis, whereas the highest concentrations are in the pons. MR spectroscopy in epileptic patients has been widely used to delineate the epileptic zone, and has shown a decrease of NAA, especially in temporal lobe epilepsy[41] and frontal lobe epilepsy.[42] However, there is currently no available literature addressing the epileptic neonate.

Nuclear Medicine

Single-photon emission CT (SPECT) with technetium-99m-hexamethylpropyleneamine (99 mTc-HmPAO) is widely used in neonatal seizures.[43,44] SPECT relies on increased perfusion during the ictal period to detect an active epileptic focus. The increased perfusion of the epileptic focus is the result of the metabolic demands placed on the cerebral tissue during an epileptic seizure. Clinical and electrical seizures in neonates are associated with a focal cerebral hyperperfusion

of the same amount as in adults. Although to a lesser degree than in adults, focal cerebral hyperperfusion in neonates corresponds with clinical seizures,

PET is a noninvasive imaging modality that has proved to be a powerful diagnostic tool for detecting neurochemical abnormalities associated with neurologic diseases. Although it has been well described in adults and pediatrics, its application in the newborn has not been extensively explored.[45] Early detection of brain injury secondary to intrauterine and perinatal insults using PET imaging can provide new insights for instituting early therapy. The most common tracer used in the imaging of epilepsy for clinical purposes is 2-deoxy-2-[18F]fluoro-D-glucose (FDG). FDG PET scans can detect areas of hypometabolism consistent with epileptogenic foci even in patients with normal MR imaging. In the neonate, when seizures are poorly controlled and there is no obvious cause for the seizures, the most likely causes are malformation of cortical development or an inborn error of metabolism. In this setting, if the MR imaging is not diagnostic, PET scanning with FDG may help in depicting an epileptic focus. If a diffuse pattern of abnormality is shown on the PET scan, a metabolic disorder is more likely.

THE DIAGNOSES
Malformations

Any type of malformation may be revealed by neonatal seizures, except Chiari II when isolated. The malformations most often involved in seizures are the malformations of cortical development (MCD). Agenesis of corpus callosum is easily diagnosed with US or CT, but only MR imaging allows a precise assessment of the brain tissue and may reveal the multiple commonly associated abnormalities.

Hemimegalencephalies (HME) are usually easy to identify. The anatomic pattern consists of an enlargement of the affected cerebral hemisphere (usually), and of the lateral ventricle, a thick-looking cortex with blurring of the cortical-subcortical junction, increased volume of white matter, and often an abnormal cortical gyral pattern, from a simplified gyral pattern to a pattern similar to polymicrogyria (PMG) (**Fig. 13**).

Focal cortical dysplasia type II (FCDII) is characterized by dysmorphic neurons with or without balloon cells, and may be difficult to identify on conventional sequences in the neonatal period because signal changes are not as conspicuous as in the infantile period (**Fig. 14**). In infant FCD, the white matter usually shows a bright signal on T1 and a low signal on T2. This pattern reflects an

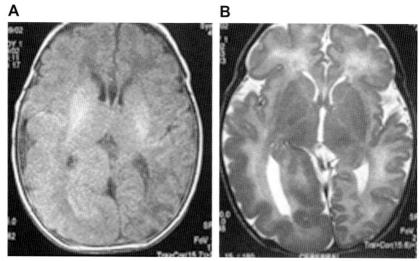

Fig. 13. Hemimegalencephaly, axial T1WI (*A*) and T2WI (*B*). Note the enlargement of the right cerebral hemisphere in the temporal and occipital area with abnormal cortical gyral pattern with poor differentiation between cortex and white matter on T1WI.

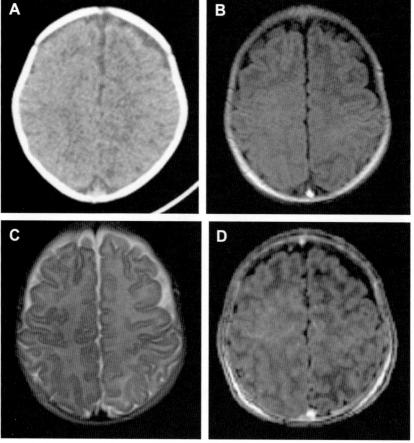

Fig. 14. FCD, CT scan (*A*), axial T1 (*B*), T2 (*C*), and postcontrast T1 (*D*). On CT, note the poor differentiation between cortex and white matter within the right frontoparietal area that is more conspicuous on MR imaging.

early myelination that is induced by the seizure activity: it suggests that the axons come from the epileptic focus, but not to the brain dysplastic tissue per se, and is lost when the whole brain becomes myelinated. In the very immature neonatal brain, the cortical ribbon is well shown on both T1 and T2, and the cortical blurring may show well: this is also lost quickly with maturation. Color maps of FA are then helpful to show the disorganization of the tissue. Tuberous sclerosis (TSC) is a syndromic, genetic form of FCD with multiple cortical tubers. Seizures may occur soon after birth. Focal cortical dysplasia type I (FCDI) may develop as secondary changes after a perinatal brain injury.[46–51]

Nodular heterotopias are either periventricular or subcortical, and easy to identify; they may be scarce and tiny, or diffuse and massive; they may be found in association with a large cistern magna; and seizures often occur later in life, not in the neonatal period. Agyria-pachygyria may be depicted in the neonatal period when early prenatal US fails to show any abnormality such as ventriculomegaly (Fig. 15).

PMG is characterized by areas of small, overfolded gyri with a loss of the normal sulcation, unilaterally or bilaterally, usually in the perisylvian regions, with loss of the normal sulcal pattern and corresponding atrophy of the underlying white matter. Usually idiopathic, PMG may be genetic (and typically symmetrically arranged), but when it is revealed in neonates it is often the result of an early fetal cytomegalovirus infection (Fig. 16); it may then be associated with schizencephaly.

Some malformations may also be seen in association with inborn error of metabolism. Agenesis of corpus callosum is encountered in several disorders such as pyruvate disorders, respiratory chain disorders, nonketotic hyperglycinemia, urea cycle disorders, cholesterol biosynthesis, and in disorders of fatty acid oxidation.[52] Heterotopias are seen in mitochondrial diseases and in peroxisomal disorders such as rhizomelic chondrodysplasia punctata.[53] Posterior sylvian PMG and frontal pachygyria are identified in peroxisomal diseases such as Zellweger disease (Fig. 17). Cobblestone brain and PMG-like cortical malformations are seen in defects of protein glycosylation (Walker-Warburg, muscle-eye-brain, Fukuyama). Enlarged subarachnoid spaces mimicking arachnoid cysts may be encountered in glutaric aciduria type 1, especially at the level of the temporal areas. Subtle enlargement of the subarachnoid spaces associated with smooth insula also suggests metabolic disorders (Fig. 18), although it is not specific to any particular disorder.

HIE

Perinatal hypoxia-ischemia is commonly revealed by seizures. It presents as an encephalopathy (HIE) that manifests either by intraperiventricular hemorrhage and leukomalacia (in early premature babies), or by focal-diffuse ischemic brain damage (in term babies). Hemorrhages are mainly seen in premature babies before 32 weeks. MR imaging is usually performed when posterior fossa

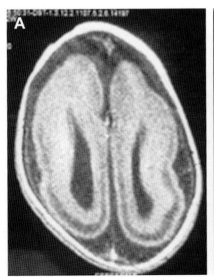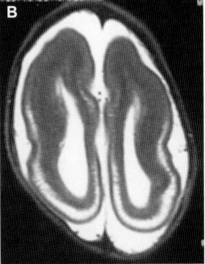

Fig. 15. Complete agyria in a 2-week-old neonate; axial T1WI (A) and T2WI (B). Note the complete absence of sulci with a shallow sylvian fissure, and a circumferential band of high signal intensity on T2 most prominent in the parietooccipital cortex corresponding with a cell-sparse zone with increased water content.

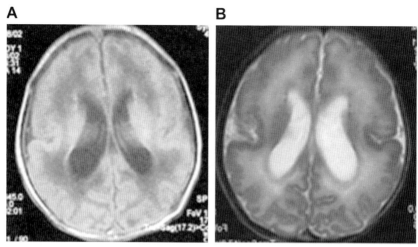

Fig. 16. Bilateral PMG in congenital cytomegalovirus infection; axial T1 (*A*) and T2 (*B*) images. Note the undulating appearance of the cerebral surface of the frontoparietal areas.

hemorrhage is suspected and in presurgical evaluation of posthemorrhagic hydrocephalus to evaluate possible brain damage and ependymal destruction. Lesions of the white matter are known as periventricular leukomalacia (PVL) and are mainly, but not exclusively, encountered in premature neonates (they may be observed in term infants when associated with severe congenital heart disease). Cystic or noncystic leukomalacia mostly involves the periventricular white matter (frontal horns and atrium) as well as the subcortical white matter where it involves the subplate and, less commonly, the corpus callosum and internal capsule. PVL might be focal, multifocal, or band-like. Commonly bilateral and symmetric, it may be unilateral or asymmetric. PVL is related in the acute stage to coagulation necrosis of the white

matter followed by astrocytic proliferation, macrophage activation, and vascular proliferation in the subacute phase; necrosis occurs within days to weeks. The acute stage of leukomalacia manifests on MR imaging as nodules of high signal on T1WI and low signal on T2WI (**Fig. 19**). Cystic cavitations display signal isointense to CSF (FLAIR imaging). Combination of acute lesions and cyst is seen, especially in cases with diffuse leukomalacia. White matter gliosis is not detectable on standard sequences, hence the development of advanced techniques to achieve this goal.

Selective neuronal necrosis is a developmental vulnerability to hypoxia that is related to age and transient increase in glutamate receptors. Particular areas of the perinatal human brain, including striatum, hippocampus, pons, and median layers

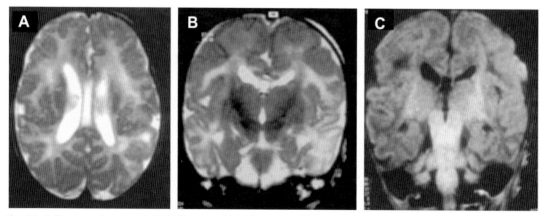

Fig. 17. Zellweger disease; axial T2 (*A*), coronal T2 (*B*), and T1 (*C*) images. Undulating appearance of the cortex in the frontal and parietal areas (*A*) suggests PMG. Gyri appear broad with poor differentiation between the cortex and white matter (*B*, *C*) especially in the medial frontal areas, compatible with pachygyria.

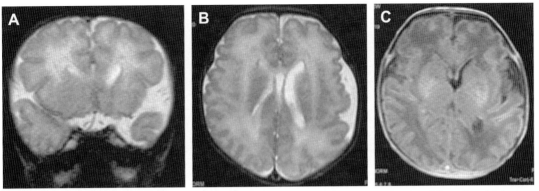

Fig. 18. Deficit in AMP (adenosine monophosphate) deaminase; coronal T2 (*A*), axial T2 (*B*), and T1 (*C*) images. Diagnosis was made in the neonatal period following polyhydramnios discovered at the end of third trimester and premature delivery at 35 weeks. Note the subtle prominence of the subarachnoid spaces over the left hemisphere with lateral ventricle asymmetry.

of the cortex, have been described as vulnerable to hypoxia and ischemia, neuronal damage being believed to involve glutamate receptor–mediated mechanisms. Standard MR imaging is still sensitive to brain injury in the first few days after injury. Restricted diffusion appears within 1 or 2 days after birth, and typically persists for about a week. T2 changes from edema begin within 12 to 18 hours after insult, with subtle loss of the gray/white contrast (**Fig. 20**), with T1 shortening appearing after 3 days (see **Fig. 20B**; **Fig. 21**), as well as restriction of diffusion (see **Fig. 20E, F**) and T2 shortening after 6 to 7 days (**Fig. 22**). Lesions characterized by T1 and T2 shortening constitute permanent injury. Cortical damage is mainly seen in the frontal, parietal, and temporal areas. Involvement of the occipital region, including the calcarine area, is rare. In contrast with animal models, damage to the hippocampus is uncommon. Damage to the basal ganglia may result in an ètat marbrè (status marmoratus), with a heterogeneous aspect of the basal nuclei especially on T2 (see **Fig. 22**). Permanent injury is uncommon within the pulvinar. Lesions of the posterior brainstem are better depicted by DWI and are usually seen in severe birth asphyxia.

Using MR spectroscopy, increase of glutamate plus glutamine (Glx) has been reported in moderate and severe HIE and correlates with the Sarnat stage of HIE (**Fig. 23**).[54,55] Increased concentration of glycine (Gly) is also correlates with the severity of the HIE.[55] For prognostic

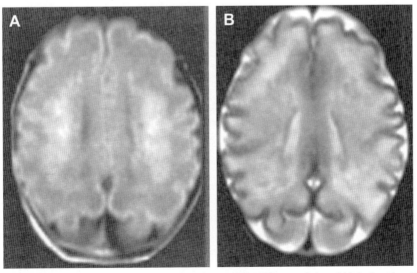

Fig. 19. Acute stage of leukomalacia, axial T1WI (*A*) and T2WI (*B*). Diffuse nodules of high signal on T1WI and low signal on T2WI in a preterm neonate exposed to bacterial maternofetal infection.

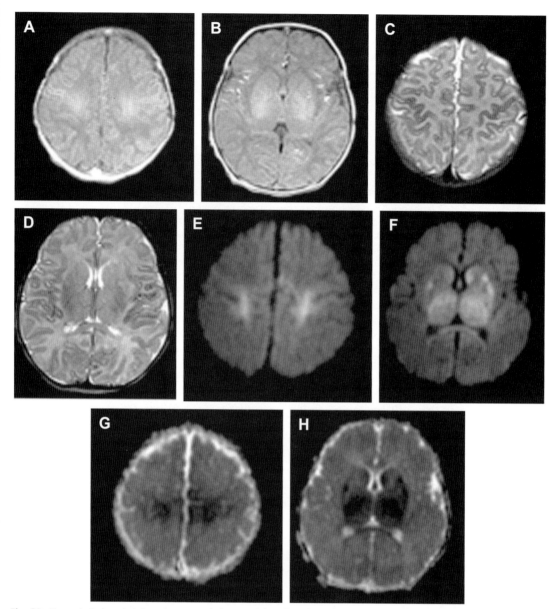

Fig. 20. Hypoxic-ischemic injury in a term infant; axial T1 (*A, B*), T2 (*C, D*), diffusion (*E, F*) images, and ADC maps (*G, H*). DWI and ADC maps show bilateral cytotoxic edema of the central area and the corresponding underlying white matter, of the basal ganglia and thalamus, and, at a lesser degree, of the splenium of the corpus callosum. T1 and T2 images are not as remarkable: note the low signal on T1 and bright signal on T2 of pulvinar thalami bilaterally; also note that globi pallidi and thalamic nuclei close to the posterior limbs of internal capsule display a higher signal than the internal capsule, suggesting basal ganglia involvement.

significance, low NAA level,[54,56] high level of myo-inositol,[57] and high concentration of lactate[56,57] (**Fig. 24**) predict a poor outcome in neonates with cerebral hypoxia-ischemia (the peak of lactate at 1.3 ppm should be differentiated from the propanediol peak at 1.1 ppm, which is associated with phenobarbital). Diffuse white matter edema is usually associated with a low level of mI (see **Fig. 24**).

HIE may induce permanent epileptogenic changes in the brain. The mechanism may be a diffuse structural alteration of the neuronal circuits but also focal changes related to the focal brain plasticity itself. Lesions of the cortex, central gray matter, or white matter may result in changes in the connectivity and cortical architectural disorganization; disconnected neurons may enlarge and develop abnormal loops with other neurons.

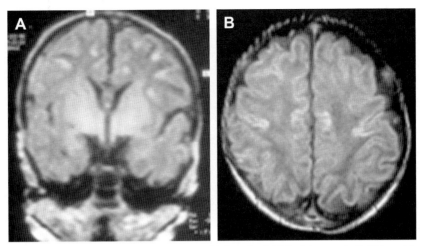

Fig. 21. Hypoxic-ischemic injury in a term infant, coronal (A) and axial (B) T1 images in 2 different term neonates. Note the bright signal of the cortex as tiny spots affecting the depth of cortex in a severe form (A) and in a mild form (B).

These changes have been analyzed by several investigators, and are described as FCD type I and may be responsible for later severe refractory localization-related epilepsy.[46–51]

Delivery may be complicated by intracranial injuries that may be expressed by neonatal seizures. Arterial stroke is uncommon, usually affecting the territory of the left middle cerebral artery: neonatal seizures are often the only manifestation of the disorder. Apart from US, early diagnosis is best accomplished by MR imaging with demonstration of restricted diffusion on DWI in the territory of the artery. Venous thrombosis is also usually expressed by neonatal seizures. US and MR would depict an hemorrhagic infarction. For various anatomic and hemodynamic reasons, MR venography at this age is difficult to interprete.[58]

Hypoglycemia is part of the acute metabolic disturbances. There are many causes of hypoglycemia in neonates and most neonates do not have primary metabolic or endocrine disorders. Hyperinsulinism is suspected if the child has recurrent severe hypoglycemic episodes. Hypoglycemia associated with metabolic acidosis suggests an organic acidemia or a defect of

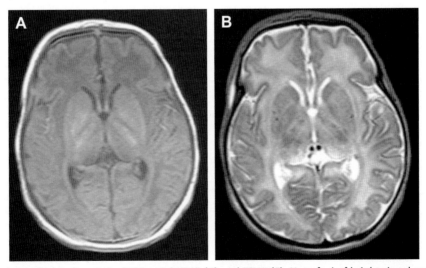

Fig. 22. Basal ganglia involvement of HIE, axial T1WI (A) and T2WI (B). Note foci of bright signal on T1 and low signal on T2 within the globus pallidus and the ventral-lateral nuclei of the thalamus giving a heterogeneous appearance on T2. Also note the low signal of posterior limbs of internal capsule on T1.

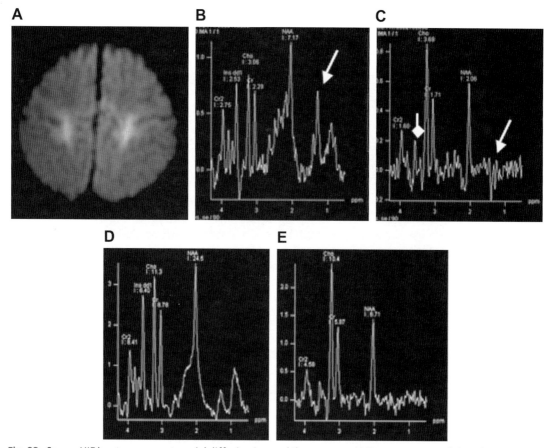

Fig. 23. Severe HIE in a term neonate, axial diffusion image (*A*), monovoxel MR spectroscopy of the white matter at short (*B*) and long echo time (*C*) compared with normal (*D, E*). Bilateral restriction of diffusion of the centrum semiovale with accumulation of lactate (*arrow* in *B* and *C*), increased Glx, and presence of glycine (*small arrow* in *C*). Note that NAA is slightly low.

gluconeogenesis. In children with cholestatic jaundice, there is the possibility of adrenal or pituitary insufficiency or defect of fatty oxidation. Diffuse cortical and white matter damage is seen in hypoglycemia, with the parietal and occipital lobes affected more severely (**Fig. 25**). Globus pallidus injury is also encountered in cases with the most severe cortical injury.[59]

Inborn Errors of Metabolism

Disorders belonging to this group are rare. Several of them may manifest at birth or soon after birth. Clinical symptoms include early onset seizures, severe hypotonia, ascites or hydrops fetalis, and dysmorphic features. Most neonates with inborn errors are born at term, initially seem to be well, and deteriorate after a symptom-free period, because they are initially protected by maternal metabolic activity. In neonates who deteriorate rapidly, it may be difficult to distinguish such a disease from birth asphyxia.

Early signs of encephalopathy are nonspecific, such as poor feeding, lethargy, vomiting, abnormalities of tone, and irritability. Seizures are mostly seen in pyridoxine dependency, peroxisomal disorders, molybdenum cofactor deficiency, nonketotic hyperglycinemia, and lactic acidosis. Neurologic deterioration is seen in previously mentioned diseases responsible for seizures but also in hyperammonemia, organic acidemias, maple syrup urine disease, and disorders of fatty acid oxidation.[60] MR imaging is efficient in showing brain damage suggesting underlying white matter disease. Specific brain anomalies are seen, such as abnormal gyration in Zellweger disease, and spongiform aspect of the brainstem and white matter in aminoacidemia (eg, maple syrup urine disease).

Mitochondrial encephalopathies are the most frequent metabolic diseases observed in the neonatal period, especially those related to deficit of the respiratory chain. Brain damage is currently believed to be the result of the glutamate-mediated

A

B

C

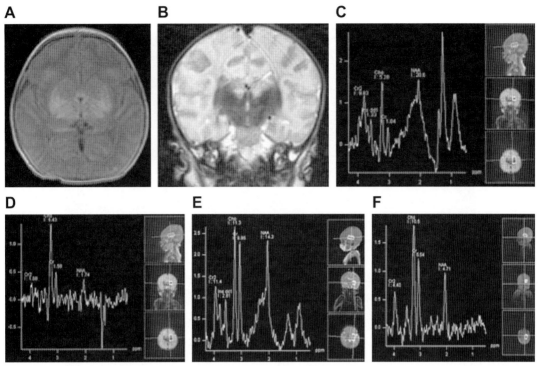

D

E

F

Fig. 24. Extremely severe HIE with poor outcome, axial T1 (*A*) and coronal T2 (*B*) images; monovoxel MR spectroscopy of basal ganglia at short (*C*) and long echo time (*D*) compared with normal at short (*E*) and long echo time (*F*). Diffuse white matter edema and basal ganglia involvement. Note high concentration of lactate, low NAA, and low level of mI within the basal ganglia.

aminoexcitotoxic cascade and of the production of free radicals[61] in response to the respiratory chain deficiency and lactic acidosis. Basal ganglia damage is rarely seen in neonates, in contrast with older infants. Various neuroradiological patterns are seen[62]: subcortical white matter swelling (edema), especially in the frontal and temporal areas (**Fig. 26**); loss of brain volume with prominent subarachnoid spaces and ventricles; absence of normal maturation (especially absence of the normal bright signal of the internal capsule on T1WI); brain malformation, especially nodular

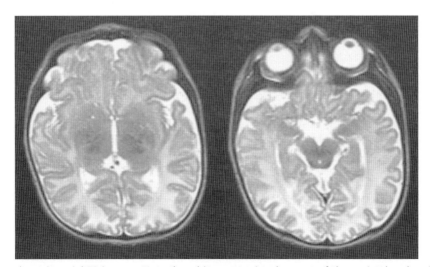

Fig. 25. Hypoglycemia, axial T2 images. Note the white matter involvement of the parietal and occipital lobes.

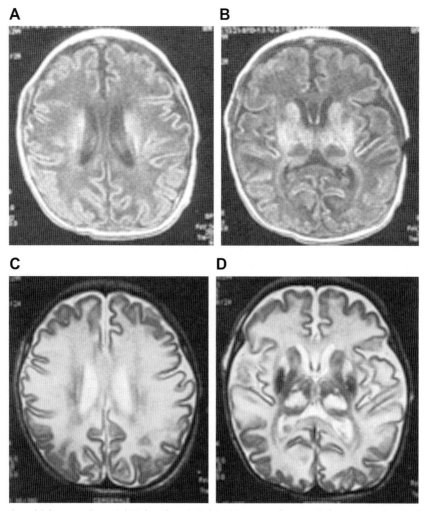

Fig. 26. Mitochondrial cytopathy, axial T1 (*A, B*) and T2 (*C, D*) images of a term infant imaged at 15 days. Note the diffuse white matter swelling with slightly enlarged lateral ventricle, which is associated with bilateral basal ganglia involvement with cystic components within the thalami and permanent injury within the putamen. Also note the absence of bright signal on T1 within the posterior limb of the internal capsules.

heterotopias; and brainstem involvement, especially of the unmyelinated areas in the anterior pons.

HIE-like lesions are encountered, usually without brain swelling, in contrast with birth asphyxia. DWI in mitochondriopathies may reveal restriction that points to cytotoxic edema. This condition lasts for approximately 2 to 4 weeks.[63] Other inborn errors of metabolism associated with free radical and amino excitotoxic cascade also show brain damage with restriction of diffusion, especially nonketotic hyperglycinemia (**Fig. 27**).[64]

Sulfite oxidase deficiency (ISOD) that is isolated or combined with xanthine oxidase deficiency and molybdenum cofactor deficiency is responsible for cortical necrosis and extensive cavitating leucoencephalopathy (**Fig. 28**) that

mimic severe birth asphyxia.[65,66] In rapid progression of brain damage with absence of criteria of neonatal asphyxia, ISOD should be considered. Hyperammonemia shows brain edema that is caused by increase of glutamine within astrocytes.

In diagnosis of other inborn disorders of metabolism, MR spectroscopy may be helpful when abnormal peaks are recognized.[14] A prominent peak in the location of myo-inositol at short echo time that persists at long echo time reflects the accumulation of glycine and is characteristic of nonketotic hyperglycinemia (**Fig. 29**). Prominent doublet peak of lactate at 1.3 ppm in the absence of ischemic lesion or in a normal-looking area of the brain suggests a failure of the energy cascade and indicates a mitochondrial disorder (although

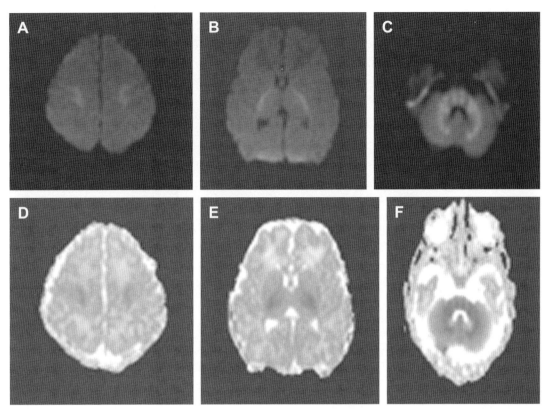

Fig. 27. Nonketotic hyperglycinemia, diffusion images (*A–C*) and ADC maps (*D–F*). Restricted diffusion is seen within the brainstem and cerebellum, internal capsules, and white matter of the central area.

there is a similar peak of phenobarb-related pro-panediol at 1.1 ppm). However, different events may lead to similar spectral patterns, and correlation with anatomic distribution and gestation history are fundamental to differentiating neonatal metabolic disease from hypoxic-ischemia: this is not always easy because neonatal metabolic disease can be associated with birth asphyxia.

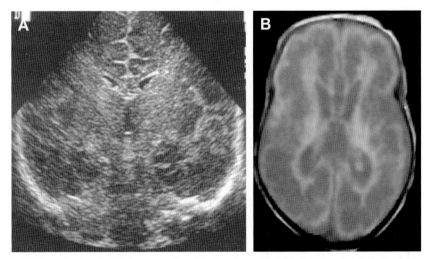

Fig. 28. Molybdenum cofactor deficiency, US (*A*) and axial T1WI (*B*). US performed at 3 days of age is unremarkable. MR imaging performed at 20 days because of secondary neurologic deterioration shows extensive cavitating leucoencephalopathy.

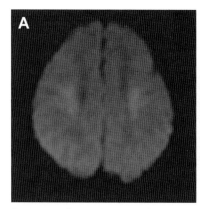 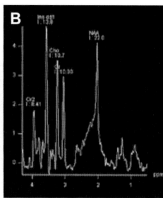 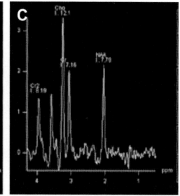

Fig. 29. Nonketotic hyperglycinemia, axial diffusion image (*A*), and monovoxel MR spectroscopy at short (*B*) and long (*C*) echo time. ml is the predominant peak at short echo time; it persists at long echo time because of the accumulation of glycine. Also note the slight accumulation of lactate.

SUMMARY

Seizure is a common and revealing clinical symptom in neonates in which the neurologic signs are usually poor. It may point to many diverse, often severe, conditions. US and MR imaging are the primary imaging techniques. CT may be performed if high-resolution MR imaging is not available. MR imaging, diffusion MR, and MR spectroscopy are the most sensitive imaging techniques in the evaluation of neonates with suspected brain injury and are especially important in neonates with seizures. The neonate can now be transported to the MR suite and imaged in a dedicated MR-compatible incubator. The normal appearance of the neonatal brain and the disorders are different from those in more mature children, and the neuroradiologist should design the sequences and read the images according to the gestational age and the different developmental stages of selective vulnerability.

REFERENCES

1. Evans D, Levene M. Neonatal seizures. Arch Dis Child Fetal Neonatal Ed 1998;78(1):F70–5.
2. Bassan H, Bental Y, Shany E, et al. Neonatal seizures: dilemmas in workup and management. Pediatr Neurol 2008;38(6):415–21.
3. Mizrahi EM, Watanabe K. Symptomatic neonatal seizures. In: Roger J, Mureau M, Dravet C, et al, editors. Epileptic syndromes in infancy, childhood and adolescence. Montrouge (France): John Libbey Eurotext; 2005. p. 17–38.
4. Tharp BR. Neonatal seizures and syndromes. Epilepsia 2002;43(Suppl 3):2–10.
5. Plouin P, Anderson VE. Benign familial and non-familial neonatal seizures. In: Roger J, Mureau M, Dravet C, et al, editors. Epileptic syndromes in infancy, childhood and adolescence. Montrouge (France): John Libbey Eurotext; 2005. p. 3–15.
6. Gourfinkel-An I, Baulac S, Nabbout R, et al. Monogenic idiopathic epilepsies. Lancet Neurol 2004; 3(4):209–18.
7. Aicardi J, Otahara S. Severe neonatal epilepsies with suppression burst. In: Roger J, Mureau M, Dravet C, et al, editors. Epileptic syndromes in infancy, childhood and adolescence. Montrouge (France): John Libbey Eurotext; 2005. p. 39–50.
8. Palmieri F. Diseases caused by defects of mitochondrial carriers: a review. Biochim Biophys Acta 2008; 1777(7–8):564–78.
9. Thibeault-Eybalin MP, Lortie A, Carmant L. Neonatal seizures: do they damage the brain? Pediatr Neurol 2009;40(3):175–80.
10. Glass HC, Glidden D, Jeremy RJ, et al. Clinical neonatal seizures are independently associated with outcome in infants at risk for hypoxic-ischemic brain injury. J Pediatr 2009;155(3):318–23.
11. Ben-Ari Y, Holmes GL. Effects of seizures on developmental processes in the immature brain. Lancet Neurol 2006;5(12):1055–63.
12. Jensen FE. Perinatal hypoxic-ischemic brain injury: maturation-dependent relation to epilepsy. Ment Retard Dev Disabil Res Rev 1997;3:85–95.
13. Johnston MV. Excitotoxicity in neonatal hypoxia. Ment Retard Dev Disabil Res Rev 2001;7:229–34.
14. Girard N, Confort-Gouny S, Schneider J, et al. Neuroimaging of neonatal encephalopathies. J Neuroradiol 2007;34(3):167–82.
15. Barkovich AJ, Hajnal BL, Vigneron D, et al. Prediction of neuromotor outcome in perinatal asphyxia: evaluation of MR scoring systems. AJNR Am J Neuroradiol 1998;19(1):143–9.
16. Barkovich AJ. The encephalopathic neonate: choosing the proper imaging technique. AJNR Am J Neuroradiol 1997;18(10):1816–20.

17. Girard N, Gambarelli D. Magnetic Resonance Imaging. Normal fetal brain. An atlas with anatomic correlations. Brunelle F, Shaw D, editors. Rickmansworth, UK, 2001.

18. Brunel H, Girard N, Confort-Gouny S, et al. Fetal brain injury. J Neuroradiol 2004;31(2):123–37.

19. Fogliarini C, Chaumoitre K, Chapon F, et al. Assessment of cortical maturation with prenatal MRI. Part I: normal cortical maturation. Eur Radiol 2005;15(8): 1671–85.

20. Maalouf EF, Duggan PJ, Counsell SJ, et al. Comparison of findings on cranial ultrasound and magnetic resonance imaging in preterm infants. Pediatrics 2001;107(4):719–27.

21. van Wezel-Meijler G, van der Knaap MS, Sie LT, et al. Magnetic resonance imaging of the brain in premature infants during the neonatal period. Normal phenomena and reflection of mild ultrasound abnormalities. Neuropediatrics 1998;29(2):89–96.

22. Girard N. Imaging brain maturation. In: Carty H, Brunelle F, Stringer D, et al, editors. Imaging children. Edinburgh (United Kingdom): Elsevier; 2005. p. 1711–34.

23. Barkovich AJ, Westmark KD, Bedi HS, et al. Proton spectroscopy and diffusion imaging on the first day of life after perinatal asphyxia: preliminary report. AJNR Am J Neuroradiol 2001;22(9):1786–94.

24. Bydder GM, Rutherford MA, Cowan FM. Diffusion-weighted imaging in neonates. Childs Nerv Syst 2001;17(4–5):190–4.

25. Forbes KP, Pipe JG, Bird R. Neonatal hypoxic-ischemic encephalopathy: detection with diffusion-weighted MR imaging. AJNR Am J Neuroradiol 2000;21(8):1490–6.

26. Neil J, Miller J, Mukherjee P, et al. Diffusion tensor imaging of normal and injured developing human brain - a technical review. NMR Biomed 2002; 15(7–8):543–52.

27. Mori S, Zhang J. Principles of diffusion tensor imaging and its applications to basic neuroscience research. Neuron 2006;51(5):527–39.

28. Powell HW, Guye M, Parker GJ, et al. Noninvasive in vivo demonstration of the connections of the human parahippocampal gyrus. Neuroimage 2004; 22(2):740–7.

29. Behrens TE, Johansen-Berg H, Woolrich MW, et al. Non-invasive mapping of connections between human thalamus and cortex using diffusion imaging. Nat Neurosci 2003;6(7):750–7.

30. Guye M, Parker GJ, Symms M, et al. Combined functional MRI and tractography to demonstrate the connectivity of the human primary motor cortex in vivo. Neuroimage 2003;19(4):1349–60.

31. Thivard L, Adam C, Hasboun D, et al. Interictal diffusion MRI in partial epilepsies explored with intracerebral electrodes. Brain 2006;129(Pt 2): 375–85.

32. Guye M, Ranjeva JP, Bartolomei F, et al. What is the significance of interictal water diffusion changes in frontal lobe epilepsies? Neuroimage 2007;35(1): 28–37.

33. Widjaja E, Mahmoodabadi SZ, Otsubo H, et al. Subcortical alterations in tissue microstructure adjacent to focal cortical dysplasia: detection at diffusion-tensor MR imaging by using magnetoencephalographic dipole cluster localization. Radiology 2009;251(1):206–15.

34. Bhardwaj RD, Mahmoodabadi SZ, Otsubo H, et al. Diffusion tensor tractography detection of functional pathway for the spread of epileptiform activity between temporal lobe and Rolandic region. Childs Nerv Syst 2010;26(2):185–90.

35. Groenendaal F, van der Grond J, Eken P, et al. Early cerebral proton MRS and neurodevelopmental outcome in infants with cystic leukomalacia. Dev Med Child Neurol 1997;39(6):373–9.

36. Hüppi PS, Lazeyras F. Proton magnetic resonance spectroscopy ((1)H-MRS) in neonatal brain injury. Pediatr Res 2001;49(3):317–20.

37. Kreis R, Ernst T, Ross BD. Development of the human brain: in vivo quantification of metabolite and water content with proton magnetic resonance spectroscopy. Magn Reson Med 1993; 30(4):424–37.

38. Bhakoo KK, Pearce D. In vitro expression of N-acetyl aspartate by oligodendrocytes: implications for proton magnetic resonance spectroscopy signal in vivo. J Neurochem 2000;74(1): 254–62.

39. Hashimoto T, Tayama M, Miyazaki M, et al. Developmental brain changes investigated with proton magnetic resonance spectroscopy. Dev Med Child Neurol 1995;37(5):398–405.

40. Kato T, Nishina M, Matsushita K, et al. Neuronal maturation and N-acetyl-L-aspartic acid development in human fetal and child brains. Brain Dev 1997;19(2):131–3.

41. Guye M, Le Fur Y, Confort-Gouny S, et al. Metabolic and electrophysiological alterations in subtypes of temporal lobe epilepsy: a combined proton magnetic resonance spectroscopic imaging and depth electrodes study. Epilepsia 2002;43(10): 1197–209.

42. Guye M, Ranjeva JP, Le Fur Y, et al. 1H-MRS imaging in intractable frontal lobe epilepsies characterized by depth electrode recording. Neuroimage 2005;26(4):1174–83.

43. Alfonso I, Papazian O, Litt R, et al. Similar brain SPECT findings in subclinical and clinical seizures in two neonates with hemimegalencephaly. Pediatr Neurol 1998;19(2):132–4.

44. Borch K, Pryds O, Holm S, et al. Regional cerebral blood flow during seizures in neonates. J Pediatr 1998;132(3 Pt 1):431–5.

45. Kannan S, Chugani HT. Applications of positron emission tomography in the newborn nursery. Semin Perinatol 2010;34(1):39–45.

46. Marin-Padilla M. Developmental neuropathology and impact of perinatal brain damage. I: hemorrhagic lesions of neocortex. J Neuropathol Exp Neurol 1996;55:758–73.

47. Marin-Padilla M. Developmental neuropathology and impact of perinatal brain damage. II: white matter lesions of the neocortex. J Neuropathol Exp Neurol 1997;56:219–35.

48. Marin-Padilla M. Developmental neuropathology and impact of perinatal brain damage. III: gray matter lesions of the neocortex. J Neuropathol Exp Neurol 1999;58:407–29.

49. Lombroso CT. Can early postnatal closed head injury induce cortical dysplasia? Epilepsia 2000;41: 245–53.

50. Marin-Padilla M, Parisi JE, Armstrong DL, et al. Shaken infant syndrome: developmental neuropathology, progressive cortical dysplasia, and epilepsy. Acta Neuropathol 2002;103:321–32.

51. Battaglia G, Becker AJ, Loturco J, et al. Basic mechanisms of MCD in animal models. Epileptic Disord 2009;11:206–14.

52. Prasad AN, Bunzeluk K, Prasad C, et al. Agenesis of the corpus callosum and cerebral anomalies in inborn errors of metabolism. Congenit Anom (Kyoto) 2007;47(4):125–35.

53. Steinberg SJ, Dodt G, Raymond GV, et al. Peroxisome biogenesis disorders. Biochim Biophys Acta 2006;1763(12):1733–48.

54. Pu Y, Li QF, Zeng CM, et al. Increased detectability of alpha brain glutamate/glutamine in neonatal hypoxic-ischemic encephalopathy. AJNR Am J Neuroradiol 2000;21(1):203–12.

55. Malik GK, Pandey M, Kumar R, et al. MR imaging and in vivo proton spectroscopy of the brain in neonates with hypoxic ischemic encephalopathy. Eur J Radiol 2002;43(1):6–13.

56. Barkovich AJ, Baranski K, Vigneron D, et al. Proton MR spectroscopy for the evaluation of brain injury in asphyxiated, term neonates. AJNR Am J Neuroradiol 1999;20(8):1399–405.

57. Scarabino T, Popolizio T, Bertolino A, et al. Proton magnetic resonance spectroscopy of the brain in pediatric patients. Eur J Radiol 1999;30(2): 142–53.

58. Widjaja E, Shroff M, Blaser S, et al. 2D time-of-flight MR venography in neonates: anatomy and pitfalls. AJNR Am J Neuroradiol 2006;27:1913–8.

59. Barkovich AJ, Ali FA, Rowley HA, et al. Imaging patterns of neonatal hypoglycemia. AJNR Am J Neuroradiol 1998;19(3):523–8.

60. Leonard JV, Morris AA. Inborn errors of metabolism around time of birth. Lancet 2000;356(9229):583–7.

61. van der Knaap MS, Jakobs C, Valk J. Magnetic resonance imaging in lactic acidosis. J Inherit Metab Dis 1996;19(4):535–47.

62. Gire C, Girard N, Nicaise C, et al. Clinical features and neuroradiological findings of mitochondrial pathology in six neonates. Childs Nerv Syst 2002; 18(11):621–8.

63. Haas R, Dietrich R. Neuroimaging of mitochondrial disorders. Mitochondrion 2004;4(5–6):471–90.

64. Khong PL, Lam BC, Chung BH, et al. Diffusion-weighted MR imaging in neonatal nonketotic hyperglycinemia. AJNR Am J Neuroradiol 2003;24(6): 1181–3.

65. Salvan AM, Chabrol B, Lamoureux S, et al. In vivo brain proton MR spectroscopy in a case of molybdenum cofactor deficiency. Pediatr Radiol 1999; 29(11):846–8.

66. Dublin AB, Hald JK, Wootton-Gorges SL. Isolated sulfite oxidase deficiency: MR imaging features. AJNR Am J Neuroradiol 2002;23(3):484–5.

MR Imaging of the Term and Preterm Neonate with Diffuse Brain Injury

Izlem Izbudak, MD[a],*, P. Ellen Grant, MD[b,c]

KEYWORDS

- Newborn • Hypoxia-ischemia encephalopathy • Brain
- Magnetic resonance imaging • Premature • Outcome

Hypoxic-ischemic encephalopathy (HIE) describes a clinical syndrome observed in neonates that may be, but is not always, associated with a pattern of global hypoxic-ischemic injury (HII) to the brain on magnetic resonance (MR) imaging; thought to result from decreased blood flow and decreased oxygen supply to the neonatal brain either before, during, or after birth.[1] HII is most likely to occur as a consequence of interruption in placental blood flow and gas exchange, often referred to as asphyxia. The clinical features and extent of injury depend on the severity and duration of the insult, although other factors such as inflammatory changes are also likely to play a role. The incidence of systemic asphyxia is estimated to be 2 to 4/1000 in full-term infants.[2] Antepartum risk factors include maternal hypotension, infertility treatment, and thyroid disease. Intrapartum risk factors include forceps delivery, breech extraction, cord prolapse, abruption placentae, and maternal fever. Postpartum risk factors include severe respiratory distress, sepsis, and shock.[3] Before therapeutic hypothermia, between 20% and 50% of asphyxiated newborn infants with HIE expired during the newborn period and, of the survivors, up to 25% had permanent neurologic handicap including sensory motor deficits and seizures as well as behavioral and cognitive deficits. These statistics were derived before the advent of therapeutic hypothermia in full-term newborn infants with moderate to severe HIE. The results of the latest Cochrane review in 2007 on cooling in newborns with HIE concluded that cooling reduces mortality or disability without increasing major neurodevelopmental disability in survivors. This reduction in death and major disability was reported as significant for severe encephalopathy, but borderline for the moderate subgroup.[4]

The likelihood of diffuse brain injury is higher in preterm infants because of low physiologic cerebral blood flow to white matter, intrinsic vulnerability of premyelinating oligodendrocytes to free radical attack, and also because of an increased frequency of events potentially causing hypoperfusion, such as respiratory distress syndrome, pneumothorax, patent ductus arteriosus, and neonatal sepsis.[1,5] The initiating mechanisms

The authors have nothing to disclose.

a Neuroradiology Division, Department of Radiology and Radiological Science, Johns Hopkins University, 600 North Wolfe Street, Phipps B-126-B, Baltimore, MD 21287-0842, USA
b Division of Newborn Medicine, Department of Medicine, Harvard Medical School, Center for Fetal Neonatal Neuroimaging & Developmental Science, Children's Hospital Boston, 300 Longwood Avenue, Boston, MA 02115, USA
c Division of Neuroradiology, Department of Radiology, Harvard Medical School, Center for Fetal Neonatal Neuroimaging & Developmental Science, Children's Hospital Boston, 300 Longwood Avenue, Boston, MA 02115, USA
* Corresponding author.
E-mail address: iizbuda1@jhmi.edu

Magn Reson Imaging Clin N Am 19 (2011) 709–731
doi:10.1016/j.mric.2011.08.014

may be a combination of ischemia and inflammation/infection; these often coexist and can potentiate each other. Major advances in neonatal intensive care have been achieved in the last decades and approximately 85% of premature infants survive in the United States; of the survivors, 5% to 15% have major spastic motor deficits, also known as cerebral palsy, and an additional 25% to 50% have less prominent developmental disabilities, including cognitive and behavioral disabilities.[6]

Extensive human and animal research in the last 30 years has shown that MR imaging is the most sensitive imaging technique for the early detection of diffuse brain injury in term neonates suffering from perinatal HII. MR imaging is also beginning to play a central role in the detection of diffuse white matter injury in preterm neonates. The focus of this article is the global patterns of brain injury seen in HII (profound and partial) typically seen at term and the diffuse white matter injury typically seen in preterm neonates. Focal injuries such as arterial ischemic infarcts or germinal matrix hemorrhages are not discussed.

MR IMAGING
Transport

MR imaging of a sick neonate is complex. Safe and successful MR imaging of the neonate requires close communication and cooperation between the radiologist, MR technologists, MR nurses, and neonatology staff. In most hospitals, MR imaging suites are far from the neonatology department, necessitating transportation of the compromised neonate. The neonate should be carefully prepared on the floor for safe transportation to the MR unit. The ears must be protected from the loud noise of the MR coils with ear muffs and ear plugs. Heart rate monitoring leads must be changed to MR-compatible leads. A physician and/or nurse experienced in neonatal resuscitation should accompany the infant during the transport and MR procedure, with the infant's heart rate and oxygen saturation continuously monitored. When ventilated, a respiratory therapist must also be present. Resuscitation equipment appropriate for neonates should be available during the transport and MR procedure.

Special MR-compatible incubators have become available in recent years. The MR-compatible incubator includes a neonatal head coil, MR-compatible monitors, intravenous fluid pumps, ventilators, oxygen tanks, and MR-compatible trolley (eg, Lammers Medical Technology, Lübeck, Germany). The baby is placed into the incubator within the head coil at the neonatal unit, MR-compatible monitors are attached, and then the neonate is transported to the MR suite, imaged, and returned to the floor without being moved out of the incubator and using the same monitors, intravenous lines, ventilator, and so forth. MR-compatible incubators remove the transfers that used to take place in the MR area, making the whole process more efficient for the staff and safer for the neonate.

Sedation

The MR scan takes approximately 30 to 45 minutes and many neonates naturally sleep throughout the scan after being fed, snugly swaddled, and having ear plugs/ear muffs placed. Some need light sedation. Chloral hydrate is used routinely in some centers.[7] The oral form is used, but the rectal form is also available. The oral dose varies between institutions and ranges from 25 mg/kg to 55 mg/kg. Another drug used in neonates for conscious sedation is nembutol, and intravenous or oral forms can be used in adjusted doses. Severely encephalopathic neonates often do not need sedation or may be already sedated by anticonvulsants. In general, sedation is avoided if possible, particularly in the preterm population. All sedation agents have immediate risks such as postsedation apnea and oxygen desaturation with chloral hydrate,[8] which are worse in young and severely injured neonates. Of increasing concern is the potential long-term risk of neurodegeneration with possible cognitive sequelae suggested in animal studies.[9]

Protocol

A field strength of 3 T is optimal for MR imaging and is recommended rather than 1.5 T and lower magnetic field strengths for optimal signal/noise ratio (SNR). A small head coil, preferably a multichannel neonatal head coil that allows image acceleration, is preferred.[10] If not available, a 32-channel adult head coil is the second choice. If only birdcage coils are available, the adult knee coil may be a better alternative, although, given the variability in coil performance, signal to noise comparisons would be needed to confirm the optimal choice. The MR imaging scanning protocol should include a volumetric T1-weighted sequence, a T2-weighted axial sequence, a susceptibility-weighted (SW) image or T2* sequence, an axial diffusion-weighted (DW) sequence with a calculated apparent diffusion coefficient (ADC) map, and at least 1 to 2 MR spectroscopy (MRS) samples in the ventrolateral thalamus/lentiform nucleus and centrum semiovale to include the corticospinal tract. For DW sequence, the b values used in pediatric centers range from 700 to 1500 s/mm^2 with higher b values providing better contrast between regions of low and high ADC on DW images. Diffusion tensor (DT) imaging is preferred in advanced centers to allow for tract-specific evaluation of diffusion parameters. Arterial spin labeling (ASL) sequences are becoming commercially available and also show great promise in the evaluation of neonatal brain injury. Resting state functional connectivity (rsFC) is being considered in advanced centers. Although DT imaging with tract-based measures, ASL, and rsFC are promising advanced techniques, their role in diagnosis and prognosis remains unproven.

In daily practice, the MR imaging studies are typically performed at variable times after birth, depending on the severity of the injury, the stability of the neonate, and the availability of scanner time.[11] Therefore, each sequence should be interpreted in reference to its sensitivity at that specific time point and the potential mechanisms of injury. In term neonates presenting with clinical findings of HIE at birth, MR imaging including ^{1}H-MRS and DT imaging should ideally be performed at less than 6 hours to allow rapid diagnosis and exclusion of risk factors such as hemorrhage before initiation of therapeutic hypothermia. However, rapid MR imaging before hypothermia is difficult and often unethical in practice because neonates transported from outside centers typically arrive hypothermic and MR imaging would delay initiation and therefore potentially decrease the beneficial effects of therapeutic hypothermia. Currently there are only a few centers that have a magnet in the neonatal intensive care unit and scan babies in the first 6 hours; most centers that use therapeutic hypothermia scan the babies while on cooling or after cooling at 4 to 10 days of life. In preterm neonates, particularly those of very low birth weight, transport to MR imaging is also difficult in the first few weeks of life because of the instability and fragility of the neonates. MR-compatible incubators are increasing the safety of these early scans but, in most centers, early MR imaging is not yet deemed clinical and therefore most MR imaging studies in preterm neonates are done near term or as part of research protocols.

TERM NEONATES
Profound HII

Pathophysiology
At the cellular level, the decrease in blood flow and oxygen delivery initiates a cascade of biochemical events.[12] Depletion of oxygen results in a switch to anaerobic metabolism, which is an energy-inefficient state resulting in (1) rapid depletion of high-energy phosphate reserves including adenosine triphosphate, (2) accumulation of lactic acid, and, when severe, (3) the inability to maintain cellular functions.[12] Transcellular ion-pump failure results in the intracellular accumulation of Na$^+$, Ca^{++}, and water (cytotoxic edema). The membrane depolarization results in excitatory neurotransmitter release, specifically glutamate from axon terminals, which causes an influx of Na$^+$ and Ca^{++} into postsynaptic neurons. There is also a decrease in the efflux of Ca^{++} across plasma membranes and release from mitochondria and endoplasmic reticulum. The intracellular calcium induces the production of nitric oxide, a free radical that diffuses into adjacent cells that are susceptible to nitric oxide toxicity. Within the cytoplasm, there is an accumulation of free fatty acids secondary to increased membrane phospholipid turnover. When cellular energy failure occurs, acidosis, glutamate release, intracellular Ca^{++} accumulation, lipid peroxidation, and nitric oxide neurotoxicity disrupt essential components of the cell and lead to necrosis.[2,12,13]

Energy failure and necrosis may occur immediately if there is severe hypoxia and ischemia but, if reperfusion occurs early enough to advert immediate energy failure, delayed energy failure and necrosis may occur. In still milder injuries, delayed apoptosis and delayed autophagosis occur.[12,14] Thus the severity and duration of the initial hypoxic-ischemic insult likely determine the mode of death; although the most severe injury results in immediate necrosis, milder insult may result in delayed necrosis, apoptosis, or autophagosis. These delayed events require ATP and are associated with activation of a genetic program.[15] Immediate cell necrosis is a passive process of cell swelling, disrupted cytoplasmic organelles, loss of membrane integrity, and eventual lysis of neuronal cells and activation of an inflammatory process. In contrast, delayed cell deaths of any type (necrosis, apoptosis, or autophagosis) are active processes requiring energy and occur in the absence of an inflammatory response. Furthermore, it has been shown that necrosis-apoptosis is a continuum of cell death variants with multiple forms of programmed cell death with different morphologic features and likely distinct molecular mechanisms.[3,16,17] It is also known that programmed cell death occurs normally during brain development and these processes might be activated more easily in the immature brain.[16–18]

Additional genetic, epigenetic, and environmental factors may play a modulating role. For example, genetic mutations resulting in mitochondrial disorders and/or inflammatory processes could increase the vulnerability of neonates to periods of hypoxia and ischemia.

MR imaging features

Specific regions of the deep gray nuclei are extremely vulnerable to damage when the hypoxia-ischemia is profound even though the duration might be short. The resulting MR imaging pattern of injury is called central pattern or thalamus/posterior limb internal capsule pattern. It is equivalent to a cardiac arrest and is seen when there is an acute severe hypoxic-ischemic event such as uterine rupture, abruption of the placenta, cord prolapse, maternal collapse that requires emergent cesarean section, or documented neonatal arrest.[19,20] These neonates usually present with Sarnat stage II or III encephalopathy, cord pH less than 7.00, first and 5-minute Apgar scores less than 5, need for resuscitation at birth, and seizures.[19,20] The injury is typically at the ventrolateral thalami and posterior limb internal capsule (PLIC) often with additional involvement of the posterior lateral putamen and the perirolandic cortex. These regions are the most metabolically active and mature areas of the brain with the most advanced myelination with high energy demands.[5] When the insult is more severe or if imaged at a later period in time, the entire thalamus and putamen, the globus pallidi, caudate head, the posterior limb of the internal capsule, hippocampi, corticospinal tracts, dorsal brainstem, and entire cortex may also be affected.

T1-weighted images

No significant signal abnormality or subtle signal change is usually present in the first 2 to 3 days (**Fig. 1**). If the neonate is scanned between 3 and 7 days of life, increased signal may be observed in bilateral ventrolateral thalami and posterolateral putamina on T1-weighted images (**Fig. 2**). This signal is graded as mild and the normal hyperintense signal of the PLIC might be preserved.[20,21] In moderate injury, extension of the T1 hyperintensity anteriorly in the putamen and posteromedially in the thalamus with equivocal or abnormal signal in PLIC is usually seen (**Fig. 3**).[20,21] In severe injury, the entire thalamus, putamen and globus pallidi might show hyperintense signal and the normal hyperintense signal of PLIC is typically lost (**Fig. 4A**).[11,20] Hyperintense T1 signal is also noted in the perirolandic cortex (**Fig. 5**) and, if the insult is more severe, the insular cortex might be added. In very severe cases, total cortical highlighting is observed, which is a predictor of a poor clinical outcome.[20]

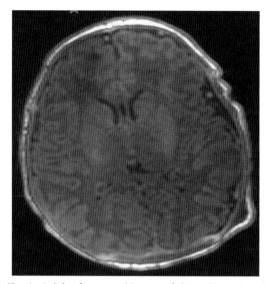

Fig. 1. Axial reformatted image of three-dimensional (3D) sagittal T1-weighted sequence in a term newborn at 16 hours of life. Patient experienced severe hypoxic-ischemic event at birth caused by uterine rupture. Normal hyperintense signal of the posterior limbs of the internal capsule on both sides are seen. No apparent abnormal signal is noted.

Barkovich and colleagues,[22] in their sequential study of HIE at term infants with DT imaging, MRS, and MR imaging showed that the lesions evolved continuously in the first 2 weeks after birth on all pulse sequences. Thus the milder injury

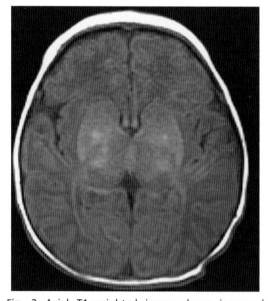

Fig. 2. Axial T1-weighted image shows increased signal in bilateral ventrolateral thalami and posterior region of bilateral putamina as well as in globus pallidi. The normal T1 hyperintense signal of PLIC is lost.

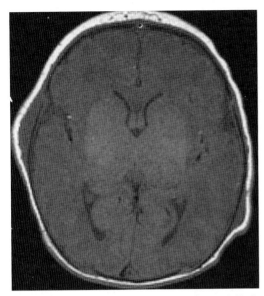

Fig. 3. Five-day-old newborn with moderate HIE. On T1-weighted axial image, subtle hyperintense signal is seen in ventrolateral thalami bilaterally and also in bilateral lentiform nuclei. The normal T1 hyperintense signal of PLIC is lost.

patterns may evolve to more severe injury patterns in the first week as delayed cell death occurs. On T1-weighted images, the hyperintense thalamus/PLIC lesions show a gradual increase in size in the first 7 days and later, in the second week,

show smaller, more focal T1 hyperintensity involving the ventrolateral thalami, posterior putamina, and perirolandic cortex.[22] T1 shortening in these areas may persist for several months (**Fig. 6**A).[23]

T2-weighted images

T2-weighted images often do not show any signal changes in the first days in central pattern; in some neonates, the deep gray nuclei may become subtly indistinct or the posterior thalami may become isointense with white matter, possibly because of vasogenic edema.[5,24] If the injury is more pronounced, larger area of thalami, lentiform nuclei, and caudate head may show T2 prolongation and the normal hypointense signal of PLIC may disappear (see **Fig. 4**B).[5,24] After the first 7 days, particularly when the injury is severe, T2 shortening develops in thalami and basal ganglia either in a diffuse or patchy pattern (**Fig. 7**A).[11,25,26] The cause of T2 shortening remains controversial. Hemorrhage, calcification, lipid release from myelin breakdown, myelin gliosis, and paramagnetic effects of free radicals are the proposed causes.[23] Hemorrhage is an unlikely cause because T2 shortening occurs several days after the initial T1 changes and these regions do not bloom on gradient echo T2-weighted images or SW images (see **Fig. 7**B). T2 shortening may persist for several months (see **Fig. 6**B). In the chronic stage, atrophy of the injured structures is seen along with T2 prolongation (**Fig. 8**).[23]

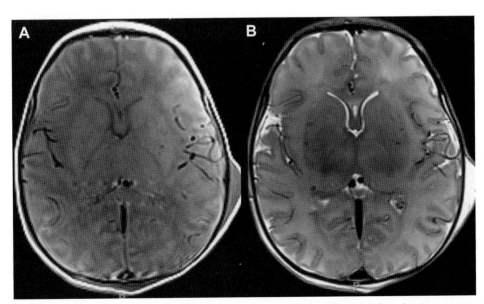

Fig. 4. Three-day-old newborn with severe HIE. On T1-weighted image (*A*) PLIC is hypointense compared with bilateral lentiform nuclei and thalami; diffuse brain edema and loss of gray-white matter differentiation is noted. (*B*) Axial T2-weighted image shows increased signal in bilateral basal ganglia and posteromedial thalami and PLIC is not seen. Diffuse brain edema is present.

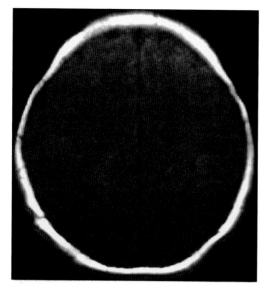

Fig. 5. Axial T1-weighted image shows increased T1 signal in bilateral perirolandic cortex.

DW imaging

DW imaging enables early demonstration of hypoxic-ischemic brain injury in the first few days when conventional MR sequences show only subtle changes. Diffusion imaging typically shows reduced diffusion in the ventrolateral thalami within the first 24 hours of life; however, because of processes of delayed cell death, the extent of

the injury may be underestimated and, rarely, may yield false-negative results at early time points (**Fig. 9**A).[11,27] It is important to review ADC maps as well as DW images because early injury typically involves regions that are actively myelinating and that are therefore low in T2 signal compared with surrounding brain. Low T2 signal drives the DW imaging signal down, sometimes masking regions of decreased ADC that are readily apparent on ADC maps (see **Fig. 9**B). DW images (and ADC values) change continuously during the first week of life, worsening until about day 5 and then pseudonormalizing at around 8 to 10 days (**Fig. 10**).[11,27] Regions of the brain with abnormal diffusivity evolve because of delayed cell death, so, for example, ventrolateral thalami may be the only affected area in the first 24 hours but decreased diffusion may become apparent in the posterolateral putamina by day 3 or 4 (see **Fig. 9**C, D) and may appear to be affected exclusively by day 8 when the thalamic injury has pseudonormalized.[11] Thus the pattern of abnormal diffusivity varies, presumably because of regional variability in timing of delayed cell death, and the pattern of injury can look different when imaging is performed at different times during this evolution.[11] After pseudonormalization, ADC maps show increased diffusion in the following week secondary to evolving cellular necrosis and vasogenic edema (**Fig. 11**). Visual analysis of DW imaging may be particularly misleading when there

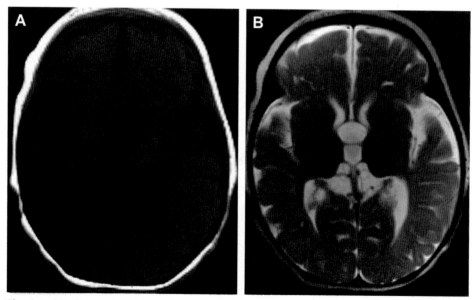

Fig. 6. Fifty-day-old infant with a history of perinatal asphyxia. On T1-weighted image (A), T1 shortening is noted in bilateral posterior putamina and ventrolateral thalami. Volume loss is also noted within these structures with ex vacuo dilatation of third ventricle. Mild diffuse cerebral volume loss is also present. T2-weighted image (B) shows T2 shortening in bilateral posterior putamina and ventrolateral thalami.

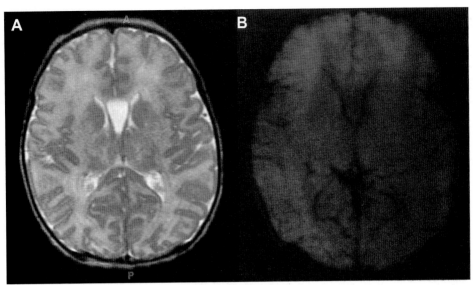

Fig. 7. Ten-day-old neonate. (*A*) T2-weighted image shows focal ill-defined areas of hypointensity within hyperintense bilateral thalami and increased T2 signal in bilateral putamina. (*B*) SW image does not show any susceptibility artifact to suggest hemorrhage within thalami.

has been widespread injury to the thalamus/PLIC and diffuse white matter/cortex, probably because there is no normal tissue for comparison. A useful clue is to compare the signal of the supratentorial brain with the cerebellar hemispheres, which are typically spared (**Fig. 12**). In these cases, measuring ADC correctly detects the presence of ischemic tissue.

DT imaging not only provides quantitative information on the brain tissue diffusivity with the ADC values but also information on the relative bias of diffusion directionality that can be assessed with fractional anisotropy (FA). This quantitative information may serve as a biomarker of the degree of tissue injury. Ward and colleagues[28] showed that, during the first week after birth, FA

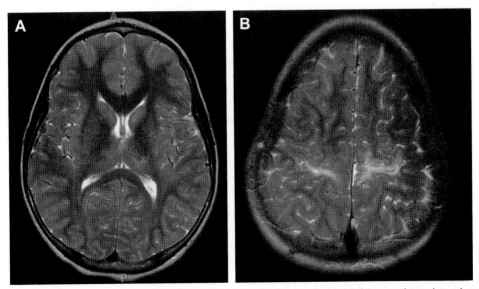

Fig. 8. Five-year-old child with a history of perinatal HIE. (*A*) T2-weighted axial image shows hyperintense ill-defined areas within bilateral thalami, bilateral posterior putamina, and possibly bilateral caudate heads; left more prominent than right. (*B*) T2-weighted axial image at a higher level shows hyperintense signal in bilateral perirolandic region.

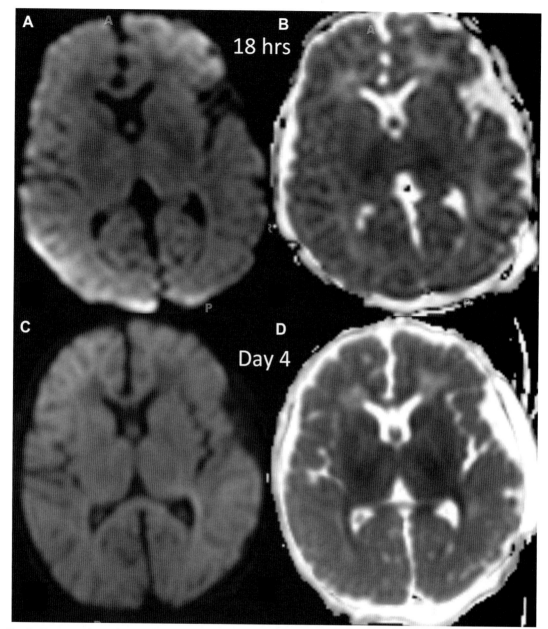

Fig. 9. Term newborn, history of uterine rupture at birth, severe asphyxia. (A) DW imaging at 18 hours of life shows no apparent bright signal to suggest ischemia. (B) ADC map shows subtle low signal in bilateral ventrolateral thalami and PLIC with quantitative values of 0.7 mm²/s, whereas the remainder of the basal ganglia show ADC values in the range of 0.9 mm²/s. (C) At 4 days of life, DW imaging shows no focal bright signal but there is diffuse hyperintense signal and swollen appearance of the brain. (D) ADC map now shows low signal in bilateral thalami, putamina, caudate heads, and bilateral optic radiations. The ventrolateral thalami measure 0.6 mm²/s, the posterolateral thalami measure 0.7 mm²/s, the posterolateral putamina measure about 0.6 mm²/s, caudate heads measure about 0.75 mm²/s, and the optic radiations measure 0.7 mm²/s.

values in the white matter were significantly decreased in neonates with moderate to severe HIE. In severe white matter injury, FA values remained significantly decreased during the second and third weeks after delivery. FA was significantly decreased in the first week in basal ganglia and thalami and became progressively more abnormal within ventrolateral thalami.[28]

^{1}H-MRS allows identification and quantification of many important brain metabolites. The most

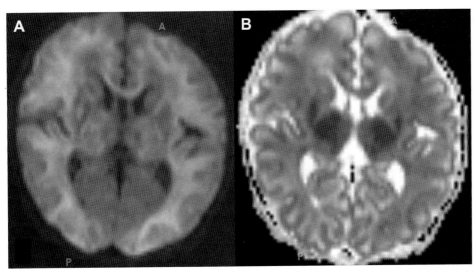

Fig. 10. Seven-day-old term neonate with severe HIE. (*A*) DW imaging shows no apparent bright signal in bilateral thalami or putamina because of pseudonormalization. (*B*) ADC map shows apparent low signal within these regions.

frequently studied metabolites are *N*-acetyl aspartate (NAA), a marker of neurons and their processes; choline (Cho), a marker of membrane turnover; and creatinine (Cr), related to brain energy metabolism. During development, NAA is also found in oligodendrocyte-type-2 astrocyte progenitor cells and immature oligodendrocytes and is therefore an ideal indicator of intact central nervous tissue.[29] Ratios of NAA/Cho and NAA/Cr have therefore been used to assess cellular metabolic integrity in neonatal brain injury.

^{1}H-MRS can also measure lactate, which occupies a special position in energy metabolism. As an end product of anaerobic glycolysis, the lactate concentration increases whenever the glycolytic rate exceeds the tissue's capacity to catabolize lactate or export it to the bloodstream. This process takes place during episodes of significant hypoxia or hypoxia-ischemia (**Fig. 13**). As in HIE, this episode occurs in utero; by the time the neonate has MR imaging, the neonate has been resuscitated and the hypoxia or

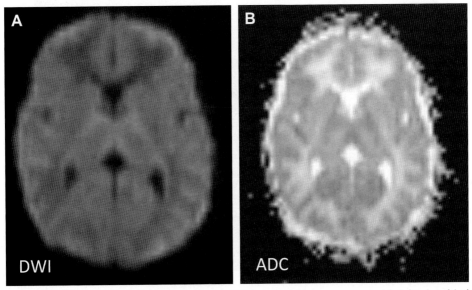

Fig. 11. Ten-day-old term infant with severe HIE. (*A*) DW imaging shows no apparent bright signal in bilateral thalami or posterolateral putamina because of pseudonormalization. (*B*) ADC map shows no low signal but higher signal in these regions, suggesting developing vasogenic edema.

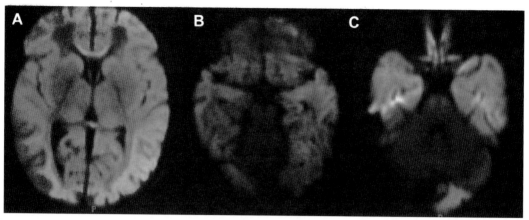

Fig. 12. Five-day-old term infant with severe HIE. (*A*) DW imaging does not show any focal bright lesion. However there is diffuse hyperintense signal in the supratentorial brain compared with cerebellum (*B* and *C*).

hypoxia-ischemia has resolved. However, lactate may be detected on these early MR studies, likely because of secondary energy failure and associated with delayed necrosis. This early lactic acidosis is followed by persistently increased lactate levels not associated with acidosis 1 to several weeks after hypoxic-ischemic event.[30] Possible mechanisms leading to persisting cerebral lactic alkalosis are a prolonged change in redox state within neuronal cells, the presence of

phagocytic cells, the proliferation of glial cells, or altered buffering mechanisms.[30] This secondary lactate accumulation is accompanied by a decrease in NAA for which the Lac/NAA ratio becomes a good marker of severity of HIE in the subacute to chronic phase.[31]

Animal and human ^{1}H-MRS studies indicate that glutamate/glutamine (Glx), which is a major excitatory amino acid neurotransmitter in the brain, is also involved in the pathogenesis of HIE.[32] The

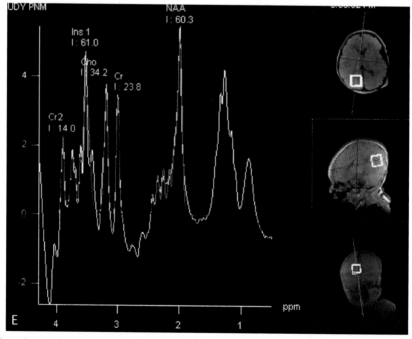

Fig. 13. MR imaging and MRS performed at 18 hours of life. Single-voxel (2×2×2 mL) proton MRS (TR/TE = 1.5 s/30 ms) in the right occipital region shows a lactate superimposed on the lipid signal at 1.3 ppm. Overall Cho levels were lower than expected for a newborn, probably reflecting disruption in normal myelination. (*Courtesy of* Doris Lin, MD.)

increased Glx in the extracellular spaces of the brain plays an important role in neuronal injury and death and may also play a role in epileptogenesis and seizure expression induced by hypoxia and ischemia.[32]

Outcome prediction

Data from several studies have shown that the extent of brain injury evident on MR imaging is an important predictor of neurodevelopmental outcome in affected newborns.[33–37] In addition, the predominant pattern of brain injury as seen on MR imaging was found to be more strongly associated with long-term outcome than the severity of injury in any given region.[38] The thalamus/PLIC pattern of injury on MR imaging predicts severely impaired motor and cognitive outcomes.[7,37–39] Children with central pattern of injury are often so severely disabled that they can not be included in long-term follow-up studies. Ability to sit by 2 years of age and walk by 5 years of age occurred in 5 of 7 children who showed involvement restricted to the lentiform nucleus and ventrolateral thalamus, whereas none of the 10 children with more extensive injury, including injury to the perirolandic cortex and hippocampus, were able to reach these goals.[40] Himmelmann and colleagues[41] studied 48 children at a mean age of 9 years (range 4–13 years) with dyskinetic cerebral palsy mostly caused by central gray matter injury and found that most children were Gross Motor Function Classification System level IV (n = 10) and level V (n = 28). The rate of learning disability (n = 35) and epilepsy (n = 30) increased with the severity of the motor disability.

Changes in metabolite ratios were shown to predict long-term neurodevelopment after HIE; better outcomes were associated with higher ratios of NAA to Cho and lower ratios of lactate to choline.[19] Early spectroscopy (18 hours after event) and measurement of high Lac/Cr ratio in ^{1}H-MRS correlated well with poor neurodevelopmental outcome at 1 year of age.[42] Late-phase lactic alkalosis is also a concern because in vitro studies show that such intracellular alkalosis is detrimental to cell survival after HIE. This information may help to define optimal resuscitation techniques after perinatal HIE to delay rebound brain alkalosis and minimize subsequent cellular injury.[43] Zhu and colleagues[44] recently showed that ^{1}H-MRS is a useful tool for evaluating the severity and prognosis of HIE noninvasively, and that higher Glx-a/Cr ratio in basal ganglia and thalamus may predict the poor prognosis of neonates with HIE.

Recently Thayyil and colleagues[45] performed a meta-analysis of the published data to reveal the most accurate MR imaging biomarker for prediction of neurodevelopmental outcome after neonatal HIE. The literature from January 1990 to July 2008 was screened in MEDLINE and Embase; to minimize the clinical heterogeneity, preterm infants (born ≤35 weeks' gestation), healthy control infants, and infants aged 12 months or less at neurodevelopmental testing were excluded from each study. Based on the MR imaging data in this literature, deep gray matter Lac/NAA and Lac/Cr are the most accurate quantitative MR biomarker for prediction of neurodevelopmental outcome after HIE in term neonates.

There has been speculation that treatment with hypothermia delays the appearance of abnormalities on MR imaging but, to date, no study has been able to confirm this.[7] Rutherford and colleagues[7] suggested that, with or without hypothermia, the second week from delivery is the best for maximum lesion detection on conventional imaging. In the recently published TOBY (Total Body Hypothermia) trial, treatment with hypothermia did not influence the ability of posttreatment neonatal MR imaging (median 8 days) to predict neurodevelopmental outcome.[46]

Partial HII

Pathophysiology

The physiologic mechanisms behind these types of injury are not completely understood, but these injuries may be associated with a protracted and difficult delivery or a history of maternal fever. Injury is thought to result from prolonged partial hypoxia-ischemia, although other factors such as inflammatory mediators may play a potentiating role. Neurologic manifestations at birth may be mild and many do not meet the clinical criteria for hypoxic-ischemic encephalopathy. In addition, the onset of neurologic signs can be delayed.

This peripheral pattern of injury seen in these cases of partial HII is characterized by injury to the cortex and the immediately adjacent white matter, with parieto-occipital regions and posterior temporal lobes typically more affected than the anterior regions.[47] One study reported that the precuneus was particularly vulnerable to damage in this pattern of injury.[24] At the cellular level, injury severity is variable, ranging from full-thickness cortical necrosis, laminar necrosis of cortical pyramidal cells, or selective cellular death.[24]

MR imaging features

MR imaging has facilitated identification of these cases compared with ultrasound (US) and computed tomography. Again, the earliest changes are identified on DW imaging within the first 24 hours and can underestimate the extent of the injury at day 2 to 4, but show the pattern of injury with decreased diffusion in peripheral cortex and subcortical white matter (**Fig. 14**). Findings on DW images might be subtle because of the high T2 signal of the unmyelinated white matter at this age; however, ADC values show approximately 30% to 50% decrease.[11] Follow-up imaging shows a spectrum of outcomes on T2-weighted and T1-weighted images, often involving smaller regions than the initial DW imaging and ADC abnormality, therefore the term stroke or infarct should be avoided when describing these lesions on DW imaging and ADC. Metabolic insult or stress may be used to imply that the tissue has an abnormal DW imaging signal. This region has experienced a severe enough insult to at least alter its energy metabolism and to allow for the possibility that some or all of the cellular elements may recover and that selective cellular death may occur instead of full-thickness injury.[16] On T1-weighted and T2-weighted images, the most obvious finding is the loss of gray-white matter differentiation in affected cerebral cortex and underlying white matter, which can be seen by 2 days. However, the extent of the white matter injury can be underestimated. The final extent of T2 and T1 signal changes in the white matter may become apparent by 4 months but may not be fully appreciable until the end of the first year (**Fig. 15**).[48] The sagittal and coronal planes are best for detection of these high-convexity lesions

(**Fig. 16**). As the injury evolves, cortical thinning and diminution of the underlying white matter occurs and may result in ulegyri (mushroom-shaped pattern; when injury is in the deeper sulcal portion of the convolutions and spares the crown).

In a prospective study of asphyxiated neonates with ^{1}H-MRS in the first week of life and correlation with neurologic and developmental status at age 12 months, 1 of the 2 MR spectra was acquired from 5.5 cm^3 of tissue including mostly white matter of the high frontal parasagittal region.[49] This study showed minimal amounts of lactate in this region, particularly in premature infants, without any evidence of asphyxia or other brain damage and it was suggested that the presence of a small amount of lactate in the neonatal brain was not, in itself, evidence of brain injury. Lactate/choline ratios were more strongly associated with neurodevelopmental status and emphasized that lactate had a long T2 relaxation time and was therefore detected and quantitated well on long trapped electron (TE) spectra (TE = 288 ms). High lactate/choline ratio but normal neurodevelopmental status at 12 months was found in 3 patients in this study.[49]

Outcome prediction
These patients may eventually evolve to proximal extremity weakness and spasticity in arms more than legs.[50] Cognitive outcome is variable, but seems worse when the frontal zones are

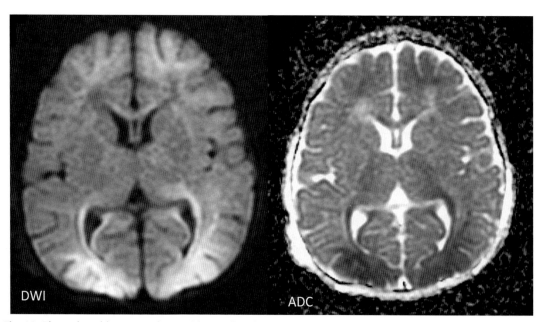

Fig. 14. Three-day-old term newborn with peripheral type HIE. DW imaging shows high signal in bilateral posterior occipital cortex and white matter also involving bilateral optic radiation. Mildly increased signal in bilateral frontal cortex and subcortical white matter is also noted. These areas show restricted diffusion on ADC map.

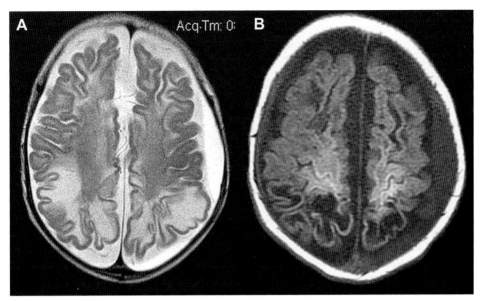

Fig. 15. One-year-old child with peripheral type HIE at term. (*A*) T2-weighted image shows hyperintense signal (encephalomalacia) in bilateral parietal white matter and also in bilateral frontal white matter. A left subdural hygroma is also noted. (*B*) T1-weighted image shows hypointense signal in the same regions. In addition, T1 hyperintense signal is noted in bilateral perirolandic cortex. (*Courtesy of* Leonardo Macedo, MD.)

involved; this impairment becomes more apparent as the child matures.[49] Severe motor impairment is uncommon in this group of infants, and they are often considered to have an early normal outcome when seen at 12 to 18 months. Miller and colleagues[19] were first able to recognize cognitive deficits associated with the peripheral pattern of injury at 30 months; more recently they also showed a correlation with verbal intelligence quotient at 4 years of age.[51] Symptomatic parieto-occipital epilepsy may occur later in childhood, often associated with reduced intelligence quotients and visuospatial cognitive functions.[52] In a recent study by Twomey and colleagues,[53] all infants with peripheral or atypical patterns on MR imaging within 10 days of

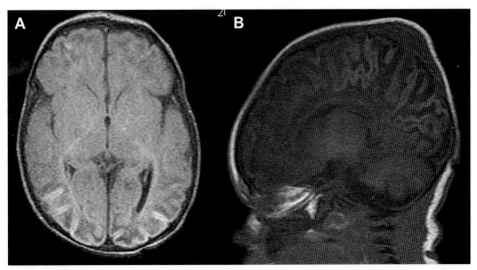

Fig. 16. Four-month-old infant with peripheral type HIE at term. (*A*) T1-weighted axial (*A*) and sagittal (*B*) images show gyriform hyperintense signal in bilateral posterior frontal, parietal, occipital, and posterior temporal cortex as well as in bilateral PLIC and frontal subcortical white matter on axial T1-weighted images. (*Courtesy of* Leonardo Macedo, MD.)

birth had a favorable outcome at 2 years of age compared with those with central patterns. DW imaging predicted outcome group, as did T1-weighted and T2-weighted sequences and cranial US.

de Vries and Jongmans,[54] in their recent review article about long-term outcome after HIE, also emphasized that childhood survivors of HIE in the absence of central patterns are at increased risk of cognitive, behavioral, and memory problems. Although most children with mild HIE studied so far were not found to significantly differ from controls, they were found to be performing between the controls and those with moderate HIE, suggesting a gradual effect. Longitudinal monitoring of educational and behavioral development into childhood and adolescence is recommended in children with both mild and moderate HIE. This recommendation also applies to the infants who participated in the multicenter trials of therapeutic hypothermia.[54]

PRETERM NEONATES
Profound Asphyxia

Pathophysiology and MR imaging features
The risk factors for development of HIE in preterm neonates are similar to those seen in term neonates. However, the likelihood of injury is higher in preterm infants because of low physiologic cerebral blood flow to cerebral white matter, intrinsic vulnerability of premyelinating oligodendrocytes to free radical attack, and also because of an increased frequency of events potentially causing hypoperfusion, such as respiratory distress syndrome, pneumothorax, patent ductus arteriosus, and neonatal sepsis.[5,50] Thus the initiating pathogenetic mechanisms may be a combination of ischemia and inflammation/infection and these often coexist and can potentiate each other. When the hypoxic-ischemic insult is acute and profound, this would cause damage once more in the deep gray matter and brainstem, similar to term infants.[55]

Few studies to date have evaluated the imaging patterns of severe asphyxia in preterm infants.[25,55–57] In these infants, the injury is predominantly in the deep gray matter nuclei and brainstem nuclei, although white matter injury accompanies this in most infants and germinal matrix hemorrhage may be seen in some infants.[25,55] In the study by Barkovich and Sargent,[25] profound asphyxia before 32 weeks' gestation resulted in injury in the thalami, basal ganglia, and brainstem. The basal ganglia are less affected and this was attributed to the later myelination of the basal ganglia at 33 to 35 weeks of gestation.[25] The thalami myelinate at 23 to 25 weeks, before the basal ganglia, and, because myelinated regions have higher metabolic activity and hence higher energy demands, they are more susceptible to acute profound hypoperfusion. However, in the study by Logitharajah and colleagues,[55] thalamic involvement co-occurred with basal ganglia injury in equal degrees, despite earlier thalamic myelination. In their study, the median gestational age of infants with cortical injury was significantly higher than that of infants without cortical injury, possibly explained by the caudocranial pattern of myelination, and by an increase in cortical glutamate receptors as term was approached.[55,58] The relative sparing of preterm cortex was also reported by Barkovich and Sargent.[25,59]

Similar to term neonates, if MR imaging is performed in the first day, T1-weighted and T2-weighted images may be normal or show subtle abnormalities. DW imaging shows decreased diffusion by 24 hours and, in 3 to 5 days, diffusion decrease in thalami becomes apparent but subsequently pseudonormalizes (**Fig. 17A**).[5] T2-weighted images show hyperintense signal in thalami by day 2 and T2 shortening develops after the first week (see **Fig. 17B**).[25] T1-weighted images show hyperintense signal in injured regions by day 3 (see **Fig. 17C**), and T1 shortening persists into the chronic stage. In the chronic stage, the thalami are small, shrunken, and often calcified, the brainstem and cerebellum are small, basal ganglia might be small or absent, and the cerebral white matter volume is reduced.[25,60–63] The reduction of cerebral white matter is possibly the result of loss of the thalamocortical, cortico-thalamic, and corticoputaminal axons.[5]

Outcome prediction
Outcome is poorer than expected for term HIE. In the study by Logitharajah and colleagues,[55] the first large neuroimaging study assessing injury patterns in preterm infants with clinical criteria consistent with HIE and the first to assess outcome beyond infancy, only one-third of infants had normal outcomes at 2 years, a third died, and nearly a quarter developed quadriplegic cerebral palsy.[55] Their study revealed a high incidence of severe central gray matter and brainstem involvement.

White Matter Injury of Prematurity

Pathophysiology
White matter injury of prematurity consists of 2 principal components, focal and diffuse, in pathologic analysis.[13,64] The focal component, located deep in the cerebral white matter, is characterized by localized necrosis of all cellular elements with

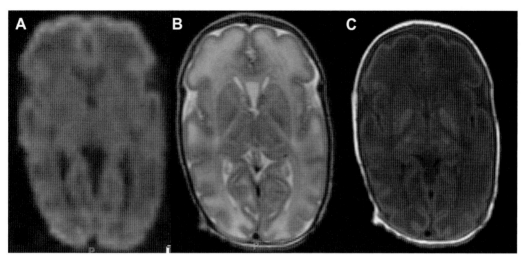

Fig. 17. Nineteen-day-old premature neonate (born at 31 weeks of gestation) with a history of maternal grand mal seizures during delivery at home. (*A*) DW imaging shows no bright signal to suggest ischemia. (*B*) T2 hypo-intense signal is seen in bilateral ventrolateral thalami and globus pallidi. The posterior limbs of internal capsules are hyperintense. (*C*) T1 hyperintense signal is noted in bilateral globus pallidi and ventrolateral thalami, and PLIC are hypointense suggesting severe HIE.

subsequent cyst formation and ventricular en-largement (classic periventricular leukomalacia [PVL]). Another focal form is noncystic with micro-scopic necrosis evolving into glial scars. A third form of cerebral white matter injury is diffuse astro-gliosis without necrosis.[13,64] Recent neuroimaging studies support that the incidence of cystic necrotic lesions is declining, whereas diffuse or focal noncystic cerebral white matter injury is emerging as the predominant lesion.[60,65–67] In these series, cystic lesions accounted for less than 5% of cases. The diffuse white matter injury is a less severe injury, with diffuse gliosis within the regions of myelination disturbance thought to represent reactive gliosis in response to damage to oligodendrocyte progenitors.[64,68]

Generally, in the acute stage, white matter injury of prematurity is clinically silent.[69] Although cranial ultrasonography can be used for screening for focal cystic necrosis of classic PVL, the cystic changes take days to appear and US is insensitive to the milder more diffuse forms of white matter injury. Correlative ultrasonographic-neuropathologic studies indicate that up to 70% of cases of PVL are missed by neonatal ultrasonography and that the undetected injury is principally the more dif-fuse component of PVL.[70–72]

Correlative studies of ultrasonography and MR imaging at term-equivalent age showed that the sensitivity of US was poor for noncystic focal or diffuse white matter injury.[31,66,67,73–76] In the study by Inder and colleagues,[66] approximately 55% of infants with extensive signal intensity abnormali-ties in the cerebral white matter, as shown with

MR imaging at term, had either entirely normal findings or only transient hyperechogenicity on neonatal cranial US. Hyperechogenicity in the posterior parietal region in cranial US has low positive predictive value for the presence of prominent white matter injury defined by means of MR imaging at term or in neuropathologic analysis.[66,75]

A recent study using sequential cranial US during the neonatal period detected severely abnormal white matter in very preterm infants but was less reliable for mildly and moderately ab-normal white matter compared with MR imaging.[77] Another study with a cohort of 72 extremely low gestational age infants performed concomitant cranial US and conventional MR imaging at term age and showed that all severe white matter abnormalities identified on MR imaging at term age were also detected by cranial US at term, providing the examinations were performed on the same day. Infants with normal cranial US at term age were found to have normal MR imaging or only mild white matter abnormalities on MR imaging at term age.[78]

MR imaging features
MR imaging shows high signal intensity foci on T1-weighted images that appear hypointense on T2-weighted images. The 2 most common loca-tions are the posterior periventricular white matter adjacent to the lateral aspect of the trigone of the lateral ventricles and the frontal white matter adja-cent to the foramina of Monro. T1 shortening is seen as early as 3 to 4 days after birth and mild

T2 shortening appears as early as 6 to 7 days.[5] The T1 and T2 abnormalities seem to represent reactive astrogliosis and they persist in the white matter for several weeks to months after injury.[79,80] The affected tissue may gradually undergo necrosis, resulting in formation of cavities in the white matter, as shown at term-equivalent age.[5,81] These cavities are seen within or adjacent to the T1 hyperintense lesions and appear hypointense on T1-weighted images. The cavities shrink in 3 to 4 weeks and the areas of signal abnormality appear closer and closer to the ventricular wall until they eventually disappear. Then the classic end-stage PVL appears with diminished white matter volume and irregular ventricular enlargement (**Fig. 18**).[5]

In the acute stage, diffusion restriction is noted in affected periventricular white matter on DW imaging (**Fig. 19**) and some of these areas might result in cystic cavities at term-equivalent age (**Fig. 20**). In some cases, DW imaging shows bilateral periventricular and deep white matter diffuse decreased diffusion.[5,81–85] In the DW imaging study of 3 premature neonates by Kidokoro and colleagues,[82] the areas of decreased diffusion were larger than the conventional MR imaging signal changes and extended to the bilateral posterior limbs of the internal capsule, cerebral peduncles, pons, and corpus callosum. This is postulated to be pre-Wallerian degeneration and was also reported in neonatal stroke and neonatal encephalopathy.[82,84] This finding might be used to predict subsequent motor impairment. Rutherford and colleagues[81] recently reported that, in infants with PVL, bilateral thalamic atrophy and abnormal delayed myelination in the posterior limb of the internal capsule are characteristic findings on MR imaging at term-equivalent age and could be used to determine whether the child would achieve independent walking. The article by Rutherford and colleagues[81] shows examples of decreased diffusion in the periventricular and deep white matter; however, decreased diffusion in the PLIC or thalami is not mentioned in this article. There are limited studies on acute MR imaging findings of white matter injury in preterm infants because of the instability of the infants around the expected time of injury, and most of the MR imaging studies are performed at term-equivalent age.

There are no animal models of punctate lesions, although they are thought to represent a milder form of PVL and are seen in a similar gestational age range. Rutherford and colleagues[81] detected clusters of activated microglia within the regions of punctate lesions in a postmortem pathologic analysis. Punctate lesions are most frequently detected along the corona radiata and along the optic radiation, and occasionally in the central gray matter. They are usually hyperintense on T1-weighted images, hypointense on T2-weighted images, and do not show blooming effect on gradient echo, which enables differentiation from hemorrhage (**Fig. 21**). Some are located in the immediate periventricular white matter and have a branching tree appearance resembling venous congestion or venous infarcts, and these show blooming on SW images (**Fig. 22**).

Diffuse extensive high signal intensity (DEHSI) is an imaging finding described on T2-weighted MR imaging at term-equivalent age in extremely preterm infants (<28 weeks' gestation). There is prolongation of both T1 and T2 diffusely in bilateral

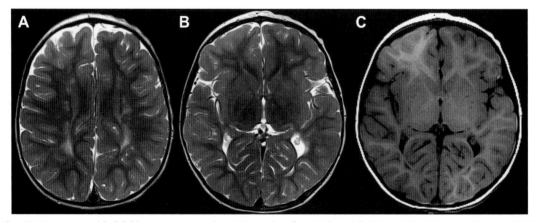

Fig. 18. Two-year- old child born prematurely at 35 weeks of gestation. (*A*) T2-weighted images show multiple small, ill-defined hyperintense foci in bilateral centrum semiovale and (*B*) in periventricular white matter resulting in irregularity and dilatation of the lateral ventricles. Decreased periventricular white matter volume is also noted. (*C*) On T1-weighted image, decrease in periventricular white matter volume is well shown. These findings are consistent with PVL.

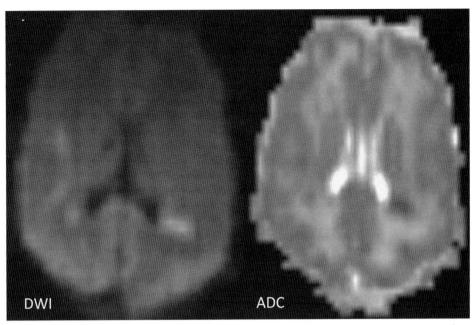

Fig. 19. Five-day-old premature neonate born at 34 weeks of gestation. DW imaging and ADC map show left greater than right bilateral posterior periventricular white matter and right temporal subcortical and deep white matter focal areas of restricted diffusion.

cerebral white matter (Fig. 23). Enlarged ventricles and thinning of the corpus callosum are noted in addition to T2 prolongation at 1 or 2 years of age. Because it is a milder injury compared with PVL and not a fatal process, postmortem neuropathology studies are not available. PLIC signal was thought to be appropriate for age in DEHSI but delayed myelination in PLIC was noted by both visual evaluation and by DT imaging analysis in a recent study from Sweden in a cohort of extremely preterm infants scanned at term-

equivalent age.[85] In this study, DEHSI was present in 56% of the infants.

Arzoumanian and colleagues[33] prospectively studied low-birth-weight preterm infants with DT imaging at near term-equivalent age, and neurologic development of the infants was followed up and assessed at 18 to 24 months of age. DT imaging showed a significant reduction of FA in the PLIC in neurologically abnormal infants compared with control preterm infants with normal neurologic outcomes. In their DT imaging study of

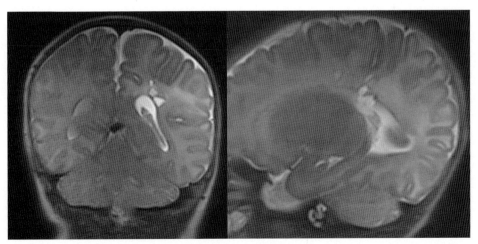

Fig. 20. The same premature neonate in Fig. 19 at term-equivalent age. Coronal and sagittal T2-weighted images show small cysts in the left posterior periventricular white matter consistent with focal PVL.

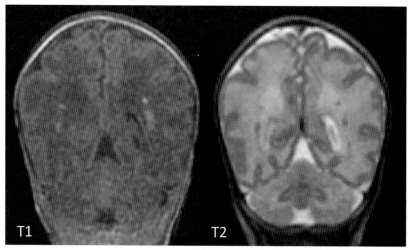

Fig. 21. A 22-day-old prematurely born neonate. Coronal T1-weighted image shows punctate hyperintense lesions in bilateral occipital white matter that appear T2 hypointense on coronal image.

preterm infants with DEHSI, Counsell and colleagues[86] reported increased radial diffusivity in the PLIC and splenium of the corpus callosum and increased axial and radial diffusivity in the white matter of the centrum semiovale, the frontal, the posterior periventricular and the occipital white matter. Axial and radial diffusivity values were similar in preterm infants with normal-appearing white matter and term control infants, suggesting that preterm birth is not necessarily associated with abnormal white matter development.[86] However, in their recent DT imaging study, Skiold and colleagues[85] showed abnormal diffusion values within the corpus callosum in their cohort of extremely preterm infants with or without white matter abnormality compared with their term-born, healthy controls.

Outcome prediction

The abnormalities of visual pathways detected on MR images obtained in late infancy in premature infants show a strong correlation with visual impairment.[87] In a study of 167 very preterm infants, moderate to severe cerebral white matter injury on MR imaging obtained at term-equivalent age, whether cystic or diffuse in nature, strongly predicted cognitive delay, motor delay, cerebral palsy, and neurosensory impairment at 2 years of age.[88] Volumetric analysis of MR imaging studies on former premature infants when they reach adolescence show reductions in overall brain volume and gray matter volume with an increase in lateral ventricular volume.[89] The presence of signal abnormalities in the white matter of former premature infants, evaluated at 15 years of age,

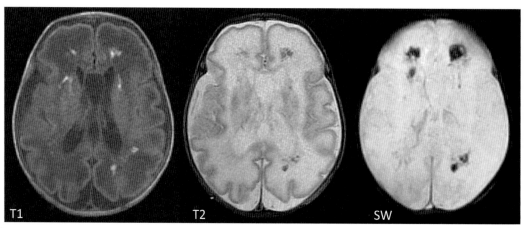

Fig. 22. In this preterm neonate, punctate T1 hyperintense lesions in the periventricular white matter are seen. On T2-weighted image, some have a branching tree appearance and show blooming on SW image.

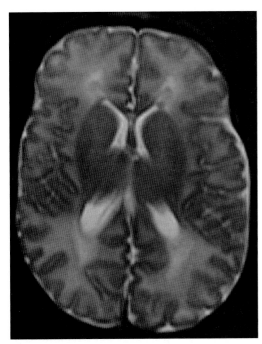

Fig. 23. Extremely preterm neonate (born at 23 2/7 weeks of gestation) who had an MR imaging study 4 months after delivery. Hyperintense T2 signal in bilateral periventricular white matter is noted.

was associated with reduced white matter volume.[90] Increased lateral ventricular size in this population was associated with cognitive and motor deficits.[91] The volumes of sensorimotor and midtemporal cortices were associated positively with full-scale, verbal, and performance intelligence quotient scores.[92]

In the presence of normal conventional MR imaging, an isolated increase in ADC values in central white matter in preterm infants at term-equivalent age correlated with a lower developmental quotient at a corrected age of 2 years.[93] One small study found that decreases in anisotropy in the internal capsule and occipital white matter correlated with poor motor outcome at a corrected age of 2 years.[94] Abnormalities of diffusion parameters of the PLIC also correlate with outcome. For preterm infants imaged at term-equivalent age, low values for diffusion anisotropy in the PLIC correlated significantly with cerebral palsy.[33,95] Analysis of DT imaging data also provides estimates of ADC values parallel to major axonal bundles (parallel diffusivity) and perpendicular to major axonal bundles (axial diffusivity). Disruption of axons is hypothesized to lead to a decrease in parallel diffusivity, possibly because the axon pathways along which water molecules diffuse are disrupted. Conversely, loss of myelin is hypothesized to be associated with an increase in axial diffusivity, possibly because there are fewer intact myelin membranes to hinder water displacement perpendicular to fiber tracts.[96] Either a reduction in parallel diffusivity or an increase in axial diffusivity leads to a decrease in overall anisotropy. Thus, some have hypothesized that injury to axons and myelin requires assessment of more than fractional or relative anisotropy values.[97] The true picture is likely more complex, but FA values from both tract-based spatial statistical analysis and probabilistic tractography indicate that visual function is correlated with FA in the optic radiation of preterm infants at term-equivalent age.[98,99]

Despite these early differences, serial neurocognitive evaluations have shown progressive improvement such that, by adolescence, language scores for preterm subjects approach those of term subjects.[62,100,101] Although there are decreases in the volume of gray and white matter at birth, there seems to be no significant difference in total volume as children reach adulthood.[102] The cognitive improvement may be attributable to the development and engagement of alternative pathways, particularly in language and memory domains.[103–105] The environment and the genome may also have a strong influence on white matter microstructure and cognitive development.[106–108]

SUMMARY

Diffuse brain injury in term and preterm neonates is a complex issue for neonatologists, radiologists, and also parents. MR imaging with advanced techniques has helped significantly and will probably continue to shed light on pathogenesis, treatment effects and new treatment potentials, and short-term and long-term neurodevelopmental outcomes in this population. There is a significant number of ongoing animal studies, clinical trials, and clinical research studies using MR imaging techniques. Radiologists, particularly pediatric radiologists and neuroradiologists, should understand and learn MR imaging findings of neonatal diffuse brain injury to improve patient care.

REFERENCES

1. Volpe JJ. Hypoxic-ischemic encephalopathy: clinical aspects. In: Vople JJ, editor. Neurology of the newborn. 4th edition. Philadelphia: WB Saunders; 2001. p. 331–94.
2. Vanucci RC, Vannucci SJ. Perinatal hypoxic-ischemic brain damage: evolution of an animal model. Dev Neurosci 2005;27(2–4):81.
3. Ferriero DM. Neonatal brain injury. N Engl J Med 2004;351:1985.

4. Jacobs SH, Hunt R, Tarnow-Mordi WO, et al. Cooling for newborns with hypoxic ischaemic encephalopathy. Cochrane Database Syst Rev 2007;4: CD003311.

5. Barkovich AJ. Pediatric neuroimaging. 4th edition. Philadelphia: Lippincott Williams & Wilkins; 2005.

6. Volpe J. Brain injury in premature infants: a complex amalgam of destructive and developmental disturbances. Lancet Neurol 2009;8:110–24.

7. Rutherford M, Malamateniou C, McGuinness A, et al. Magnetic resonance imaging in hypoxic-ischaemic encephalopathy. Early Hum Dev 2010;86:351–60.

8. Litman RS, Soin K, Salam A. Postoperative hypoxemia in term and preterm infants after chloral hydrate sedation. Anesth Analg 2010;110:739–46.

9. Mellon RD, Simone AF, Rappaport BA. Use of anesthetic agents in neonates and young children. Anesth Analg 2007;104:509–20.

10. Keil B, Alagappan V, Mareyam A, et al. Size-optimized 32-channel brain arrays for 3T pediatric imaging. Magn Reson Med 2011. DOI:10.1002/mrm.22961.

11. Barkovich A. MRI of the neonatal brain. Neuroimaging Clin N Am 2006;16:117–35.

12. Perlman J. Summary proceedings from the neurology group on hypoxic-ischemic encephalopathy. Pediatrics 2006;117:S28–33.

13. Volpe JJ. Neurology of the newborn. 5th edition. Philadelphia: Elsevier; 2008.

14. Calvert J, Zhang JH. Pathophysiology of the hypoxic-ischemic insult during the perinatal period. Neurol Res 2005;27:246–60.

15. Banasiak KJ, Xia Y, Haddad GG. Mechanisms underlying hypoxia-induced neuronal apoptosis. Prog Neurobiol 2000;62:215–49.

16. Grant PE, Yu D. Acute injury to the immature brain with hypoxia with or without hypoperfusion. Radiol Clin North Am 2006;44:63–77.

17. Yakovlev AG, Faden AI. Mechanisms of neural cell death: implications for development of neuroprotective treatment strategies. NeuroRx 2004;1:5–16.

18. Kitanaka C, Kuchino Y. Caspase independent cell death with necrotic morphology. Cell Death Differ 1999;6(6):508–15.

19. Miller SP, Newton M, Ferriero D, et al. Predictors of 30-month outcome following perinatal depression: role of proton MRS and socioeconomic factors. Pediatr Res 2002;52:71–7.

20. Okereafor A, Allsop J, Counsell SJ, et al. Patterns of brain injury in neonates exposed to perinatal sentinel events. Pediatrics 2008;121:906–14.

21. Mercuri E, Ricci D, Cowan FM, et al. Head growth in infants with hypoxic-ischaemic encephalopathy: correlation with neonatal magnetic resonance imaging. Pediatrics 2000;106(2):235–43.

22. Barkovich AJ, Miller SP, Bartha A. MR imaging, MR spectroscopy, and diffusion tensor imaging of sequential studies in neonates with encephalopathy. AJNR Am J Neuroradiol 2006;27:533–47.

23. Barkovich AJ. MR and CT evaluation of profound neonatal and infantile asphyxia. AJNR Am J Neuroradiol 1992;13:959–72.

24. Rennie JM, Hagmann CF, Robertson NJ. Neonatal cerebral investigation. Cambridge (United Kingdom): Cambridge University Press; 2008.

25. Barkovich AJ, Sargent SK. Profound asphyxia in the premature infant: imaging findings. AJNR Am J Neuroradiol 1995;16:1837–46.

26. Huang BY, Castillo M. Hypoxic-ischemic brain injury: imaging findings from birth to adulthood. Radiographics 2008;28:417–39.

27. Rutherford M, Srinivasan L, Dyet L, et al. Magnetic resonance imaging in perinatal brain injury: clinical presentation, lesions and outcome. Pediatr Radiol 2006;36:582–92.

28. Ward P, Counsell S, Allsop J, et al. Reduced fractional anisotropy on diffusion tensor magnetic resonance imaging after hypoxic-ischemic encephalopathy. Pediatrics 2006;117(4):e619–30.

29. Bhakoo K, Pearce D. In vitro expression of N-acetyl-aspartate by oligodendrocytes: implications for proton magnetic resonance spectroscopy signal in vivo. J Neurochem 2000;74:254–62.

30. Robertson N, Cox IJ, Cowan F, et al. Cerebral intracellular lactic alkalosis persisting months after neonatal encephalopathy measured by magnetic resonance spectroscopy. Pediatr Res 1999;46:287–96.

31. Roelants-van Rijn A, van der Gront J, de Vries L, et al. Value of 1H-MRS using different echo times in neonates with cerebral hypoxia-ischemia. Pediatr Res 2001;49:356–62.

32. Pu Y, Li QY, Zeng CM, et al. Increased detectability of alpha-brain glutamate/glutamine in neonatal hypoxic-ischemic encephalopathy. AJNR Am J Neuroradiol 2000;21:203–12.

33. Arzoumanian Y, Mirmiran M, Barnes PD, et al. Diffusion tensor brain imaging findings at term-equivalent age may predict neurologic abnormalities in low birth weight preterm infants. AJNR Am J Neuroradiol 2003;24:1646–53.

34. Belet N, Belet U, Incesu L, et al. Hypoxic-ischemic encephalopathy: correlation of serial MRI and outcome. Pediatr Neurol 2004;31:267–74.

35. Boichot C, Walker PM, Durand C, et al. Term neonate prognoses after perinatal asphyxia: contributions of MR imaging, MR spectroscopy, relaxation times, and apparent diffusion coefficients. Radiology 2006;239:839–48.

36. Chau V, Poskitt KJ, Miller SP. Advanced neuroimaging techniques for the term newborn with encephalopathy. Pediatr Neurol 2009;40:181–8.

37. Kuenzle C, Baenziger O, Martin E, et al. Prognostic value of early MR imaging in term infants with

severe perinatal asphyxia. Neuropediatrics 1994; 25:191–200.

38. Miller SP, Ramaswamy V, Michelson D, et al. Patterns of brain injury in term neonatal encephalopathy. J Pediatr 2005;146:453–60.

39. Barkovich AJ, Hajnal BL, Vigneron D, et al. Prediction of neuromotor outcome in perinatal asphyxia: evaluation of MR scoring systems. AJNR Am J Neuroradiol 1998;19:143–9.

40. Krägeloh-Mann I, Helber A, Mader I, et al. Bilateral lesions of thalamus and basal ganglia: origin and outcome. Dev Med Child Neurol 2002; 44:477–84.

41. Himmelmann K, Hagberg G, Wiklund LM, et al. Dyskinetic cerebral palsy: a population based study of children born between 1991 and 1998. Dev Med Child Neurol 2007;49:246–51.

42. Hanrahan J, Cox I, Azzopardi D, et al. Relation between proton magnetic resonance spectroscopy within 18 hours of birth asphyxia and neurodevelopment at 1 year of age. Dev Med Child Neurol 1999;41(2):76–82.

43. Robertson NJ, Cowan FM, Cox IJ, et al. Brain alkaline intracellular pH after neonatal encephalopathy. Ann Neurol 2002;52(6):732–42.

44. Zhu W, Zhong W, Qi J, et al. Proton magnetic resonance spectroscopy in neonates with hypoxic-ischemic injury and its prognostic value. Transl Res 2008;152:225–32.

45. Thayyil S, Chandrasekaran M, Taylor A, et al. Cerebral magnetic resonance biomarkers for predicting neurodevelopmental outcome following neonatal encephalopathy: a meta-analysis. Pediatrics 2010; 125(2):e382–95.

46. Rutherford M, Ramenghi L, Edwards AD, et al. Assessment of brain tissue injury after moderate hypothermia in neonates with hypoxic-ischaemic injury: a nested substudy of a randomized controlled trial. Lancet Neurol 2010;9:39.

47. Volpe JJ, Pasternak JF. Parasagittal cerebral injury in neonatal hypoxic-ischaemic encephalopathy. J Pediatr 1977;91:472–6.

48. Byrne P, Welch R, Johnson MA, et al. Serial magnetic resonance imaging in neonatal hypoxic-ischemic encephalopathy. J Pediatr 1990;117: 694–700.

49. Barkovich AJ, Baranski K, Vigneron D, et al. Proton MR spectroscopy in the evaluation of asphyxiated term neonates. AJNR Am J Neuroradiol 1999;20: 1399–405.

50. Volpe JJ. Hypoxic-ischemic encephalopathy. In: Volpe JJ, editor. Neurology of the newborn. 4th edition. Philadelphia: WB Saunders; 2001. p. 331.

51. Steinman KJ, Gorno-Tempini ML, Glidden DV, et al. Neonatal watershed brain injury on magnetic resonance imaging correlates with verbal IQ at 4 years. Pediatrics 2009;123(3):1025–30.

52. Oguni H, Sugawa M, Osawa M. Symptomatic parieto-occipital epilepsy as sequela of perinatal asphyxia. Pediatr Neurol 2008;38(5):345–52.

53. Twomey E, Twomey A, Ryan S, et al. MR imaging of term infants with hypoxic-ischaemic encephalopathy as a predictor of neurodevelopmental outcome and late MRI appearances. Pediatr Radiol 2010;40(9):1526–35.

54. de Vries LS, Jongmans MJ. Long-term outcome after neonatal hypoxic-ischaemic encephalopathy. Arch Dis Child Fetal Neonatal Ed 2010;95(3): F220–4.

55. Logitharajah P, Rutherford MA, Cowan F. Hypoxic-ischemic encephalopathy in preterm infants: antecedent factors, brain imaging and outcomes. Pediatr Res 2009;66(2):222–9.

56. Keeney SE, Adcock EW, McArdle CB. Prospective observations of 100 high-risk neonates by high-field (1.5 Tesla) magnetic resonance imaging of the central nervous system. II. Lesions associated with hypoxic-ischemic encephalopathy. Pediatrics 1991;87(4):431–8.

57. Sie LT, van der Knaap MS, Oosting J, et al. MR patterns of hypoxic-ischemic brain damage after prenatal, perinatal, or postnatal asphyxia. Neuropediatrics 2000;31(3):128–36.

58. Talos DM, Follett PL, Folkerth RD, et al. Developmental regulation of alpha-amino-3-hydroxy-5-methyl-4-isoxazole-propionic acid receptor subunit expression in the forebrain and relationship to regional susceptibility to hypoxic/ischemic injury. II. Human cerebral white matter and cortex. J Comp Neurol 2006;497:61–77.

59. Hasegawa M, Houdou S, Mito T, et al. Development of myelination in the human fetal and infant cerebrum: a myelin basic protein immunohistochemical study. Brain Dev 1992;14:1–6.

60. Dyet LE, Kennea R, Counsell SJ, et al. Natural history of brain lesions in extremely preterm infants studied with serial magnetic resonance from birth and neurodevelopmental assessment. Pediatrics 2006;118:536–48.

61. Nosarti C, Giouroukou E, Healy E, et al. Grey and white matter distribution in very preterm adolescents mediates neurodevelopmental outcome. Brain 2008;131:205–17.

62. Ment LR, Vohr B, Allan W, et al. Change in cognitive function over time in very low-birth-weight infants. JAMA 2003;289(6):705–11.

63. Inder TE, Warfield SK, Wang H, et al. Abnormal cerebral structure is present at term in premature infants. Pediatrics 2005;115:286–94.

64. Khwaja O, Volpe JJ. Pathogenesis of cerebral white matter injury of prematurity. Arch Dis Child Fetal Neonatal Ed 2008;93:F153–61.

65. Counsell SJ, Allsop J, Harrison M, et al. Diffusion-weighted imaging of the brain in preterm infants

with focal and diffuse white matter abnormality. Pediatrics 2003;112:176–80.

66. Inder TE, Andersen NJ, Spencer C, et al. White matter injury in the premature infant: a comparison between serial cranial ultrasound and MRI at term. AJNR Am J Neuroradiol 2003;24:805–9.

67. Miller SP, Cozzio CC, Goldstein RB, et al. Comparing the diagnosis of white matter injury in premature newborns with serial MR imaging and transfontanel ultrasonography findings. AJNR Am J Neuroradiol 2003;24:1661–9.

68. Kinney HC, Back SA. Human oligodendroglial development: relationship to periventricular leukomalacia. Semin Pediatr Neurol 1998;5:180–9.

69. Perlman JM, Risser R, Broyles RS. Bilateral cystic periventricular leukomalacia in the premature infant: associated risk factors. Pediatrics 1996;97:822–7.

70. Rodriguez J, Claus D, Verellen G, et al. Periventricular leukomalacia: ultrasonic and neuropathologic correlations. Dev Med Child Neurol 1990;32:347–52.

71. Paneth N, Rudelli R, Monte W, et al. White matter necrosis in very low birth weight infants: neuropathologic and ultrasonographic findings in infants surviving six days or longer. J Pediatr 1990;116:975–84.

72. Hope PL, Gould SJ, Howard S, et al. Precision of ultrasound diagnosis of pathologically verified lesions in the brains of very preterm infants. Dev Med Child Neurol 1988;30:457–71.

73. Maalouf EF, Duggan PJ, Counsell S, et al. Comparison of findings on cranial ultrasound and magnetic resonance imaging in preterm infants. Pediatrics 2001;107:719–27.

74. Roelants-van Rijn AM, Groenendaal F, Beek FJ, et al. Parenchymal brain injury in the preterm infant: comparison of cranial ultrasound, MRI and neurodevelopmental outcome. Neuropediatrics 2001;32:80–9.

75. van Mezel-Meijler G, van der Knaap MS, Oosting J, et al. Predictive value of neonatal MRI as compared to ultrasound in premature infants with mild periventricular white matter changes. Neuropediatrics 1999;30:231–8.

76. Childs AM, Cornette L, Ramenghi LA, et al. Magnetic resonance and cranial ultrasound characteristics of periventricular white matter abnormalities in newborn infants. Clin Radiol 2001;56:647–55.

77. Leijser LM, de Bruïne FT, van der Grond J, et al. Is sequential cranial ultrasound reliable for detection of white matter injury in very preterm infants? Neuroradiology 2010;52(5):397–406.

78. Horsch S, Skiöld B, Hallberg B, et al. Cranial ultrasound and MRI at term age in extremely preterm infants. Arch Dis Child Fetal Neonatal Ed 2010;95(5):F310–4.

79. Felderhoff-Mueser U, Rutherford MA, Squier WV, et al. Relationship between MR imaging and histopathologic findings of the brain in extremely sick preterm infants. AJNR Am J Neuroradiol 1999;20:1349–57.

80. Schouman-Claeys E, Henry-Feugeas MC, Roset F, et al. Periventricular leukomalacia: correlation between MR imaging and autopsy findings during the first 2 months of life. Radiology 1993;189:59–64.

81. Rutherford MA, Supramaniam V, Ederies A, et al. Magnetic resonance imaging of white matter diseases of prematurity. Neuroradiology 2010;52(6):505–21.

82. Kidokoro H, Kubota T, Ohe H, et al. Diffusion-weighted magnetic resonance imaging in infants with periventricular leukomalacia. Neuropediatrics 2008;39:233–8.

83. Inder TE, Huppi PS, Warfield SK, et al. Periventricular white matter injury in the premature infant is followed by reduced cerebral cortical gray matter volume at term. Ann Neurol 1999;46(5):755–60.

84. Domi T, deVeber G, Shroff M, et al. Corticospinal tract pre-wallerian degeneration: a novel outcome predictor for pediatric stroke on acute MRI. Stroke 2009;40(3):780–7.

85. Skiold B, Horsch S, Hallberg B, et al. White matter changes in extremely preterm infants, a population-based diffusion tensor imaging study. Acta Paediatr 2010;99:842–9.

86. Counsell SJ, Shen Y, Boardman JP, et al. Axial and radial diffusivity in preterm infants who have diffuse white matter changes on magnetic resonance imaging at term-equivalent age. Pediatrics 2006;117(2):376–86.

87. Lanzi G, Fazzi E, Uggetti C, et al. Cerebral visual impairment in periventricular leukomalacia. Neuropediatrics 1998;29:145–50.

88. Woodward LJ, Anderson PJ, Austin NC, et al. Neonatal MRI to predict neurodevelopmental outcomes in preterm infants. N Engl J Med 2006;355:685–94.

89. Nosarti C, Al-Asady MH, Frangou S, et al. Adolescents who were born very preterm have decreased brain volumes. Brain 2002;125:1616–23.

90. Panigrahy A, Barnes PD, Robertson RL, et al. Volumetric brain differences in children with periventricular T2-signal hyperintensities: a grouping by gestational age at birth. AJR Am J Roentgenol 2001;177:695–702.

91. Melhem ER, Hoon AH, Ferrucci JT Jr, et al. Periventricular leukomalacia: relationship between lateral ventricular volume on brain MR images and severity of cognitive and motor impairment. Radiology 2000;214:199–204.

92. Peterson BS, Vohr B, Staib LH, et al. Regional brain volume abnormalities and long-term cognitive outcome in preterm infants. JAMA 2000;284:1939–47.

93. Krishnan ML, Dyet LE, Boardman JP, et al. Relationship between white matter apparent diffusion coefficients in preterm infants at term-equivalent age and developmental outcome at 2 years. Pediatrics 2007;120:e604–9.

94. Drobyshevsky A, Bregman J, Store P, et al. Serial diffusion tensor imaging detects white matter changes that correlate with motor outcome in premature infants. Dev Neurosci 2007;29:289–301.

95. Rose J, Mirmiran M, Butler EE, et al. Neonatal microstructural development of the internal capsule on diffusion tensor imaging correlates with severity of gait. Dev Med Child Neurol 2007;49:745–50.

96. Song SK, Sun SW, Ju WK, et al. Diffusion tensor imaging detects and differentiates axon and myelin degeneration in mouse optic nerve after retinal ischemia. Neuroimage 2003;20:1714–22.

97. Mathur AM, Neil JJ, Inder TE. Understanding brain injury and neurodevelopmental disabilities in the preterm infant: the evolving role of advanced magnetic resonance imaging. Semin Perinatol 2010;34(1):57–66.

98. Bassi L, Ricci D, Volzone A, et al. Probabilistic diffusion tractography of the optic radiations and visual function in preterm infants at term equivalent age. Brain 2008;131:573–82.

99. Berman JI, Glass HC, Miller SP, et al. Quantitative fiber tracking analysis of the optic radiation correlated with visual performance in premature newborns. AJNR Am J Neuroradiol 2009;30:120–4.

100. Saigal S, Doyle LW. An overview of mortality and sequela of preterm birth from infancy to adulthood. Lancet 2008;371(9608):261–9.

101. Scafidi J, Fagel DM, Ment LR, et al. Modeling premature brain injury and recovery. Int J Dev Neurosci 2009;27(8):863–71.

102. Allin M, Henderson M, Suckling J, et al. Effects of very low birthweight on brain structure in adulthood. Dev Med Child Neurol 2004;46(1):46–53.

103. Ment LR, Constable RT. Injury and recovery in the developing brain: evidence from functional MRI studies of prematurely born children. Nat Clin Pract Neurol 2007;3:558–71.

104. Ment LR, Peterson BS, Vohr B, et al. Cortical recruitment patterns in children born prematurely compared with control subjects during a passive listening functional magnetic resonance imaging test. J Pediatr 2006;149:490–8.

105. Schafer RJ, Lacadie C, Vohr B, et al. Alterations in functional connectivity for language in prematurely born adolescents. Brain 2009;132:661–70.

106. Thompson PM, Cannon TD, Narr KL, et al. Genetic influences on brain structure. Nat Neurosci 2001;4:1253–8.

107. Als H, Duffy FH, McAnulty GB, et al. Early experience alters brain function and structure. Pediatrics 2004;113:846–57.

108. Chiang MC, Barysheva M, Shattuck DW, et al. Genetics of brain fiber architecture and intellectual performance. J Neurosci 2009;29:2212–24.

MR Imaging Workup of Inborn Errors of Metabolism of Early Postnatal Onset

Zoltán Patay, MD, PhD[a,b,*]

KEYWORDS

- Inborn errors of metabolism • Magnetic resonance imaging
- Diffusion-weighted imaging
- Magnetic resonance spectroscopy

Inborn errors of metabolism may present clinically with systemic metabolic abnormalities (eg, acidosis, ketosis, ketoacidosis, or hypoglycemia) or clinical signs and symptoms related to the involvement of one or more of the organ systems, such as the central and the peripheral nervous system (white matter disease, gray matter disease, or most commonly a combination of the two), the musculoskeletal system (myopathy, dysostosis), some of the visceral organs (cardiomyopathy, hepatosplenomegaly), the anterior visual system (cataract, retinal degeneration), or even the skin (alopecia, dermatitis, petechiae).[1] Diseases in which the clinical manifestations are exclusive to or dominated by signs and symptoms of central nervous system (CNS) involvement are referred to as neurometabolic diseases.

The age of onset of the clinically manifesting disease is a significant confounder in the remarkable clinical phenotypic variability of inborn errors of metabolism. (Please note: in inborn errors of metabolism, the enzyme deficiency may be compensated by maternal [in utero] or other mechanisms for a variable amount of time before the clinically manifesting disease actually develops.) Most metabolic disorders are known to have early (neonatal, infantile) or later (juvenile,

adult) onsets, as a function of effective (residual) enzyme activity. As a general rule, early onset indicates a more profound enzymatic dysfunction and severe, often therapy-resistant disease, whereas later-onset forms are typically associated with a more benign and manageable clinical course, but of course many exceptions to this "rule of thumb" are known too.

In addition to the typically more severe clinical systemic manifestations, early-onset metabolic disorders are important from a different point of view. The developing brain (both in utero and postnatally) is particularly vulnerable to any noxious process that may interfere with its normal development.[2,3] In the context of metabolic decompensation, patients often present in critical conditions, and the underlying disease may not be known or may mimic other more common diseases (infection, gastrointestinal problems); hence, prompt and efficient diagnostic workup strategies are needed to prevent serious sequelae. Diagnostic imaging has a significant and well-established role in that scheme; nonetheless, it is important that available modalities and techniques be used judiciously, adequately, and efficiently. At present, the diagnostic imaging workup of CNS involvement in inborn errors of metabolism heavily relies

The author has nothing to disclose.

[a] Section of Neuroimaging, Department of Radiological Sciences, MS 220, St. Jude Children's Research Hospital, 262 Danny Thomas Place, Memphis, TN 38105-3678, USA

[b] College of Medicine, University of Tennessee Health Science Center, 262 Danny Thomas Place, Memphis, TN 38105-3678, USA

* Section of Neuroimaging, Department of Radiological Sciences, MS 220, St. Jude Children's Research Hospital, 262 Danny Thomas Place, Memphis, TN 38105-3678.

E-mail address: zoltan.patay@stjude.org

Magn Reson Imaging Clin N Am 19 (2011) 733–759
doi:10.1016/j.mric.2011.09.001

on magnetic resonance (MR) imaging, which includes conventional ("anatomic") and advanced ("physiologic" or "functional") techniques (diffusion-weighted and diffusion tensor imaging, proton MR spectroscopy). The comprehensive MR imaging evaluation of inborn errors of metabolism takes into account all structural and "functional" lesion pattern elements revealed by anatomic and pathophysiologic MR imaging data to enhance the sensitivity and specificity of the diagnostic workup process.

GENERAL CONSIDERATIONS

The most severe inborn errors of metabolism of neonatal onset fall into the category of devastating metabolic diseases (**Box 1**).

Many of these conditions belong to organic acidurias and aminoacidopathies. Especially in this subgroup of the entities, clinically, affected neonates may be normal at birth but the severely altered metabolic processes lead to rapid onset of severe metabolic decompensation, resulting in global brain toxicity presenting with diffuse brain edema and neurologic manifestations of dysfunction of white or gray matter or both. Clinical hallmarks of these conditions are poor feeding, vomiting (these may mimic pyloric stenosis), seizures, changes in muscle tone, stupor, and lethargy (these may mimic CNS infection), rapidly leading to deep coma and death (or severe neurologic impairment in survivors).

The time of onset of the clinical disease may somewhat vary. Some entities present immediately at birth; those include primary lactic acidosis, type 2 glutaric aciduria, very long-chain acyl coenzyme A dehydrogenase, 3-hydroxy-3-methylglutaryl–coenzyme A (HMG-CoA) lyase, ornithine transcarbamylase, and carbamyl phosphatase synthetase deficiencies. In some others, clinical presentation is delayed by a few days after birth, such as in isovaleric acidemia, methylmalonic acidemia, propionic acidemia, nonketotic hyperglycinemia, citrullinemia, argininosuccinic aciduria, and maple syrup urine disease (MSUD). Again in others, although the metabolic derangement is present immediately after birth, actual clinical manifestations may not be obvious or severe until a few weeks or months later (eg, Canavan disease, Menkes disease).

CLINICAL SIGNS AND SYMPTOMS

Physical examination of patients with inborn errors of metabolism of neonatal onset may reveal abnormalities that may be suggestive or characteristic of certain entities, awareness of which may be helpful to the attending radiologist too. Those include dysmorphic features of the midfacial structures, head circumference changes, notably microcephaly (pyruvate dehydrogenase deficiency, Menkes disease, methylmalonic aciduria [cblC], pyroglutamic aciduria) or macrocephaly (neonatal-onset forms of multiple sulfatase deficiency, pyruvate carboxylase deficiency, vanishing white matter disease—which usually develops somewhat later in life, such as in macrocephalic leukodystrophies and storage disorders), or malformations of the brain.

Abnormal metabolites may be excreted into urine or sweat and may cause an abnormal odor, such as "sweaty feet" in glutaric aciduria type 2 and isovaleric acidemia, "burnt sugar" in MSUD, or "cat urine" in multiple carboxylase deficiency.

Ophthalmologic abnormalities affecting various components of the eye are very common in inborn errors of metabolism, and these may be present at birth already or shortly after and may include:

- Cataract (eg, in galactosemia, Zellweger syndrome, rhizomelic chondrodystrophia punctata)
- Lens dislocation (eg, isolated and the molybdenum cofactor-deficient forms of sulfite oxidase deficiency, homocystinuria).

Box 1
Devastating metabolic diseases of the newborn

Organic acidurias

   Propionic acidemia

   Methylmalonic acidemia

   Isovaleric acidemia

   3-Hydroxy-3-methylglutaryl–coenzyme A lyase deficiency

   Multiple carboxylase deficiency

   Pyroglutamic aciduria

   Canavan disease

Amino acidemias

   Urea cycle defects

   Maple syrup urine disease

   Nonketotic hyperglycinemia

Others

   Primary lactic acidosis

   Fatty acid oxidation disorders

   Zellweger disease

   Neonatal adrenoleukodystrophy

   D-bifunctional protein deficiency

   Menkes disease

   Sulfite oxidase deficiency

   Galactosemia

It is noteworthy that the so-called zonular fibers (inserting on the lens capsules and connecting it to the ciliary body, thereby keeping it in its place) are composed of glycoprotein with a high concentration of cysteine; therefore, diseases characterized by abnormal sulfur metabolism lead to abnormal formation of those proteins with resultant weakening and the potential of lens dislocation later during the course of the disease[4]

- Retinal degeneration (eg, in Zellweger syndrome, neonatal adrenoleukodystrophy, combined methylmalonic aciduria and homocystinuria).

Organomegaly (hepatosplenomegaly, cardiomyopathy) may be seen in fatty acid oxidation disorders, Zellweger disease, respiratory chain disorders, and galactosemia.

Tonus abnormalities include hypotonia in urea cycle defects, primary lactic acidosis, nonketotic hyperglycinemia, peroxisomal disorders, propionic acidemia and hypertonia in methylmalonic acidemia, and isovaleric acidemia (and rhizomelic chondrodystrophia punctata, due to contractures). Alternating hypotonia and hypertonia (opisthotonus) may be seen in MSUD.

Epileptic seizures (usually myoclonic in neonates) are seen in urea cycle defects, nonketotic hyperglycinemia, and fatty acid oxidation disorders (related to hypoglycemia).

Acute metabolic crises often mimic infection (meningoencephalitis) of the CNS, but patients with organic acidemia, urea cycle defect, and MSUD are also prone to infectious complications (this may result in confusing clinical presentations, potentially leading to a delay in diagnosis and treatment).

MALFORMATIONS OF THE CENTRAL NERVOUS SYSTEM IN INBORN ERRORS OF METABOLISM

Metabolic disorders of prenatal onset (or maternal metabolic disorders) are often associated with in utero derangement of normal brain development.[5] Malformation of the CNS is most commonly seen in profound peroxisomal and energy metabolism disorders; therefore, their recognition by imaging may be a helpful clue in the differential diagnostic process.[6,7] Some of the malformations may be detectable both prenatally and postnatally by anatomic imaging techniques (ultrasonography, computed tomography [CT], MR imaging). The most common CNS malformations are listed in **Table 1**.

DIAGNOSTIC IMAGING CONCEPTS IN NEUROMETABOLIC DISEASES
Prenatal Imaging Workup of Inborn Errors of Metabolism in Neonates

With the increasing use of fast MR imaging sequences, diseases presenting with malformations or robust morphologic abnormalities of the brain, such as corpus callosum abnormalities, open Sylvian fissures, cortical dysgenesis, and so forth may be depicted in utero too.[8–10] Early results suggest that in some of the metabolic disorders of prenatal onset, MR spectroscopy may also be of value.[11,12]

Postnatal Diagnostic Imaging Management of Neonatal Neurometabolic Disorders

Ultrasonography and computed tomography
Historically these imaging techniques have been found to be useful in the demonstration of morphologic changes suggestive of neurometabolic disease (eg, bilateral Sylvian fissure abnormalities in glutaric aciduria type 1 or germinolytic cysts in Zellweger syndrome). These techniques have a definite role in ruling out other nonmetabolic pathologies, such as hydrocephalus in neonates with a progressive increase of head size and intracerebral bleeding. It is well documented now in the literature that patients with various inborn errors of metabolism, such as organic acidurias (isovaleric aciduria, methylmalonic aciduria, propionic aciduria) and urea cycle defects are prone to strokes, both hemorrhagic and ischemic and, somewhat surprisingly, it seems that these may occur in the absence of metabolic decompensation.[13,14]

Conventional MR imaging in metabolic diseases in the neonate
In general, conventional imaging findings are nonspecific or unremarkable in neonates with neurometabolic disorders. In patients presenting with acute metabolic decompensation, brain swelling is common and, if the patient survives the metabolic crisis, may lead to rapidly developing brain atrophy afterward. Occasionally, peculiar lesion pattern elements may be encountered, some of which reflect in utero damage (eg, hypoplasia/dysplasia of the corpus callosum in nonketotic hyperglycinemia), or selective vulnerability of specific structures or substances (eg, selective damage to myelinated white matter structures in MSUD), which may be useful in narrowing down differential diagnostic options from the imaging point of view. The relatively inconclusive appearance of many neurometabolic diseases by conventional MR imaging highlights the importance of the use of advanced MR imaging techniques (see later in this article).

Table 1
Malformations of the central nervous system[a]

Abnormality	Metabolic Disorder
Cerebellar dysgenesis	Nonketotic hyperglycinemia (cerebellar hypoplasia) Respiratory chain deficiencies involving complex IV (hypoplasia of cerebellar hemispheres with relative sparing of the vermis, pontocerebellar hypoplasia) Pyruvate dehydrogenase deficiency Glutaric aciduria type 2 (dysgenesis of cerebellar vermis) Zellweger syndrome (abnormal layering of cerebellum) Pseudoneonatal adrenoleukodystrophy (cerebellar dysplasia) Menkes disease (cerebellar dysplasia, vermian hypoplasia/agenesis) Sulfite oxidase deficiency (pontocerebellar hypoplasia)
Dentate nucleus abnormalities	Pyruvate dehydrogenase deficiency (dysplasia) Zellweger syndrome (dysplasia)
Inferior olivary nucleus abnormality	Pyruvate dehydrogenase deficiency (ectopic inferior olives) Zellweger syndrome (dysplasia) Pseudoneonatal adrenoleukodystrophy (dysplasia) Bifunctional enzyme deficiency (dysplasia)
Corpus callosum abnormality (dysgenesis, hypotrophy)	Nonketotic hyperglycinemia (agenesis, dysgenesis, hypogenesis) Neonatal lactic acidosis, including pyruvate dehydrogenase deficiency, complex I/IV deficiency (agenesis, hypoplasia) Glutaric aciduria type 2 (hypoplasia) Zellweger syndrome (agenesis, partial dysgenesis) Neonatal adrenoleukodystrophy Menkes disease (dysgenesis)
Cerebral dysgenesis	Glutaric acidemia type 2 (warty protrusion of the surface of the cerebral cortex)
Gray matter heterotopia	Neonatal lactic acidosis, including pyruvate dehydrogenase deficiency, complex I/IV deficiency, and fetal cerebral disruption Neonatal carnitine palmitoyl transferase 2 deficiency Glutaric acidemia type 2 Zellweger syndrome (periventricular heterotopia, band heterotopia) Menkes disease
Pachygyria	Nonketotic hyperglycinemia Pyruvate dehydrogenase deficiency Glutaric aciduria type 2 D-bifunctional enzyme deficiency (pachygyria/lissencephaly)
Polymicrogyria	Carnitine palmitoyl transferase II deficiency Zellweger syndrome (perisylvian pseudopolymicrogyria) Neonatal adrenoleukodystrophy D-bifunctional enzyme deficiency

[a] Described in the literature in the context of "devastating neurometabolic disorders" of the newborn (note: terminology used here corresponds to the descriptions of abnormalities in the original reports).

Indeed, data arising from such techniques may sometimes allow the radiologist to propose a specific diagnosis (eg, diffusion-weighted [DW] imaging in MSUD, MR spectroscopy in Canavan disease). At other times, the advanced MR findings may be nonspecific too, yet more or less suggestive to one or a limited number of entities (eg, MR spectroscopy in nonketotic hyperglycinemia or in urea cycle defects). Such data may also improve our understanding of underlying biochemical and histopathologic processes.

Organic acid disorders
Propionic acidemia (MIM ID #606054)
   Enzyme deficiency Propionyl coenzyme A carboxylase.

   Inheritance Autosomal recessive: Gene map locus: 13q32, 3q21-q22.

   Metabolic features The neonatal form presents with ketoacidosis, hypoglycemia, and hyperammonemia; the latter may erroneously suggest urea cycle defect. Increased glycine levels in serum (and urine) are also present; hence the disease is sometimes referred to "ketotic hyper-glycinemia." The cofactor of the enzyme is biotin; therefore, other enzyme deficiencies (multiple carboxylase deficiency) related to impairment of the biotin cycle (holocarboxylase synthetase, biotinidase) may cause differential diagnostic problems.

Clinical features The disease has a severe neonatal (80%–90%) and a somewhat milder infantile (10%–20%) onset variant. In the neonatal form, lethargy, hypotonia, episodic vomiting, neutropenia, thrombocytopenia, hypogamma-globulinemia, rashes, seizures, and irregular breathing are the main clinical signs and symp-toms before severe acidosis leads to coma and death.

Imaging In the neonate, MR imaging findings may be unremarkable. If metabolic decompensa-tion occurs in early postnatal life, MR imaging changes include swelling and abnormal T2 hyper-signal of the dentate nuclei, the basal ganglia, and the cerebral cortex. In the chronic phase, necrosis of the basal ganglia, diffuse brain atrophy and, occasionally, patchy white matter lesions are present (**Fig. 1**).

Spectroscopy No disease-specific metabolites have been identified. Of interest, abnormal glycine levels have not been described as yet. As a nonspe-cific finding, increased lactate may be present at the 1.3 ppm level in conjunction with decreased N-acetyl aspartate (NAA) and myoinositol. Increased glutamate/glutamine have also been found with short echo-time MR spectroscopy.

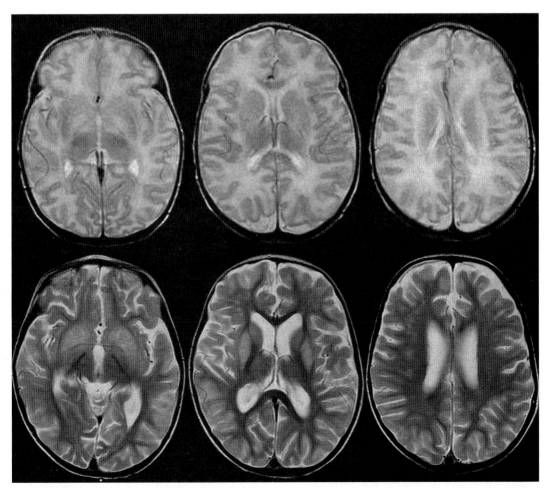

Fig. 1. Propionic aciduria. (*Upper row*) Axial T2-weighted images in a 16-day-old female infant showing diffuse swelling but no focal lesion within brain parenchyma. (*Lower row*) Different female patient at the age of 3 years after metabolic decompensation presenting with typical (although nonspecific) bilateral basal ganglia abnormalities.

Isovaleric acidemia (MIM ID #243500)

Enzyme deficiency Isovaleryl coenzyme A dehydrogenase.

Inheritance Autosomal recessive, gene map locus 15q14-q15.

Metabolic features As the third step on the L-leucine pathway (see also MSUD, multiple carboxylase deficiency, 3-methylglutaconic aciduria, HMG-CoA lyase deficiency), isovaleryl coenzyme A is converted into 2-methylcrotonyl coenzyme A. Deficiency of the isovaleryl coenzyme A dehydrogenase results in isovaleric acidemia. The excess metabolite is isovaleryl coenzyme A, which is believed to be directly toxic to the CNS, but in addition the disease is characterized by severe systemic metabolic disturbances, such as ketosis, metabolic acidosis, and hypoglycemia (due to the lack of gluconeogenesis).

Clinical features The disease has a severe early neonatal and a more benign (intermittent) chronic form. The acute neonatal form accounts for about half the cases. Affected patients present between days 3 and 6 with vomiting, dehydration, tachypnea, metabolic acidosis, hepatomegaly, and stupor. The often associated thrombocytopenia may present clinically with disseminated intravascular coagulopathy. In many ways, isovaleric acidemia may mimic propionic and methylmalonic acidemias, but the distinctive "sweaty feet" urinary odor of the patients often makes diagnosis possible by physical examination.

Imaging Imaging data are sparse. In a case of a 20-day-old neonate, atrophy of the brain with frontotemporal predominance was noted, and delayed myelination was suggested. On the T2-weighted images bilateral symmetric signal abnormalities were seen within the posterior parts of the putamen (Zoltán Patay, unpublished data).

Spectroscopy In a 5-month-old patient with isovaleric acidemia and normal MR imaging findings, no abnormality was revealed by proton MR spectroscopy using 135-ms and 270-ms echo times (Zoltán Patay, unpublished data).

3-Methylcrotonylglycinurias (MIM ID #210200, #210210) and multiple carboxylase deficiencies (MIM ID #253270, #253260)

Enzyme deficiency 3-Methylcrotonyl coenzyme A carboxylase (MCC) deficiency 1 (MCCD 1) and 2 (MCCD 2) in isolated 3-methylcrotonylglycinuria, HLCS, and biotinidase deficiencies in multiple carboxylase deficiency (MCD).

Inheritance Autosomal recessive, 3q25-q27 (MCCD 1), 5q12-q13 (MCCD 2), 21q22.1 (HLCSD), 3p25 (BTD).

Metabolic features As the fourth step in the L-leucine breakdown pathway, 3-methylcrotonyl coenzyme A is converted into 3-methylglutaconyl coenzyme A. Isolated deficiency of 3-methylcrotonyl coenzyme A carboxylase catalyzing this process is one of the more common organic acidopathies in the newborn (note that there are very significant clinical phenotypic variations, including asymptomatic cases), but it is also encountered in conjunction with multiple other carboxylase (pyruvate carboxylase, propionyl coenzyme A carboxylase, acetyl coenzyme A carboxylase; see also primary lactic acidosis, propionic aciduria) deficiencies.[15] Because biotin is an essential cofactor for all 4 carboxylases (also known as biotin-dependent carboxylases), MCD develops if biotin is unavailable[16]; this happens in deficiencies of holocarboxylase synthetase (attaches biotin to the active center of MCC and other carboxylases) or biotinidase (involved in the "recycling" of biotin). Holocarboxylase synthetase deficiency (also known as MCD of early onset) may present in neonates as a devastating metabolic disorder, whereas biotinidase deficiency (also known as MCD of late onset) manifests with an insidiously developing progressive encephalopathy usually later in infancy. In isolated MCCD, the resultant "organic aciduria" consists of increased excretion of 3-hydroxyisovaleric acid and 3-methylcrotonyl glycine. In MCD, severe metabolic acidosis, moderate hyperammonemia and, rarely, hypoglycemia may develop, while large quantities of 3-hydroxyisovaleric acid and 3-hydroxypropionic acid are excreted in the urine.

Clinical features Clinical manifestations of isolated MCCD are hypotonia, seizures, and Reye-like symptoms. In MCD, multiple critical metabolic processes, such as fatty acid synthesis, gluconeogenesis, and amino acid catabolism are impaired; therefore, the clinical picture is somewhat confusing, with manifestations of involvement of the CNS (hypotonia and sometimes seizures), the respiratory system (tachypnea), the digestive system (vomiting), and the skin (rashes), but great individual phenotypic variations often make the clinical diagnosis difficult. Because biotin supplementation may result in dramatic improvement, early diagnosis and treatment are essential to prevent severe sequelae of metabolic acidosis, including irreversible damage to the CNS.

Imaging Imaging findings in the neonatal form of isolated MCCD are not available. In an infant with holocarboxylase synthetase (HLCS) deficiency, subependymal cysts have been found by cranial ultrasonography and then confirmed by MR imaging. Six months after biotin treatment, follow-up MR imaging showed complete resolution of the cysts (the patient was neurologically normal too).[17]

Spectroscopy In biotinidase deficiency of infantile onset, a decreased NAA/creatine (Cr) ratio and abnormal lactate within the brain parenchyma were noted prior to biotin supplementation. Six weeks after treatment, these abnormalities disappeared (while cerebrospinal fluid [CSF], 3-hydroxyvaleric acid, and lactate levels returned to normal too).[18]

3-Methylglutaconic acidurias (MIM ID #250950, #302060, #258501, #250951, #610198)

Enzyme deficiency 3-Methylglutaconyl coenzyme A (3-MGC) hydratase (in type 1 MGA), not known in the other types.

Inheritance Autosomal recessive in MGA1, gene map locus chromosome 9. X-linked in MGA2, gene map locus Xq28, autosomal recessive in MGA3, gene map locus 19q13.2-q13.3, gene map locus is unknown in MGA4, gene map locus 3q26.3 in MGA5.

Metabolic features 3-Methylglutaconic aciduria is a heterogeneous group of several biochemically and clinically distinct entities, all "characterized" by abnormal urinary excretion of 3-methylglutaconic acid and 3-methylglutaric acid. In MGA1, 3-MGC hydratase deficiency leads to impaired conversion of 3 methylglutaconyl coenzyme A into 3-hydroxy-3-methylglutaryl coenzyme A, which is the fifth step on the L-leucine breakdown pathway. In the other clinical phenotypes (types 2, 3, 4, and 5), the underlying metabolic derangements are obscure, and it is believed that the "characteristic" organic aciduria pattern may be considered a biochemical marker or epiphenomenon only.[19] Because in most forms of 3-MGA the target organs are usually the brain and heart and sometimes liver and skeletal muscles, it is possible that the primary defect is an unspecified energy metabolism disorder in the mitochondrial respiratory chain, but as yet the source of the excreted 3-methylglutaconic acid remains undetermined.

Clinical features Most entities within the 3-methylglutaconic acidurias are characterized by delayed onset with their first clinical manifestations in infancy or later (including adulthood).[20] However, rare exceptions are also known. In MGA2 (Barth syndrome), although the disease does not have neurologic manifestations, it may still be fatal in early infancy as a result of cardiac failure. The so-called unspecified type 4 MGA comprises several different clinical-biochemical phenotypes, the only common feature of which is that they do not fit into the 3 other categories.

This subtype of the disease is probably the most poorly understood. One form may present in the neonate with severe acidosis and hypoglycemia. In this subtype, mitochondrial adenosine triphosphate (ATP) synthetase deficiency and multiple respiratory chain abnormalities have been proposed as possible causes. It is noteworthy that in Pearson syndrome, which is a respiratory chain defect, increased excretion of 3-methylglutaconic acid has been found to be a consistent marker of the disease. This disease usually has an infantile onset, presenting with severe hematologic disorders, exocrine pancreatic insufficiency, and occasionally with episodes of severe lactic acidosis and hypoglycemia. The complexity of the "entity" is well illustrated by the continuous emergence of new 3-MGA "subtypes" (eg, 3-MGA associated with hypermethioninemia without hepatic failure and severe early-onset 3-MGA in conjunction with hypertrophic cardiomyopathy, cataract, hypotonia/developmental delay, lactic acidosis, and normal 3-methylglutaconyl coenzyme A hydratase activity).[21] Type 4 MGA has been found to manifest clinically as Leigh syndrome too, again supporting the "respiratory chain defect" hypothesis.[22]

Imaging No reports are available on the MR imaging findings in the neonatal age group in 3-methylglutaconic acidurias. Later-onset disease typically presents with progressive cerebellar atrophy and bilateral lesion involvement of the deep gray matter nuclei. Initially, the basal ganglia are swollen and exhibit high signal on DW images, consistent with cytotoxic edema. This pattern is commonly encountered in the context of metabolic crisis with lactic acidosis but may also be observed in clinically insidious forms. During the metabolic crisis, the cerebellar cortex and dentate nuclei may also show swelling and signal abnormalities. In an appropriate clinical setting the association of progressive cerebellar atrophy and basal ganglia disease, if present, may be suggestive imaging pattern of 3-methylglutaconic aciduria, but again, this is typically not present in the neonate or young infant.

HMG-CoA lyase deficiency (MIM ID #246450)

Enzyme deficiency HMG-CoA lyase.

Inheritance Autosomal recessive, gene map locus: 1pter-p33.

Metabolic features The last step in the L-leucine breakdown pathway is the conversion of HMG-CoA into acetoacetate + acetyl coenzyme A. HMG-CoA lyase deficiency has multiple adverse biochemical consequences, including impairment of ketone body synthesis and intrinsic gluconeo-genesis, resulting in global metabolic fuel deple-tion. This process leads to a life-threatening acute encephalopathy if extrinsic alimentary supply is insufficient (eg, fasting, vomiting) or glucose use is high (eg, intercurrent illness). During acute decompensations, hypoglycemia and acidosis (without ketosis) are the key metabolic features of the condition. Because patients with HMG-CoA lyase deficiency accumulate 3-hydroxyisovaleric, 3-methylglutaconic, and 3-methylglutaric acids and HMG in tissues and blood, the characteristic "organic aciduria" in this disease consists of the urinary excretion of high concentrations of carnitine esters of these compounds, which may be de-tected by tandem mass spectrometry.

Clinical features Some phenotypes (eg, Saudi) of the disease typically present in neonates; else-where the disease is characterized by later infantile onset.[23] In general, metabolic decompensations occur mainly during the first 5 years of life and are rare later, although these may be lethal at any age. If treated promptly, patients recover rapidly and grow normally.

Imaging In neonates, imaging may be deceiv-ingly unremarkable, except for "generic" abnor-malities typically present during metabolic crisis in the neonatal brain (swelling and T2 hypersignal consistent with vasogenic edema). If hypoglycemia is severe and treatment is delayed, a "character-istic" post-hypoglycemia lesion pattern (bilateral parieto-occipital T2 hyperintensities) may also develop. In patients undergoing MR imaging examination later in life, a combination of gray and white matter abnormalities may be found.[24] Bilateral basal ganglia and dentate nucleus in-volvement as well as multiple patchy, somewhat confluent white matter lesions are typically seen.

Spectroscopy Spectroscopy may be diagnostic in HMG-CoA lyase deficiency, because it shows, in all ages, abnormal peaks at 1.3 and 2.4 ppm, which should not be mistaken for lactate and glutamine/glutamate.[25]

Methylmalonic acidemia (MIM ID: isolated forms #251000, #25110, #251110; combined forms #277400, #277410, #277380)
Enzyme deficiency Methylmalonyl coenzyme A mutase (mut−, mut0), cobalamin adenosyltransfer-ase (cblA, cblB), methylmalonyl coenzyme A mutase, and methyltetrahydrofolate: homocys-teine methyltransferase (cblC), N^5-methyltetrahy-drofolate-homocysteine S-methyltransferase, and cobalamin reductase (cblD), "putative" lysosomal cobalamin exporter (cblF).

Inheritance Autosomal recessive, gene map locus: 6p21 in mut(−) and mut(0), 4q31 in cblA, 12q24 in cblB, 1p34.1 in cblC, 2q23.2 in cblD, 6q13 in cblF.

Metabolic features From the biochemical perspective, methylmalonic acidemia (MMA) may develop as a result of defects of either the methyl-malonate or cobalamin metabolism.[26] Isolated and combined disease forms are known. In isolated MMA the most common underlying enzyme dysfunction is methylmalonyl coenzyme A mutase deficiency, which can be either partial (mut−) or complete (mut 0); these are related to mutations on the MUT gene. On the other hand, because cobalamin, in the form of adenosylcobalamin (AdoCbl, located in mitochondria), is a cofactor of methylmalonyl coenzyme A mutase, reduced availability of adenosylcobalamin (due to cobal-amin adenosyltransferase deficiency, caused by mutation in the MMAA and MMAB genes) may also lead to isolated methylmalonic acidemias, which are labeled according to complementation groups, such as cblA and cblB. Finally, because cobalamin, in the form of methylcobalamin (MeCbl, located in cytosol), is also a cofactor of methionine synthetase (involved in the remethyla-tion of homocysteine from methionine), combined AdoCbl and MeCbl deficiencies (the defect here is believed to be proximal to the separation of the AdoCbl and MeCbl synthesis pathways) may result in a "dual disease," notably methylmalonic aciduria and homocystinuria, referred to as cblC. Additional similar "combined" disease entities, labeled as cblD and cblF are also known, and the latter is believed to be related to impaired lyso-somal release of cobalamin due to a defective transport mechanism.

Excess methylmalonyl coenzyme A inhibits multiple other critical metabolic pathways such as gluconeogenesis (pyruvate carboxylase), the urea cycle (*N*-acetylglutamate synthetase), and the hepatic glycine cleavage system. Neonates with early-onset forms of the isolated disease present therefore with ketoacidosis, hyperammo-nemia, and hyperglycinemia during the first few days of life or in early infancy.

Clinical features Quite logically, in mut(−) and mut(0), the clinical presentation, including onset and severity of the disease, varies with the enzy-matic defect, ranging from a relatively benign condition to fatal neonatal disease. Most infants with mut(0) present within 7 days after birth. The most common presenting manifestations are vom-iting, dehydration, stupor, hypotonia, respiratory distress (tachypnea), and occasionally seizures. In cblA/cblB, the disease may also have early postnatal and later infantile onset forms, and clinical presentation is quite similar. In the early postnatal form of cblC, patients have complex metabolic, hematologic, neurologic, ophthalmologic, and dermatologic problems, which include failure to thrive, hepatic dysfunction, pancytopenia, renal failure consistent with hemolytic-uremic syndrome, respiratory insufficiency, rashes, hypotonia, and lethargy. Postnatal hydrocephalus is relatively common too.

Imaging Literature data regarding the imaging manifestations are somewhat inconsistent. In the neonate, the disease may present with unremarkable or nonspecific MR imaging findings. As a sign of acute metabolic neurotoxicity, mild brain swelling may be seen, in conjunction with T2 prolongation within the nonmyelinated white matter structures, which are most probably related to vasogenic edema. The myelinated white matter structures (in the brainstem, the posterior limbs of the internal capsules, and so forth) appear to be spared, somewhat similarly to urea cycle defects. After the acute phase, diffuse brain atrophy may ensue.[27] In the later-onset forms of the disease, bilateral globus pallidus lesions are found without involvement of other deep gray matter nuclei.[28] This, when present, is a fairly characteristic imaging finding, but unfortunately it is usually not seen in the neonate.

5-Oxoprolinuria (also known as pyroglutamic aciduria) (MIM ID #266130)
Enzyme deficiency Glutathione synthetase (classic form).

Inheritance Autosomal recessive, gene map locus: 20q11.2.

Metabolic features Glutathione is produced by glutathione synthetase from the amino acids cysteine, glutamate, and glycine.[29] It has multiple important biological roles, including protection of cells from oxidative damage and membrane transport. In the severe form of the disease, lack of glutathione within neurons seems to have a very damaging effect on the CNS. A milder form of the same mutation may cause glutathione synthetase deficiency within erythrocytes (glutathione synthetase deficiency of erythrocytes, MIM ID #231900), in which the unavailability of glutathione causes membrane fragility, leading to hemolytic anemia and jaundice. The disease is characterized by metabolic acidosis without ketosis or lactic acidosis and massive urinary excretion of 5-oxoproline. The latter is caused by the upregulation of the synthesis of γ-glutamylcysteine by γ-glutamylcysteine synthetase and its subsequent conversion to 5-oxoproline.

5-oxoproline is actually a nonspecific biochemical marker of the disease, because symptomatic 5-oxoprolinuria may also occur without a defect in the γ-glutamyl cycle (eg, in GM2 gangliosidosis, urea cycle defects, tyrosinemia type 1, and methylmalonic and propionic acidemias).

Clinical features Based on clinical presentation, classic 5-oxoprolinuria (glutathione synthetase deficiency) can be classified into 3 phenotypes: mild (hemolytic anemia), moderate (metabolic acidosis), and severe (neurologic involvement). Severe, potentially lethal hemolytic acidotic crisis situations with CNS damage may be seen both in neonates and later in life.[30,31]

Imaging Imaging findings in 5-oxoprolinuria have not been reported as yet. In a personal observation of 5-oxoprolinuria in a 13-year-old boy, both conventional MR imaging and proton MR spectroscopy were normal.

Canavan disease (MIM ID #271900)
Enzyme deficiency Aspartoacylase.

Inheritance Autosomal recessive, gene map locus: 17pter-p13.

Metabolic features NAA is a brain-specific metabolite. It is synthesized from acetyl coenzyme A and aspartate, and is metabolized into acetate and aspartate by aspartoacylase enzyme. Deficiency of aspartoacylase enzyme causes accumulation of NAA in brain, which subsequently enters the blood pool and is eventually eliminated through urine as N-acetylaspartic acid. Hence, technically, Canavan disease is an organic acidemia and aciduria. The function of N-acetylaspartic acid is not fully understood; it is likely involved in maintaining normal water homeostasis, notably the fluid balance between intracellular (axon-glial) and extracellular (interlamellar) spaces within myelinated white matter. As an abundant low molecular weight intracellular compound, it perhaps functions as a water transporter, but it is critical to myelin synthesis.[32,33] NAA is synthesized in neurons, but its hydrolytic breakdown takes place in the periaxonal space by the myelin-associated aspartoacylase. Accumulation of NAA in the periaxonal space entails excess water buildup (intramyelinic edema), possibly causing a rupture of the sealed interlamellar spaces (vacuolating myelinopathy), which eventually leads to demyelination and loss of glial cells. This condition has been traditionally described in the histopathology literature as spongy degeneration of the CNS.

Clinical features The actual clinical phenotype of the disease is modulated by residual aspartoacylase activity, explaining variations in age of onset and possibly the course and length of survival too. Although the biochemical abnormality is present in the neonate, neonatal onset of the disease is rare. In most cases the clinical manifestations develop in early infancy, just a few months after birth. The characteristic neurologic signs and symptoms include poor development and loss of milestones, generalized hypotonia and, in particular, atonia of neck muscles, hyperextension of legs and flexion of arms, blindness, and macrocephaly.

Imaging In the neonate, conventional MR imaging findings may be normal, but no data are available on the actual neonatal form of the disease. By the time the neurologic deterioration warrants a complete diagnostic workup, including imaging, the MR imaging findings are usually quite dramatic. Conventional MR imaging shows obvious and extensive "leukodystrophy" with some sparing of the deeper white matter structures. White matter within posterior fossa structures initially may be less involved too. One of the hallmark imaging features of the disease is the involvement of globi pallidi and thalami, and the sparing of caudate nuclei and putamina. These differences in selective vulnerability constitute an important pattern recognition element which, together with the white matter lesions, leads to a virtually pathognomonic pattern in the full-blown stage of the disease.

Spectroscopy Canavan disease is one of the few metabolic disorders in which MR spectroscopy findings are pathognomonic too. There is a very prominent elevation of the NAA peak on spectra obtained by either short or long echo times. This elevation is already present in the neonate, hence allowing for confident diagnosis even in the absence of conclusive conventional or DW imaging findings (**Fig. 2**).

Disorders of amino acid metabolism
Urea cycle defects (MIM ID #237300) carbamoyl phosphate synthetase deficiency, #311250 ornithine transcarbamylase deficiency, #207800 hyperargininemia, #207800 argininosuccinic aciduria (also known as argininosuccinate lyase deficiency), #215700 citrullinemia (also known as argininosuccinate synthetase deficiency)

Enzyme deficiencies Carbamoyl phosphate synthetase (CPS), ornithine transcarbamylase (OTC), arginase (ARG), argininosuccinate lyase (ASL), and argininosuccinate synthetase (ASS).

Inheritance X-linked recessive in OTC deficiency, gene map locus: Xp21.1; autosomal recessive in all others, notably CPS deficiency, gene map locus: 2q35; hyperargininemia, gene map locus: 6q23; ASL deficiency, gene map locus: 7cen-q11.2; and citrullinemia, gene map locus: 9q34.1.

Metabolic features Because the urea cycle is involved in the biosynthesis of arginine in the various forms of defects of the urea cycle (except in hyperargininemia), arginine becomes an essential amino acid. Furthermore, the integrity of the

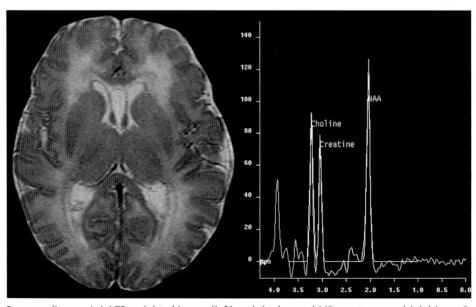

Fig. 2. Canavan disease. Axial T2-weighted image (*left*) and single-voxel MR spectroscopy (*right*) in an 8-day-old female infant. Conventional imaging is normal, but MR spectroscopy shows a prominent *N*-acetyl aspartate (NAA) peak. Note that in the neonate both choline and creatine peaks should be higher than NAA.

urea cycle is critical in the elimination of excess nitrogen from the body (through the formation of urea); therefore, impairment of the urea cycle leads to severe hyperammonemia. Hyperammonemia is known to be directly toxic to brain parenchyma, but because it promotes the synthesis of glutamate from glutamine and ammonia at the presynaptic level too, it also leads to a disequilibrium between excitatory (glutamate) and inhibitory (γ-aminobutyric acid [GABA]) neurotransmitters, which is believed to be one of the major factors behind the development of the devastating effects on the brain parenchyma (often referred to as "glutamate suicide") in urea cycle defects.

Clinical features In the neonate, OTC deficiency, CPS deficiency, and citrullinemia are the most commonly encountered entities.[34] Argininosuccinic aciduria usually, but not always, develops a few weeks later (whereas in hyperargininemia the typical clinical presentation is slowly progressive encephalopathy). Urea cycle defects are characterized by the classic triad of hyperammonemia, encephalopathy, and respiratory alkalosis. Hyperammonemia leads to diffuse brain swelling and raised intracranial pressure, with resultant clinical signs and symptoms of acute encephalopathy (hypotonia, vomiting, hypothermia, seizures, bulging fontanel, and rapidly increasing head circumference). Hyperventilation causes the distinctly characteristic respiratory alkalosis.

Imaging The direct toxic effect of hyperammonemia in all neonatal forms of the urea cycle defects manifests itself through diffuse and prominent vasogenic edema (**Fig. 3**). Nonmyelinated white matter appears to be severely affected, whereas myelinated areas are relatively spared. This situation allows easy imaging differentiation from MSUD, especially when DW imaging is also used. The underlying pathophysiologic mechanism of brain swelling in urea cycle defects (vasogenic edema) is different from that in MSUD (combined vacuolating myelinopathy and vasogenic edema), which is well demonstrated by the distinctly different presentations on DW images. Gray matter structures (basal ganglia, cortex) may also be involved in the most severe cases. Indeed, T1 hypersignal of the globi pallidi (with or without similar changes of the insular cortex) in a neonate suggests urea cycle disorder. Urea cycle defects may also present with stroke or stroke-like imaging manifestations.

Spectroscopy In urea cycle defects, an increase of glutamate and glutamine and a decrease of myoinositol are typical. These changes are easier to see with a short echo time (20 milliseconds), but higher concentrations may be detectable at longer echo times (135 milliseconds).[35] Additional

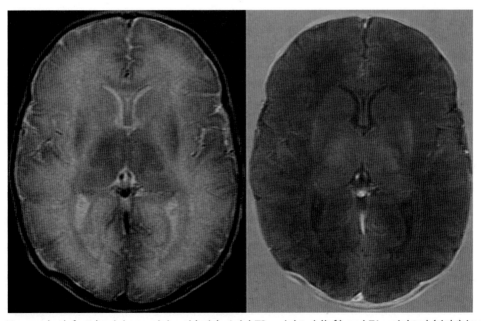

Fig. 3. Urea cycle defect (argininosuccinic aciduria). Axial T2-weighted (*left*) and T1-weighted (*right*) inversion recovery images of a 4-day-old male infant showing very prominent and extensive brain swelling, secondary to vasogenic edema (induced by hyperammonemia).

abnormal findings include a decrease of NAA, choline, and creatinine. All of these abnormalities are nonspecific (note that similar changes may be encountered in hepatic encephalopathy or after nearly drowning), but in the given clinical setting and when interpreted together with conventional imaging findings, they may be highly suggestive and hence useful (**Fig. 4**).

Maple syrup urine disease (MIM ID #248600)

Enzyme deficiency Branched-chain α-keto acid dehydrogenase (BCKD).

Inheritance Autosomal recessive, gene map locus: 19q13.1-q13.2, 6q14, 1p31, 7q31-q32 (all of these genes are involved in the coding of the catalytic center of BCKD).

Metabolic features Deficiency of BCKD interrupts the metabolism of α-ketoisocaproic, α-keto-β-methylvaleric, and α-ketoisovaleric acids (intermediate metabolites in the breakdown of L-leucine, L-isoleucine, and L-valine). Elevation of branched-chain ketoacids in all body fluids adversely affects the metabolism of neurotransmitters and energy (pyruvate and glucose), and the synthesis of proteins and myelin.

Clinical features The most severe, classic form of MSUD occurs in neonates (other clinical phenotypes include the intermediate, intermittent, thiamine responsive, and E3-deficient form with lactic acidosis). It usually presents 5 to 7 days after birth with the classic set of clinical signs and symptoms of a neonatal "devastating neurometabolic disorder," notably poor feeding, vomiting, hypoglycemia, seizures, coma, and a characteristic odor of maple syrup.

Imaging This disease presents with a highly characteristic MR imaging pattern and, if DW images are also available, a practically pathognomonic pattern presenting with restricted water diffusion within myelinated white matter structures (**Fig. 5**). Because of the vasogenic edema involving the nonmyelinated white matter, diffuse brain swelling is observed.[36] Prolongation of the T2 relaxation time is seen within the cerebral white matter and is more pronounced within the myelinated (due to vacuolating myelinopathy) than the nonmyelinated (due to vasogenic edema) white matter (**Fig. 6**).

Spectroscopy The protons of the methyl groups of the branched-chain amino acids resonate at 0.9 to 1.0 ppm; hence, in MSUD during metabolic decompensation, an abnormal positive peak may be detected at this level using proton MR spectroscopy with either short or long echo time.[37] As an indicator of impaired use of pyruvate in the citric acid cycle, a lactate peak may also be present at

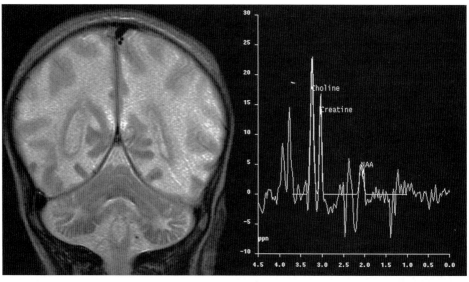

Fig. 4. Urea cycle defect (carbamoyl-phosphate synthetase deficiency). Axial T2-weighted image (*left*) and MR spectroscopy (*right*) of the brain in a 12-day-old male infant. The supratentorial brain is markedly swollen. The MR spectroscopy spectrum (short echo time acquisition mode [STEAM]; echo time [TE]: 20 milliseconds) shows decreased NAA and gross normal choline and creatine peaks. The baseline is "noisy," but two abnormal peaks at 2.4 and 3.8 ppm levels are well identified, which correspond to glutamate (produced from glutamine and excess ammonia).

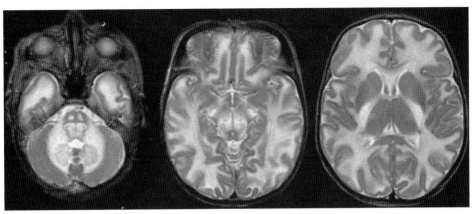

Fig. 5. Maple syrup urine disease. Axial T2-weighted images of a 35-day-old male infant (already on treatment). White matter structures that are myelinated at this age (eg, cerebellar white matter, pyramidal tracts, posterior limbs of the internal capsules) exhibit abnormal hypersignal.

1.3 ppm. Both peaks may improve or disappear after successful management of the metabolic crisis (**Fig. 7**).

Nonketotic hyperglycinemia (MIM ID #605899, also known as glycine encephalopathy)

Enzyme deficiency Lipoic acid–containing H protein (GCSH), pyridoxal phosphate–dependent glycine decarboxylase P protein (GLDC), aminomethyltransferase T protein (AMT).

Inheritance Autosomal recessive, gene map locus: 16q24 (H protein), 9p22 (P protein), 3p21.2-p21.1 (T protein).

Metabolic features The mitochondrial glycine cleavage system has 4 components (H, L, P, and T protein). Mutations of the H, P, or T, proteins are known. A defect of the glycine cleavage system (expressed in liver, kidney, and brain) results in the accumulation of glycine in body fluids, but hyperglycinemia is particularly detrimental to the CNS. There are two neurotransmitter roles for glycine in the CNS—one inhibitory and one excitatory. The glycine receptors in the spinal cord and brain stem are inhibitory. Glycine receptors elsewhere are associated with the *N*-methyl-D-aspartate receptor channel complex and are excitatory, potentiating the action of glutamate, leading to glutamate excitotoxicity and ultimately to cell death.

Clinical features Nonketotic hyperglycinemia has 4 known clinical phenotypes: neonatal, infantile, late-onset, and transient. The neonatal form (often referred to as "classic," whereas the others are "atypical") is the most common (>70%), and GLDC or AMT mutations have been found to be most commonly associated with it. The neonatal form of nonketotic hyperglycinemia presents within the first 2 days of life with severe encephalopathy, hypotonia (possibly related to the inhibitory effect of glycine on anterior horn cells within the spinal cord), lethargy, respiratory failure, multifocal myoclonic seizures, and hiccups.[38] It is a severe, potentially life-threatening condition.[39]

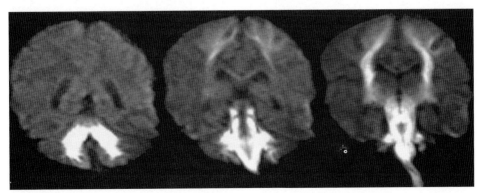

Fig. 6. Maple syrup urine disease. Coronal diffusion-weighted images in a 20-day-old male patient. All myelinated structures within cerebellum, brainstem, and cerebral hemispheres exhibit markedly restricted water diffusion. In an appropriate clinical setting, these findings are pathognomonic to maple syrup urine disease.

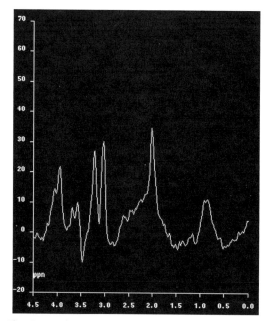

Fig. 7. Maple syrup urine disease. MR spectroscopy (STEAM; TE: 30 milliseconds) during metabolic crisis in a 4-month-old male infant. The broad peak at the 0.8 to 1.1 ppm level corresponds to branched-chain amino acids.

Imaging Diffuse cerebral atrophy, callosal hypoplasia/hypotrophy, and disturbed/delayed myelination constitute the imaging hallmarks of nonketotic hyperglycinemia. Atrophy and myelination disorders progress with age. (It is important to remember that atrophy and delayed myelination are also quite common findings in other metabolic disorders, in particular in organic acidurias.) In a subset of patients the disease is rapidly progressive, resulting in severe devastation of brain

parenchyma (**Fig. 8**). Assessment of the corpus callosum may be challenging in the neonate (due to its small size and lack of myelin), but the underdevelopment of the corpus callosum also becomes increasingly evident later. Occasionally, a true malformation (agenesis, dysgenesis) of the corpus callosum may also be encountered.

Spectroscopy Proton MR spectroscopy allows direct imaging of increased amounts of glycine in brain parenchyma in patients with in nonketotic hyperglycinemia. This aspect is important because actual cerebral glycine concentrations seem to correspond more reliably with the clinical presentation than plasma or even CSF levels. The glycine peak at 3.56 ppm, however, overlaps with that of myoinositol, and at short (eg, 20 milliseconds) echo times the two substances may not be confidently differentiated from each other. (In fact, glycine accounts for less than 20% of the 3.56 ppm signal in normal subjects on short echo-time spectra.) However, as the signal from myoinositol more rapidly decays with longer echo times, a prominent "residual" signal at 135 milliseconds or longer allows for the reliable identification of glycine (**Fig. 9**).

Primary lactic acidosis (disorders of oxidative phosphorylation) Lactic acid is the product of anaerobic metabolism of glucose. In lactic acidosis (a distinct form of metabolic acidosis), tissue and blood pH levels are lowered and lactate accumulates. Lactic acidosis indicates hypoxia, hypoperfusion, or impaired glucose metabolism. Accordingly, several types of lactic acidosis are distinguished, notably lactic acidosis caused by tissue hypoxia/hypoperfusion (type A), underlying

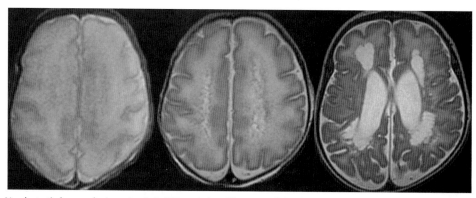

Fig. 8. Nonketotic hyperglycinemia. Axial T2-weighted images of the same patient. The first study (*left*) was done shortly after birth (32 weeks premature newborn) and shows diffuse brain swelling. The second study (*center*) was performed 6 weeks later and shows early periventricular abnormalities, whereas the third study (*right*) another 6 weeks later shows obvious cystic encephalomalacia. The images illustrate the rapidly progressive devastating consequences of the disease on brain parenchyma. (*Courtesy of* Dr C. Hoffmann, Sheba Medical Center, Tel Hashomer, Sackler School of Medicine, Tel Aviv University, Israel.)

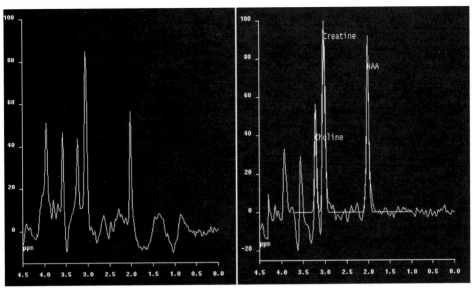

Fig. 9. Nonketotic hyperglycinemia. MR spectroscopy spectra of the brain in a 9-month-old female patient using short (STEAM; TE: 30 milliseconds) and long (point-resolved spectroscopy; TE: 135 milliseconds) echo times. The short TE spectrum (*left*) shows a prominent peak at the 3.6 ppm level, which does not disappear on the 135-ms spectrum; this indicates that the metabolite producing the signal is glycine rather than myoinositol (both resonate at the same ppm level, but have different T2 relaxation times).

disease (type B1), medication or intoxication (type B2), or inborn errors of metabolism (type B3). Another way to classify lactic acidosis is primary versus secondary. The most common causes of severe primary lactic acidosis (type B3) in neonates are pyruvate carboxylase deficiency, pyruvate dehydrogenase deficiency, and mitochondrial complex IV (also known as cytochrome *c* oxidase [COX]) deficiency.[40] However, lactic acidosis may be encountered in a host of other inborn errors of metabolism, notably in organic acidemias and in urea cycle and fatty acid oxidation defects. Common causes in the acquired, secondary forms of lactic acidosis are cardiopulmonary disease, diabetes mellitus, hepatic failure, severe anemia, malignancy, and postconvulsion status or medication (eg, metformin).

Pyruvate carboxylase deficiency (MIM ID #266150)
Enzyme deficiency Pyruvate carboxylase.

Inheritance Autosomal recessive, gene map locus: 11q13.4-q13.5.

Metabolic features Laboratory findings are dominated by lactic and pyruvic acidosis, as well as ketosis. Hyperalaninemia, hyperammonemia, citrullinemia, and hyperlysinemia are believed to be secondary to an associated disturbance of the urea cycle. Despite the role of pyruvate carboxylase in hepatic gluconeogenesis, hypoglycemia is not a consistent feature of the condition.

Clinical features There are 2 or more clinical forms: fulminant neonatal and additional later-onset, increasingly benign forms. The fulminant neonatal form presents with acidosis, seizures, hypotonia, tachypnea, and stupor, rapidly leading to coma.

Pyruvate dehydrogenase deficiency (MIM ID E1a #312170, E1b #179060, E2 #245348, E3 #238331)
Enzyme deficiency Pyruvate dehydrogenase complex (the enzyme has 3 subunits, E1, E2, and E3, all of which are prone to mutations).

Inheritance X-linked (E1-α subunit defect), gene map locus: Xp22.2-p22.1, autosomal recessive (in all others), gene map locus: 3p13-q23 (E1-beta), 11q23.1 (E2), 7q31-q32 (E3).

Metabolic features The pyruvate dehydrogenase enzyme (PDH) is part (in fact the first component) of the pyruvate dehydrogenase complex. It is a tetramer and has 4 subunits: 2 α and 2 β. Besides pyruvate dehydrogenase (E1), the PDH complex includes dihydrolipoyl transacetyltransferase (E2) and dihydrolipoyl dehydrogenase (E3). The PDH complex is involved in the first step in oxidative decarboxylation, converting pyruvate to acetyl coenzyme A and CO_2. The resultant energy metabolic derangement presents with lactic and pyruvic acidosis and hyperalaninemia.

Clinical features There are 4 clinical phenotypes of PDH deficiency: (1) severe neonatal form presenting during the first week (often during the first 24 hours of life) with lactic acidosis, tachypnea, hypotonia, seizures, and stupor; (2) infantile form (usually heterozygous females with the X-linked form) presenting with nonprogressive encephalopathy (milder acidosis and hypotonia), but often with dysmorphic craniofacial features (and cerebral malformations); (3) infantile form presenting with early-onset Leigh disease (hypotonia, oculomotor abnormalities, respiratory difficulties, and seizures); and (4) infantile form with relapsing ataxia.[41]

Mitochondrial complex IV (also known as cytochrome c oxidase) deficiency (MIM ID #220110)

Enzyme deficiency COX (1 of the 5 multi-subunit enzyme complexes forming the so-called respiratory chain).

Inheritance COX consists of 13 polypeptide subunits, 3 of which (MTCO1, MTCO2, and MTCO3) are encoded by mitochondrial DNA (mtDNA) and form the actual catalytic site of complex IV; the other 10 (IV, Va, Vb, Via, VIb, Vic, VIIa, VIIb, VIIc, and VIII) are encoded by nuclear DNA. Therefore, inheritance may be maternal mitochondrial or autosomal recessive. The best known COX mutations affect the following subunits: MTCO1, MTCO2 (genes for both mapped to the heavy strand of mtDNA), SURF1 (gene map locus: 9q34), COX10 (gene map locus: 17p12-p11.2), COX15 (gene map locus: 10q24), and LRPPRC (gene map locus: 2p21-p16).

Metabolic features The so-called respiratory chain is located within the inner membrane of the mitochondrion and is responsible for electron transport (converting molecular oxygen into water) during the end stage of oxidative phosphorylation. The released energy is critical to the formation of ATP. In conditions leading to impairment of the oxidative phosphorylation process, due to the compensatory upregulation of anaerobic glycolysis, systemic lactic acidosis (with mild pyruvic acidosis) develops.

Clinical features The clinical presentation is dominated by dysfunction of organs with high energy needs (brain, heart, muscle). Neonatal forms present with severe hypotonia, weakness, and respiratory failure. Later-onset forms present with cardiomyopathy, visual and auditory problems, seizures, leukodystrophy, Leigh syndrome, and so forth.

Imaging Imaging in all forms of primary lactic acidosis of neonatal or early infantile onset is often deceivingly unremarkable or nonspecific. Diffuse brain swelling with T2 prolongation within the white matter throughout the entire brain may be seen. At the early stage, no definite structural or signal abnormality is seen within the basal ganglia, although they may appear somewhat swollen. In survivors, the disease leads to prominent manifest basal ganglia disease (suggestive of necrosis), cerebral atrophy (sometimes asymmetric, suggesting a stroke-like pathomechanism), or delayed myelination (**Fig. 10**). Infants with the less severe neonatal form of pyruvate dehydrogenase deficiency may show congenital malformations such as callosal agenesis or neuronal migration disorders.

Spectroscopy Disruption of the oxidative phosphorylation process causes increase in glycolysis to cover energy requirements, with a corresponding accumulation of lactate in the brain parenchyma. Lactate is easy to detect by proton MR spectroscopy. It presents as a peak doublet at the 1.3 ppm level. With 20 and 135 milliseconds echo time, the lactate peak is negative; with 270 milliseconds echo time, it is positive. Abnormal concentrations of lactate, however, are not limited to manifest lesion areas but may be present within normal-appearing brain parenchyma, especially gray matter structures (cortex, basal ganglia). Lactate, however, is not specific to primary energy metabolism disorders and may be present in many other inborn errors of metabolism (organic acidurias, amino acidopathies), which indirectly affect the integrity of the oxidative phosphorylation process. In a case of pyruvate dehydrogenase deficiency, excess pyruvate has been demonstrated in vivo by MR spectroscopy.[42]

Fatty acid oxidation disorders Fatty acid oxidation disorders include: (1) carnitine cycle defects (carnitine-palmitoyl transferase [CPT] deficiency: MIM ID #608836, carnitine translocase [CACT] deficiency: MIM ID #212138); (2) mitochondrial β-oxidation disorders (very long-chain acyl coenzyme A dehydrogenase [VLCAD] deficiency: MIM ID #201475, long-chain acyl coenzyme A dehydrogenase [LCAD] deficiency: MIM ID #201460, medium-chain acyl coenzyme A dehydrogenase [MCAD] deficiency: MIM ID #201450, and short-chain acyl coenzyme A dehydrogenase [SCAD] deficiency: MIM ID #201470); (3) long-chain 3-hydroxyacyl coenzyme A dehydrogenase [LCHAD] deficiency: MIM ID #609016; and (4) electron transfer flavoprotein (ETF) dehydrogenase deficiency (MIM ID #231680, also known as glutaric aciduria type 2, GA2). CPT2, VLCAD, and LCHAD deficiencies and glutaric aciduria type 2 have neonatal-onset forms. The other entities are usually encountered later in infancy, childhood,

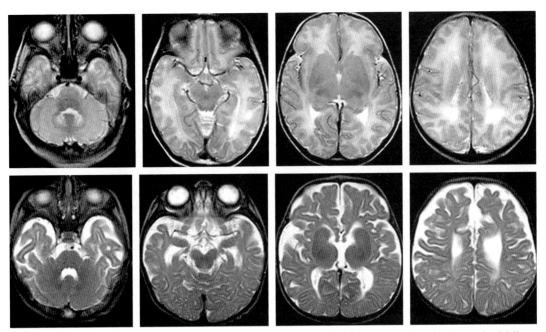

Fig. 10. Primary lactic acidosis. Axial T2-weighted images in a 5-day-old (*upper row*) and a 3-month-old (*lower row*) female patient. In the patient examined in the early postnatal period diffuse brain swelling is seen. In the other child prominent brain atrophy is shown in conjunction with delayed myelination.

or even adulthood, and are therefore not discussed here.

Enzyme deficiency CPT, VLCAD, LCHAD, multiple coenzyme A dehydrogenases (in GA2).

Inheritance Autosomal recessive, gene map locus: 1p32 (in CPT2), 17p13 (in VLCAD), 2p23 (in LCHAD), 15q23-q25 (in GA2-ETFA), 19q13.3 (in GA2-ETFB), 4q32-qter (in GA2-ETF-DH).

Metabolic features In humans, metabolic fuels include glucose, lactate, fatty acids, and ketone bodies. In the brain, glucose and ketone bodies are the most important energy providers. In muscle (especially in heart), fatty acids and ketone bodies are the dominant sources of energy. Therefore, the integrity of the fatty acid metabolism pathways, which include catabolic processes (to produce energy through mitochondrial β-oxidation of fatty acids) and anabolic processes (to synthesize ketone bodies from fatty acids), is critical for the proper functioning of these organs.[43] The fatty acid oxidation pathway is particularly important for the entire organism when the availability of glucose is limited, such as during fasting.

From the metabolic perspective, fatty acid oxidation disorders are characterized by a combination of acidosis, hypoglycemia, and hyperammonemia, as well as lipid accumulation in parenchymal organs. GA2 is somewhat different, because it is caused by a deficiency of the electron transfer flavoprotein located either in the mitochondrial matrix (ETF-A and ETF-B) or the mitochondrial inner membrane (ETF-DH). Dysfunction of the ETF leads to impaired electron transport from intramitochondrial dehydrogenase enzymes to the respiratory chain. It therefore also represents a profound mitochondrial metabolic-energetic disorder (this, however, needs to be distinguished from glutaric aciduria type 1, which is an isolated glutaryl-coenzyme A deficiency with later onset).

Clinical features Literature data based on post-mortem screening for fatty acid oxidation disorders suggests that up to 5% of sudden deaths during the first year of life may be caused by a fatty acid oxidation disorder.[44] Indeed, profound impairment of aerobic energy metabolism at the mitochondrial level in fatty acid oxidation disorders leads to multiorgan (primarily heart) failure, which may be the most common cause of sudden death. Metabolic decompensations, however, may lead to secondary CNS damage too, which is secondary to the unavailability of metabolic fuels (glucose and ketone bodies). Brain involvement may present with signs of acute encephalopathy, which may be related to a putative direct toxic effect of long- and medium-chain acyl coenzyme A and acylcarnitines but also to prolonged hypoglycemia, lactic acidosis (due to inhibition of the tricarboxylic cycle), and hyperammonemia (due to the inhibition of the urea cycle).

The lethal neonatal form of CPT2 may present with signs and symptoms of global energy deprivation (hypoglycemia, hypothermia, and lethargy) and multisystem organ involvement (hepatomegaly, cardiomegaly). Neurologic signs include hypotonia, hyperreflexia, and seizures.[45] Patients develop cardiac arrhythmias and may die suddenly of cardiac failure during the first days of life. Patients with the severe early-onset form VLCAD deficiency present with hyperammonemia, hypoglycemia, lactic acidosis, cardiac arrhythmia, and high mortality. Patients with LCHAD have hypoglycemia, early-onset cardiomyopathy, neuropathy, focal pigmentary aggregation or retinal hypopigmentation, or cholestatic liver disease, often leading to sudden death in early postnatal period of life. In the neonatal form of GA2 there is a high incidence of premature birth, and dysmorphic features are common, but malformations of the CNS or other organs may also be encountered. Metabolic decompensation usually occurs between 24 and 48 hours of age, presenting with metabolic acidosis, organic (glutaric, 2-hydroxyglutaric, isovaleric, isobutyric, ethylmalonic) aciduria, and nonketotic hypoglycemia, and clinically with stupor, hypotonia, tachypnea, and seizures.

Imaging In CPT 2, periventricular calcifications and cystic dysplasia with foci of hyperechogenicity within the basal ganglia have been found by prenatal ultrasonography, and polymicrogyria has also been described on postmortem autopsy.[46] No published imaging data are available in neonatal VLCAD deficiency, but in his own practice the author has encountered a case of bihemispheric, predominantly frontal, cortical dysplasia. In LCHAD, atrophy and periventricular and parieto-occipital infarction–like lesions have been described, the latter probably related to perinatal hypoglycemia. In a case report of neonatal GA2, underdeveloped frontal and temporal lobes with enlarged Sylvian fissures (somewhat similar to glutaric aciduria type 1), delayed myelination, and hypoplasia of the corpus callosum have been described. Cortical dysplasia and gray matter heterotopia appear to be common autopsy findings in GA2, but these have not been reported yet on neuroradiologic studies.

Spectroscopy In GA2, normal NAA in conjunction with an increased choline/creatine ratio has been described and interpreted as a sign of dysmyelination.

Peroxisomal disorders Peroxisomes are ubiquitous cellular organelles, and peroxisomal enzymes are involved in multiple anabolic, catabolic, and metabolic pathways, in particular lipid metabolism.

Peroxisomes are abundant in the CNS, particularly in the developing brain. During early development, proper peroxisomal function within neuronal precursors and immature neurons is critical to normal neuronal migration and organization. Similarly, normal peroxisomal function in oligodendrocytes is an essential prerequisite of normal myelin buildup (in the developing brain) and myelin maintenance (in the mature brain). Therefore, peroxisomal diseases typically (but obviously not exclusively) present with involvement of the CNS.

Peroxisomal diseases represent a continuum. At least 40 enzymes are known to reside in the peroxisomes, which explain the remarkable genotypic and phenotypic heterogeneity of the resultant clinical entities. Schematically, peroxisomal disorders caused by total absence of peroxisomal activity (peroxisomal biogenesis disorders) are characterized by prenatal, neonatal, or early infantile onset, and represent the most severe forms with involvement of both gray and white matter (neuronal migration disorders, hypomyelination, or dysmyelination). Other forms with multiple peroxisomal dysfunctions or loss of a single peroxisomal function are characterized predominantly by white matter abnormalities (dysmyelination, and subsequent demyelination) of infantile, childhood, or even adult onset, and the disease course is more prolonged and often more benign too. Profound peroxisomal disorders affecting biogenesis are relevant to the neonatal patient populations because several entities belong to the group of devastating neurometabolic disorders of the newborn.

Zellweger (cerebrohepatorenal) syndrome (MIM ID #214100)

Enzyme deficiency Practically all peroxisomal functions are absent (bifunctional enoyl coenzyme A hydratase/3-hydroxyacyl coenzyme A dehydrogenase, acyl coenzyme A oxidase, and β-ketothiolase).

Inheritance Autosomal recessive, gene map locus: 1p36.2, 1q22, 12p13.3, 7q21-q22, 6q23-q24, 1p36.32, 2p15, 22q11.21 (the disease may be caused by mutation of any of the genes involved in the biogenesis of the peroxisomes).

Metabolic features Elevated levels of very long-chain fatty acids (VLCFA) in the plasma and fibroblasts, impairment of plasmalogen biosynthesis, and abnormal patterns of bile acids are characteristic to Zellweger syndrome.

Clinical features Facial dysmorphic features (dolichocephaly, triangular face, hypertelorism, prominent epicanthic folds, and a high, broad forehead, congenital glaucoma, malformed ears, small mandible) are typical, but the most severe abnormalities are seen at the level of the brain (cortical dysplasia and hypomyelination), liver (intrahepatic biliary dysgenesis), and kidneys (polycystic renal disease). Affected patients present with poor sucking, prolonged icterus, seizures, and failure to thrive, and typically die during the first year of life.[47]

Imaging In an appropriate clinical setting, conventional MR imaging findings are virtually pathognomonic of this disease. Analysis of the cerebral cortex, in particular in the temporoparietal regions, reveals extensive bilateral, but not necessarily symmetric, polymicrogyria-like changes (**Fig. 11**). Sometimes more severe neuronal migration abnormalities may also be present.[48] Delayed myelination is easily recognized in both the T1-weighted and the T2-weighted images. Subependymal, so-called germinolytic, cysts are very common along the frontal horns of the lateral ventricles.[49] In keeping with the profound metabolic abnormality of prenatal onset, several additional malformative (callosal dysgenesis, cerebellar cortical dysplasia) or dysmorphic developmental changes (incomplete opercularization, verticalization of the Sylvian fissures, colpocephaly) may also be encountered, although less consistently, and some of those (hypoplasia or dysplasia of the inferior olives, dentate nuclei) may not be detectable by currently available conventional imaging techniques. Additional imaging workup shows calcification ("chondrodysplasia punctata") within the patella and acetabulum (plain radiograph) and cysts within the kidneys (ultrasonography, CT).

Spectroscopy Infants with variants of Zellweger syndrome may present with marked decrease of NAA in white and gray matter. Cerebral glutamine may increase and myoinositol decrease in the gray matter, reflecting the concomitant effect on hepatic function. In severe cases, mobile lipids in the white matter may be detected in conjunction with some increase in lactate levels. These findings are not specific to peroxisomal disorders but give insight into the metabolic effects on the developing brain.

Neonatal adrenoleukodystrophy (MIM ID #202370)

Enzyme deficiency Practically all peroxisomal functions are absent (including bifunctional enoyl coenzyme A hydratase/3-hydroxyacyl coenzyme A dehydrogenase).

Inheritance Autosomal recessive, gene map locus: 12p13.3, 7q21-q22, 1p36.32, 2p15, 22q11.21 (the disease may be caused by mutation of any of the genes involved in the biogenesis of the peroxisomes).

Metabolic features Typical laboratory findings in neonatal adrenoleukodystrophy (NALD) include increased plasma pipecolic acid, phytanic acid, and VLCFA levels. There is some clinical overlap with Zellweger syndrome, in that both have elevated saturated VLCFAs, but patients with NALD have adrenal atrophy, whereas those with Zellweger syndrome do not. In addition, in Zellweger syndrome, chondrodysplasia, glomerulocystic disease of the kidney, CNS dysmyelination, and elevations of unsaturated and saturated VLCFAs are present too.

Clinical features Infants with neonatal adrenoleukodystrophy (ALD) may also have dysmorphic features but, in contrast to Zellweger syndrome, not skeletal abnormalities (cartilaginous calcifications). Involvement of the CNS (severe hypotonia, hearing loss, retinal degeneration, and seizures) is obvious at birth. In one reported case, seizure was the first clinical manifestation of the condition shortly after birth.[50]

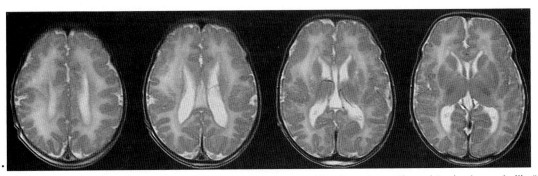

Fig. 11. Zellweger disease. Axial T2-weighted images in a 2-day-old male patient. Bilateral "polymicrogyria-like" changes in perisylvian and frontal locations are observed.

Imaging Similarly to Zellweger syndrome, neuronal migration abnormalities and white matter disease (dysmyelination or demyelination within the cerebellum and cerebrum) constitute the hallmark imaging features of NALD. Contrast uptake described on CT images suggests an active, perhaps inflammatory process, similar to that seen in X-linked ALD within the active inflammation zone.

D-bifunctional protein deficiency (DBP, also known as peroxisomal bifunctional enzyme deficiency, MIM ID #261515)

Enzyme deficiency 17β-Hydroxysteroid dehydrogenase IV.

Inheritance Autosomal recessive, gene map locus: 5q2.

Metabolic features Similarly to peroxisomal acyl coenzyme A oxidase deficiency (see also Zellweger syndrome), DBP deficiency is a peroxisomal fatty acid β-oxidation disorder. Unlike in NALD and Zellweger syndrome, peroxisomes are present within tissues. In fact, not all peroxisomal functions are lost (eg, acyl coenzyme A:dihydroxyacetone-phosphate acyltransferase, acyl coenzyme A oxidase, and β-ketothiolase have been found normal in DBP deficiency), whereas those are deficient in Zellweger syndrome. In DBP deficiency VLCFAs are elevated, but pipecolic and phytanic acids are normal.

Clinical features The clinical phenotypic manifestations of DBP may not be distinguishable from those of peroxisomal biogenesis disorders. Dysmorphic facial features may be quite similar to those seen in NALD and Zellweger syndrome (large fontanel, high forehead, low nasal bridge, micrognathia, low-set ears) and characterize the clinical phenotype in conjunction with hypotonia, seizures, loss of vision and hearing, generalized osteopenia, adrenal cortical abnormalities, and failure to thrive.

Imaging MR imaging may show white matter disease, suggesting delayed myelination or demyelination.[51] Polymicrogyria has been described through both biopsy and MR imaging studies.[52–54] Germinolytic cysts, ventriculomegaly, and cerebellar atrophy may be encountered too.

Miscellaneous
Menkes disease (also known as kinky/steely hair disease, trichopoliodystrophy, MIM ID #309400)

Enzyme deficiency All enzymes requiring copper as a cofactor ("cuproenzymes"), such as dopamine-β-hydroxylase (involved in catecholamine synthesis), COX (oxidative phosphorylation), lysyl oxidase (elastin-collagen formation), tyrosinase (pigment formation), peptidylglycine α-amidating monooxygenase (peptide amidation), and superoxide dismutase (antioxidant defense).

Inheritance X-linked, gene map locus: Xq12-q13.

Metabolic features Menkes disease is a disorder caused by a defect in intracellular-intercompartmental copper transport, which includes failure to absorb copper from the gastrointestinal tract, resulting in global copper deficiency (this is in contrast to Wilson disease, which represents an extracellular copper transport abnormality and leads to copper overload).[55]

Clinical features The disease has neonatal (more severe) and infantile (milder) onset forms. Patients present with hyperbilirubinemia, hypothermia, and failure to thrive. Impairment of catecholamine (neurotransmitter) synthesis and oxidative phosphorylation may explain the neurologic manifestations (hypotonia, hypothermia, seizures); the elastin-collagen formation disorder possibly causes skin/joint laxity as well as intimal fragility and the characteristic tortuosity of cerebral arteries, and defective pigment formation causes hair/skin hypopigmentation. The typical hair abnormalities may not be apparent in the newborn. Characteristic laboratory findings include low serum levels of copper and ceruloplasmin.

Imaging MR imaging studies during the early postnatal period usually do not reveal significant abnormalities. Subtle signal abnormalities within the cerebral cortex may be seen. The youngest patient in whom MR imaging showed evidence of neurodegeneration (cerebellar atrophy and hypomyelination) was 5 weeks old. Later scans typically show progressive white matter disease with frontal and temporal predominance. Prominent cerebral and cerebellar atrophy ensues. If global brain atrophy develops, patients with Menkes disease are prone to spontaneous, ex vacuo subdural hematomas. MR angiography is useful at any age in revealing the characteristic tortuosity of the cerebral vessels. In a patient treated with copper histidine from 4 weeks of age, cerebral atrophy and white matter abnormalities did not develop; tortuosity of the cerebral arteries was, however, still conspicuous. Ischemic stroke has also been reported as a complication of Menkes disease. In another patient with 2383C to T mutation in ATP7A who was treated with copper chloride injections, the initially quite severe cerebral white matter and deep gray matter changes were found to be reversible. Additional characteristic imaging features of the disease include the so-called wormian bones. Wormian bones are extra bone pieces within a cranial suture, also present, however, in other entities summarized by the PORKCHOPS mnemonic (Pyknodysostosis, Osteogenesis imperfecta, Rickets, Kinky hair syndrome, Cleidocranial dysostosis, Hypothyroidism/hypophosphatasia, Otopalatodigital syndrome, Primary osteoacrolysis, Syndrome of Down).

Sulfite oxidase deficiency (isolated, also known as sulfocysteinuria: MIM ID #272300, combined: MIM ID #252150)

Enzyme deficiency Sulfite oxidase or sulfite oxidase/xanthine oxidase (also known as xanthine dehydrogenase) in combined molybdenum cofactor deficiency (molybdenum is an essential cofactor of both enzymes).

Inheritance Autosomal recessive, gene map locus: chromosome 12 (in isolated sulfite oxidase deficiency), 6p21.3, 5q11, and 14q24 (in molybdenum cofactor deficiency type A, B, and C).

Metabolic features Sulfite oxidase catalyzes the terminal step of the oxidative degradation of sulfur-containing amino acids (cysteine, methionine). Sulfite oxidase deficiency may occur as an isolated enzyme defect (rare) or in combination with xanthine oxidase deficiency (more common) as part of molybdenum cofactor deficiency. The so-called molybdenum cofactor is indispensable to the proper functioning of sulfite oxidase and xanthine oxidase; therefore, in the combined form of the disease, both are deficient. Sulfite oxidase (isolated or combined) deficiency leads to excretion of excessive amounts of sulfite, S-sulfocysteine, thiosulfate, taurine, and xanthine (in molybdenum cofactor deficiency only) in the urine. Lactic acidosis may also be present.

Clinical features Features comprise feeding difficulties, vomiting, and intractable seizures within the first few days or weeks evolving toward a severe encephalopathy, which in many ways resembles hypoxic-anoxic encephalopathy (which is further supported by the deceivingly similar imaging findings). Later, global failure to thrive and progressive, acquired microcephaly become increasingly obvious. Dysmorphic features and lens dislocation are common. The severe form of the disease leads to death in infancy; with the milder clinical phenotypes, longer survivals are possible.

Imaging During the acute clinical manifestations, MR imaging shows severe brain swelling. Within deep gray matter structures (globi pallidi, subthalamic nuclei in particular), DW images may show restricted water diffusion (**Fig. 12**). This and other findings are usually symmetric. Follow-up studies (or studies performed in later stages of

the disease) show progressive destruction of cortex, basal ganglia, thalami, cerebellum, and white matter. Pontocerebellar hypoplasia/atrophy may be present early on, but it is also progressive. Ultimately cystic encephalomalacia-type changes (with severe cavitations within the subcortical white matter), global brain atrophy, and ventriculomegaly are characteristic. At this stage, the imaging findings alone are indistinguishable from those caused by severe global hypoxia, but the underlying pathomechanism is different. Indeed, damage to brain parenchyma in isolated or combined sulfite oxidase deficiency is more likely secondary to global energy deficiency at the tissue level (somewhat reminiscent, perhaps, of that seen in "mitochondrial" encephalopathies) and represent "pseudostroke" or "stroke-like" changes.[56]

Galactosemia (MIM ID #230400)

Enzyme deficiency Galactose-1-phosphate uridylyl transferase.

Inheritance Autosomal recessive, gene map locus: 9p13.

Metabolic features In galactosemia, galactose-1-phosphate is not further metabolized into uridine diphosphogalactose (the second step of galactose metabolism after intestinal absorption); therefore, galactose-1-phosphate, galactose, and its alternative catabolite, galactitol, accumulate.

Clinical features The hallmark clinical stigmata of galactosemia are hepatomegaly and cataracts, recognizable at birth, and subsequent mental retardation. The disease has two clinical phenotypes. The classic form is related to complete enzyme deficiency. The first clinical signs and symptoms (diarrhea, vomiting, and icterus) develop shortly after birth following milk ingestion but may disappear after dietary restriction. In the partial enzyme deficiency, affected patients are typically asymptomatic. Neurotoxicity in galactosemia is probably secondary to the adverse osmolar effects of galactitol, leading to water accumulation and swelling. The synthesis of galactocerebrosides may be impaired too, leading to myelination abnormalities, which are probably responsible for the late neurocognitive changes.

Imaging In the acute postnatal stage, diffuse vasogenic brain edema may be seen. Later, as expected, white matter abnormalities dominate, notably delayed myelination or hypomyelination, with additional focal patchy white matter lesions within cerebral hemispheric white matter, predominantly in periventricular locations. During the course of the disease, diffuse cerebral and

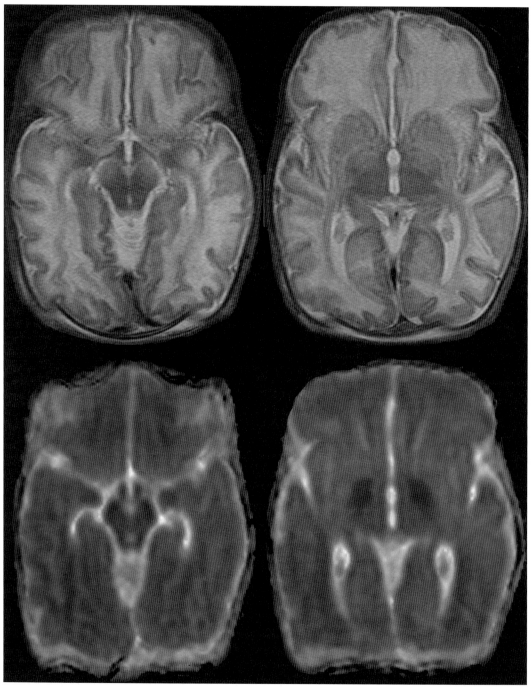

Fig. 12. Molybdenum cofactor deficiency. Axial T2-weighted (*upper row*) and apparent diffusion coefficient (ADC; *lower row*) images in an 11-day-old female patient. There is diffuse brain swelling and increased T2 signal within hemispheric white matter in conjunction with focal lesions within cerebral peduncles and globi pallidi bilaterally, the latter exhibiting restricted water diffusion on ADC map images, suggesting cytotoxic edema. (*Courtesy of* Dr K. Chong, Great Ormond Street Hospital, London.)

cerebellar atrophy with secondary enlargement of the lateral ventricles develops.

Spectroscopy One of the excess metabolites, notably galactitol, resonates at the 3.7 ppm level and may be detected in vivo in patients with galactosemia.[57,58]

Advanced imaging techniques in the diagnostic imaging workup

MR imaging findings in neonates with metabolic disorders are often nonspecific, even in diseases that eventually present with fairly characteristic lesion patterns in later stages. In fact, very few diseases present with suggestive or pathogno-monic conventional imaging abnormalities in the immediate postnatal period or during the first episode of metabolic decompensation. Because advanced MR imaging techniques such as DW imaging and proton MR spectroscopy capture different histopathologic or biochemical features of the processes, their systematic use is not only justified but recommended, because the combination of conventional imaging, DW imaging, and MR spectroscopy data may lead to more complete patterns and hence may enhance diagnostic sensitivity or even specificity.

Diffusion-weighted MR imaging in neurometabolic disorders DW imaging of the brain already has many well-established indications, including stroke and the assessment of normal and abnormal mye-lination. In nonmyelinated white matter, some but not significant water diffusion anisotropy is present, and the apparent diffusion coefficient is higher than in the mature brain. As the myelination process progresses prominent diffusion anisotropy develops, characterized by relatively free water diffusion along the fiber tracts and restricted diffusion across the myelin sheaths.

DW imaging has a unique ability to differentiate between the various edema types, all of which are associated with decreasing anisotropy but affect water mobility in different ways. Some of them are associated with restricted water diffusion (cytotoxic edema and intramyelinic edema); others are characterized by increased diffusivity (vaso-genic edema, interstitial edema). DW imaging, however, also provides information about the integrity of the tissue matrix (histoarchitecture). Loss of tissue matrix leads to decreasing anisot-ropy and increasing diffusivity.

In cytotoxic (intracellular) edema, water accu-mulates within the cells, where its diffusion is restricted in all directions. The resultant isotropi-cally restricted water diffusion presents with hy-persignal on DW images. In intramyelinic edema (related to vacuolating myelinopathy), water is probably trapped within vacuoles between the myelin sheet layers, leading to isotropically restricted water diffusion and markedly increased DW imaging signal intensities in areas of active va-cuolating myelinopathy. Cytotoxic and intramye-linic edemas are similar in appearance, although the underlying pathologic mechanisms are distinctly different. In vasogenic edema, excess water moves into the extracellular space. As a result, the apparent water diffusivity increases (hyposignal on DW and hypersignal on apparent diffusion coefficient images) isotropically in the gray matter and with some residual anisotropy along the fiber tracts in the affected white matter. These 3 edema types are relevant to the histopath-ologic processes developing in neurometabolic disorders with neonatal onset.

Intramyelinic edema Histopathologically, vacuo-lating myelinopathy is found in several neurometa-bolic diseases such as neonatal MSUD, nonketotic hyperglycinemia, and Canavan disease (but also in megalencephalic leukodystrophy with subcortical cysts and L-2-hydroxyglutaric aciduria) (see **Fig. 6**).

In MSUD, the selective involvement of myelin-ated or myelinating white matter structures makes the DW imaging findings virtually pathognomonic to the disease. Edema within nonmyelinated white matter is distinctly different (vasogenic, presenting with hyposignal on DW images), but both are important because they contribute to global brain swelling during acute metabolic decompensation. In the clinically full-blown stage of Canavan disease, DW imaging shows rather uniform hyper-signal within all affected white matter structures.[59] In the burned-out phase of the disease, this signif-icantly decreases and in some areas totally disap-pears, consistent with concomitant disintegration of the tissue matrix. In the immediate postnatal period, changes may not yet be seen on DW imaging (although biochemically the disease is already present; see later in the MR spectroscopy section).

Cytotoxic edema Cytotoxic edema is classically seen in acute stroke. However, cellular swelling in nonischemic conditions may also lead to signif-icant anisotropic water diffusion restriction and present with hypersignal on DW images (hyposig-nal on apparent diffusion coefficient maps). This phenomenon is not infrequently encountered in active metabolic diseases (in particular, organic acidemias and energy metabolism disorders), indi-cating an ongoing energy-deficient cellular dysfunction, potentially leading to cell death and extensive tissue necrosis. For example, such find-ings seem to be present in sulfite oxidase deficiency within globi pallidi and subthalamic nuclei during early presentation (see **Fig. 12**). It is nonetheless equally important to confirm or confidently rule out true ischemic cerebrovascular accident in neonates presenting with confusing clinical signs and symptoms; therefore, DW imaging should be part of the routine diagnostic imaging workup in all neonates or young infants presenting with encephalopathy or focal neurologic deficit.

Vasogenic edema This edema is the most common type encountered in patients with acute metabolic decompensation in the early postnatal period of life. It may be seen in a wide variety of entities, either as the sole imaging abnormality or in combination with others. Excessive vasogenic edema, however, is quite characteristic to urea cycle defects and sulfite oxidase deficiency.

Single-voxel proton MR spectroscopy in neonates with inborn errors of metabolism Earlier in this article, whenever relevant data in the literature have been available, reference has been made under the headings of the specific entities. Here, only some technical and conceptual issues are reviewed.

When performing an MR spectroscopic experiment, several special considerations should be made. The technique of choice is single-voxel spectroscopy, based on the assumption that the metabolic derangement affects the brain parenchyma uniformly. Nonetheless, careful positioning of the sampling voxel is important. Pulsating structures, hemorrhages, CSF, and bone should be avoided. Obvious lesion areas should also be avoided, because the metabolic profile of those may be somewhat generic and less specific, hence less representative of the underlying disease. The volume of the sampling voxel may range anywhere between 1 and 12 cm^3. The proper choice of editing techniques, notably echo time, is another important consideration. Short echo-time (20–40 milliseconds) spectra show more metabolites, but the baseline is usually noisy. The use of longer echo time (135–290 milliseconds) allows more accurate peak identification. Some metabolites, such as NAA, choline, creatine, and lactate, are well assessed on both short and long echo-time spectra. Lactate, however, has a peculiar presentation on MR spectroscopy as a function of the applied echo time. With a 135-ms echo time it presents as a negative peak doublet, whereas with a 270-ms echo time it presents as a positive peak doublet. Detection of myoinositol, glutamine, and glutamate is best achieved by short echo-time acquisitions. Glycine is best identified on the 135-ms spectrum. To confidently assess myoinositol, glutamine, glutamate, and branched-chain amino acids, a short echo-time (20–30 milliseconds) MR spectroscopy is the technique of choice.

Quantitative MR spectroscopy is very helpful, and a significant body of evidence suggests that clinical manifestations and outcome in neurometabolic disorders correlate best with the actual CNS tissue concentrations of pathologic/toxic metabolites and much less with serum, urine, or even CSF concentrations. However, quantitative analysis is possible but not always practically feasible in routine clinical settings.

Proton MR spectroscopy is increasingly recognized as a valuable tool in the diagnostic management of inborn errors of metabolism, in all stages of the disease.[60] In general, MR spectroscopic abnormalities in the brain may be divided into two major groups: process-specific and disease-specific metabolic changes. This concept may be applicable to neurometabolic disorders too.

Process-specific findings Alterations of normal constituents of the spectra, NAA, choline, and creatine, may reflect various degrees of loss of neuronal integrity, myelin breakdown, and impairment of basic energetic processes (and as such, indirectly cellular density too). These changes may be seen in almost all conditions with sufficiently significant global neurotoxicity. However, such changes in the metabolic profile of the sampled tissue are not pathognomonic of a given disease but reflect underlying "generic" biochemical (energy failure) and histopathologic (demyelination, neuroaxonal degeneration, osmotic disturbances, and so forth) processes. The role of myoinositol is less well understood; it may be an osmolar regulator, but it is quite commonly increased in pathologic processes characterized by demyelination and astrogliosis. Because many different metabolic disorders may lead to similar, stereotypical histopathologic or biochemical changes, the resultant metabolic profile by MR spectroscopy may be nonspecific. However, when interpreting an MR spectrum of the immature brain, age-related metabolic variations should be taken into account. This aspect is particularly true when comparing several follow-ups performed during infancy. In neonates, choline is the highest peak and NAA is low; the mature pattern is reached by the age of approximately 6 months.

Abnormal metabolites may also be detected in brain parenchyma. Some of these are actually present in the normal brain too, but in such small quantities that under standard conditions they are undetectable by in vivo proton MR spectroscopy. Their "conspicuity" on the spectra, therefore, may be an indicator of a pathologic biochemical process. Some of these "abnormal" metabolites are nonspecific (such as lactate and glutamine-glutamate) but in certain settings may be suggestive of metabolic disorders. For example, increased glutamine concentrations may be found in acute or chronic hepatic encephalopathy or after hypoxic-anoxic brain damage, but in a newborn without a history of birth asphyxia but with rapid neurologic deterioration it would be suggestive of a urea cycle defect (see **Fig. 4**).

Lactate is a nonspecific indicator of deficient aerobic energy metabolism. It is therefore present in a wide variety of conditions affecting oxidative phosphorylation, fatty acid oxidation, gluconeogenesis, and glucose use in general. Because lactate is almost always present in acute focal destructive brain lesions, whenever energy metabolism disorders are suspected the sampling voxel should be placed on normal-appearing parenchyma, if possible, because "positivity" would have more specific diagnostic value. It is noteworthy that in the neonate, particularly in the preterm neonate, a small amount of lactate may be a normal finding.

Disease-specific findings Some other metabolites appear only in specific disease entities; therefore their detection by MR spectroscopy may be pathognomonic. Inborn errors of metabolism of neonatal onset in which MR spectroscopy may provide more or less specific findings are few; those include Canavan disease (pathologic increase of NAA, see **Fig. 2**), nonketotic hyperglycinemia (glycine, see **Fig. 9**), galactosemia (galactitol), HMG-CoA lyase deficiency, phenylketonuria (phenylalanine), MSUD (branched-chain amino acids, see **Fig. 7**), or GABA in succinic semialdehyde dehydrogenase deficiency (the latter, however, does not belong to the group of devastating neurometabolic diseases of the newborn).

SUMMARY

1. Management of neonates with clinically manifesting inborn errors of metabolism requires a multidisciplinary approach and close collaboration of obstetricians, pediatricians, geneticists, biochemists, and radiologists.
2. The age of onset, the presence or absence of dysmorphic features and malformations of the central nervous system, skin manifestations, robust laboratory changes, neurologic signs and symptoms, visceral and musculoskeletal abnormalities, and MR imaging (including DW imaging as well as spectroscopic alterations)

are all important, potentially conclusive clues in the diagnostic workup.
3. Devastating metabolic disorders of the newborn or young infant may present with confusingly similar or distinctly different clinical, biochemical, and imaging abnormalities, some of which are therefore nonspecific; others may be characteristic, suggestive, or even pathognomonic of a disease entity.
4. The set of detectable abnormalities defines the clinical-radiologic pattern, which is a function of the varying degree of resistance or vulnerability of the various organ systems to the noxious metabolic changes.
5. Recognition of the clinical and imaging substrates of selective vulnerability constitutes a prerequisite of the clinical-radiologic pattern recognition, which is the single most important concept to be applied in the diagnostic management of inborn errors of metabolism.

REFERENCES

1. Leonard JV, Morris AA. Diagnosis and early management of inborn errors of metabolism presenting around the time of birth [review]. Acta Paediatr 2006;95:6–14.
2. Kanaumi T, Takashima S, Hirose S, et al. Neuropathology of methylmalonic acidemia in a child. Pediatr Neurol 2006;34:156–9.
3. Kolodny EH. Dysmyelinating and demyelinating conditions in infancy [review]. Curr Opin Neurol Neurosurg 1993;6:379–86.
4. Streeten BW. The nature of the ocular zonule. Trans Am Ophthalmol Soc 1982;80:823–54.
5. Nissenkorn A, Michelson M, Ben-Zeev B, et al. Inborn errors of metabolism: a cause of abnormal brain development [review]. Neurology 2001;56: 1265–72.
6. van Straaten HL, van Tintelen JP, Trijbels JM, et al. Neonatal lactic acidosis, complex I/IV deficiency, and fetal cerebral disruption. Neuropediatrics 2005;36:193–9.
7. Kyllerman M, Blomstrand S, Mansson JE, et al. Central nervous system malformations and white matter changes in pseudo-neonatal adrenoleukodystrophy. Neuropediatrics 1990;21:199–201.
8. Paupe A, Bidat L, Sonigo P, et al. Prenatal diagnosis of hypoplasia of the corpus callosum in association with non-ketotic hyperglycinemia. Ultrasound Obstet Gynecol 2002;20:616–9.
9. Mellerio C, Marignier S, Roth P, et al. Prenatal cerebral ultrasound and MRI findings in glutaric aciduria Type 1: a de novo case. Ultrasound Obstet Gynecol 2008;31:712–4.
10. Mochel F, Grebille AG, Benachi A, et al. Contribution of fetal MR imaging in the prenatal diagnosis of

Zellweger syndrome. AJNR Am J Neuroradiol 2006; 27:333–6.

11. Garel C. New advances in fetal MR neuroimaging [review]. Pediatr Radiol 2006;36:621–5.

12. Girard N, Gouny SC, Viola A, et al. Assessment of normal fetal brain maturation in utero by proton magnetic resonance spectroscopy. Magn Reson Med 2006;56:768–75.

13. Kalidas K, Behrouz R. Inherited metabolic disorders and cerebral infarction [review]. Expert Rev Neurother 2008;8:1731–41.

14. Testai FD, Gorelick PB. Inherited metabolic disorders and stroke part 2: homocystinuria, organic acidurias, and urea cycle disorders [review]. Arch Neurol 2010;67:148–53.

15. Dantas MF, Suormala T, Randolph A, et al. 3-Methylcrotonyl-CoA carboxylase deficiency: mutation analysis in 28 probands, 9 symptomatic and 19 detected by newborn screening. Hum Mutat 2005;26:164.

16. Baumgartner ER, Suormala T. Multiple carboxylase deficiency: inherited and acquired disorders of biotin metabolism [review]. Int J Vitam Nutr Res 1997;67:377–84.

17. Squires L, Betz B, Umfleet J, et al. Resolution of subependymal cysts in neonatal holocarboxylase synthetase deficiency. Dev Med Child Neurol 1997; 39:267–9.

18. Schurmann M, Engelbrecht V, Lohmeier K, et al. Cerebral metabolic changes in biotinidase deficiency. J Inherit Metab Dis 1997;20:755–60.

19. Gunay-Aygun M. 3-Methylglutaconic aciduria: a common biochemical marker in various syndromes with diverse clinical features [review]. Mol Genet Metab 2005;84:1–3.

20. Wortmann SB, Kremer BH, Graham A, et al. 3-Methylglutaconic aciduria type I redefined: a syndrome with late-onset leukoencephalopathy. Neurology 2010;75:1079–83.

21. Di Rosa G, Deodato F, Loupatty FJ, et al. Hypertrophic cardiomyopathy, cataract, developmental delay, lactic acidosis: a novel subtype of 3-methylglutaconic aciduria. J Inherit Metab Dis 2006;29:546–50.

22. Jareno NM, Fernandez-Mayoralas DM, Silvestre CP, et al. 3-methylglutaconic aciduria type 4 manifesting as Leigh syndrome in 2 siblings. J Child Neurol 2007;22:218–21.

23. Ozand PT, al Aqeel A, Gascon G, et al. 3-Hydroxy-3-methylglutaryl-coenzyme A (HMG-CoA) lyase deficiency in Saudi Arabia. J Inherit Metab Dis 1991; 14:174–88.

24. van der Knaap MS, Bakker HD, Valk J. MR imaging and proton spectroscopy in 3-hydroxy-3-methylglutaryl coenzyme A lyase deficiency. AJNR Am J Neuroradiol 1998;19:378–82.

25. Yalcinkaya C, Dincer A, Gunduz E, et al. MRI and MRS in HMG-CoA lyase deficiency [review]. Pediatr Neurol 1999;20:375–80.

26. Tanpaiboon P. Methylmalonic acidemia (MMA) [review]. Mol Genet Metab 2005;85:2–6.

27. Radmanesh A, Zaman T, Ghanaati H, et al. Methylmalonic acidemia: brain imaging findings in 52 children and a review of the literature [review]. Pediatr Radiol 2008;38:1054–61.

28. Michel SJ, Given CA 2nd, Robertson WC Jr. Imaging of the brain, including diffusion-weighted imaging in methylmalonic acidemia. Pediatr Radiol 2004;34: 580–2.

29. Ristoff E, Larsson A. Inborn errors in the metabolism of glutathione [review]. Orphanet J Rare Dis 2007;2:16.

30. Divry P, Roulaud-Parrot F, Dorche C, et al. 5-Oxoprolinuria (glutathione synthetase deficiency): a case with neonatal presentation and rapid fatal outcome. J Inherit Metab Dis 1991;14:341–4.

31. Mitanchez D, Rabier D, Mokhtari M, et al. 5-Oxoprolinuria: a cause of neonatal metabolic acidosis. Acta Paediatr 2001;90:827–8.

32. Baslow MH. Brain N-acetylaspartate as a molecular water pump and its role in the etiology of Canavan disease: a mechanistic explanation [review]. J Mol Neurosci 2003;21:185–90.

33. Namboodiri AM, Peethambaran A, Mathew R, et al. Canavan disease and the role of N-acetylaspartate in myelin synthesis [review]. Mol Cell Endocrinol 2006;252:216–23.

34. Gordon N. Ornithine transcarbamylase deficiency: a urea cycle defect [review]. Eur J Paediatr Neurol 2003;7:115–21.

35. Choi CG, Yoo HW. Localized proton MR spectroscopy in infants with urea cycle defect. AJNR Am J Neuroradiol 2001;22:834–7.

36. Righini A, Ramenghi LA, Parini R, et al. Water apparent diffusion coefficient and T2 changes in the acute stage of maple syrup urine disease: evidence of intramyelinic and vasogenic-interstitial edema. J Neuroimaging 2003;13:162–5.

37. Jan W, Zimmerman RA, Wang ZJ, et al. MR diffusion imaging and MR spectroscopy of maple syrup urine disease during acute metabolic decompensation. Neuroradiology 2003;45:393–9.

38. Demirel N, Bas AY, Zenciroglu A, et al. Neonatal nonketotic hyperglycinemia: report of five cases. Pediatr Int 2008;50:121–3.

39. Tada K, Kure S, Takayanagi M, et al. Non-ketotic hyperglycinemia: a life-threatening disorder in the neonate [review]. Early Hum Dev 1992;29: 75–81.

40. van der Knaap MS, Jakobs C, Valk J. Magnetic resonance imaging in lactic acidosis [review]. J Inherit Metab Dis 1996;19:535–47.

41. Barnerias C, Saudubray J-M, Touati G, et al. Pyruvate dehydrogenase complex deficiency: four neurological phenotypes with differing pathogenesis. Dev Med Child Neurol 2010;52:e1–9.

42. Zand DJ, Simon EM, Pulitzer SB, et al. In vivo pyruvate detected by MR spectroscopy in neonatal pyruvate dehydrogenase deficiency. AJNR Am J Neuroradiol 2003;24:1471–4.

43. Moczulski D, Majak I, Mamczur D. An overview of beta-oxidation disorders [review]. Postepy Hig Med Dosw (Online) 2009;63:266–77.

44. Boles RG, Buck EA, Blitzer MG, et al. Retrospective biochemical screening of fatty acid oxidation disorders in postmortem livers of 418 cases of sudden death in the first year of life. J Pediatr 1998;132:924–33.

45. Sharma R, Perszyk AA, Marangi D, et al. Lethal neonatal carnitine palmitoyltransferase II deficiency: an unusual presentation of a rare disorder. Am J Perinatol 2003;20:25–32.

46. Meir K, Fellig Y, Meiner V, et al. Severe infantile carnitine palmitoyltransferase II deficiency in 19-week fetal sibs. Pediatr Dev Pathol 2009;12:481–6.

47. Grayer J. Recognition of Zellweger syndrome in infancy. Adv Neonatal Care 2005;5:5–13.

48. Young S, Rabi Y, Lodha AK. Band heterotopia in Zellweger syndrome (cerebro-hepato-renal syndrome). Neurol India 2007;55:93.

49. Unay B, Kendirli T, Atac K, et al. Caudothalamic groove cysts in Zellweger syndrome. Clin Dysmorphol 2005;14:165–7.

50. Chang YC, Huang CC, Huang SC, et al. Neonatal adrenoleukodystrophy presenting with seizure at birth: a case report and review of the literature. Pediatr Neurol 2008;38:137–9.

51. van Grunsven EG, van Berkel E, Ijlst L, et al. Peroxisomal D-hydroxyacyl-CoA dehydrogenase deficiency: resolution of the enzyme defect and its molecular basis in bifunctional protein deficiency. Proc Natl Acad Sci U S A 1998;95:2128–33.

52. Ferdinandusse S, Denis S, Mooyer PA, et al. Clinical and biochemical spectrum of D-bifunctional protein deficiency. Ann Neurol 2006;59:92–104.

53. Kaufmann WE, Theda C, Naidu S, et al. Neuronal migration abnormality in peroxisomal bifunctional enzyme defect. Ann Neurol 1996;39:268–71.

54. Watkins PA, Chen WW, Harris CJ, et al. Peroxisomal bifunctional enzyme deficiency. J Clin Invest 1989;83:771–7.

55. de Bie P, Muller P, Wijmenga C, et al. Molecular pathogenesis of Wilson and Menkes disease: correlation of mutations with molecular defects and disease phenotypes [review]. J Med Genet 2007;44:673–88.

56. Hoffmann C, Ben-Zeev B, Anikster Y, et al. Magnetic resonance imaging and magnetic resonance spectroscopy in isolated sulfite oxidase deficiency. J Child Neurol 2007;22:1214–21.

57. Otaduy MC, Leite CC, Lacerda MT, et al. Proton MR spectroscopy and imaging of a galactosemic patient before and after dietary treatment. AJNR Am J Neuroradiol 2006;27:204–7.

58. Berry GT, Hunter JV, Wang Z, et al. In vivo evidence of brain galactitol accumulation in an infant with galactosemia and encephalopathy. J Pediatr 2001;138:260–2.

59. Srikanth SG, Chandrashekar HS, Nagarajan K, et al. Restricted diffusion in Canavan disease. Childs Nerv Syst 2007;23:465–8.

60. Cakmakci H, Pekcevik Y, Yis U, et al. Diagnostic value of proton MR spectroscopy and diffusion-weighted MR imaging in childhood inherited neurometabolic brain diseases and review of the literature [review]. Eur J Radiol 2010;74:e161–71.

MR Imaging of Neonatal Brain Infections

Jacques F. Schneider, MD[a],*, Sylviane Hanquinet, MD[b],
Mariasavina Severino, MD[c], Andrea Rossi, MD[c]

KEYWORDS

- MRI • Neonate • Brain • Infection

Infection of the central nervous system (CNS) in neonates may be caused by a variety of bacteria, viruses, fungi, or parasites. The late sequels of CNS insult vary with the amount and virulence of the pathogen agent, the timing of infection in relation to the degree of cerebral maturation, the amount of immunologic protection transmitted from the mother, and the ability of the neonate's immune and inflammatory system to respond to the infection. Neuroimaging patterns not only reflect changes related to selective tissue injury as in many viral infections, but also result from nonspecific changes caused by a more generalized reaction of the host as seen mainly in bacterial infections. Furthermore, there is a growing body of evidence implicating infection during the perinatal and neonatal periods as an important contributor to an increased risk of adverse neurodevelopmental outcome in the preterm compared with the term population. In the neonatal period, because of the good visualization of cerebral parenchymal structures and ventricular system through the open fontanels, ultrasound still is the primary imaging modality of the neonatal brain. It allows also the depiction of enlarged subarachnoidal or subdural spaces, although not all of the convexity can be assessed. It easily demonstrates hemorrhagic or purulent components in the parenchyma, the ventricles, and parts of the extracerebral spaces, and can be repetitively used for follow-up.

However, MR imaging better depicts white matter and cortical edematous or ischemic changes, delivers a complete assessment of the extracerebral spaces, and allows exact depiction of the posterior fossa, including brainstem, the latter two being almost blind spots for ultrasound. Besides delivering a complete anatomic coverage of the brain, MR imaging gives supplementary information by demonstrating contrast enhancement in inflammatory areas, or on tissue viability and metabolic processes by the use of diffusion-weighted imaging (DWI) and MR spectroscopy.

BACTERIAL INFECTION
Epidemiology

Neonatal sepsis has been divided into early onset (within the first 7 days of life) and late-onset sepsis. Clinical signs for meningitis and early onset sepsis in the newborn are essentially similar and nonspecific. The incidence of early onset sepsis or meningitis is higher in infants weighing less than 1500 g compared with term neonates (15–19 vs 1–8 per 1000 live births), and is related to intrapartal infection from the maternal rectovaginal flora.[1] Late-onset diseases present with a less fulminant course and meningitis is the most common presentation.[2] During the last 10 years there has been an increased incidence of neonatal late-onset sepsis, predominantly caused by coagulase-negative

[a] Department of Pediatric Radiology, University Children's Hospital Basel, UKBB, Spitalstrasse 33, 4056 Basel, Switzerland
[b] Department of Pediatric Radiology, University Children's Hospital Geneva, Rue Willy Donzé 6, 1205 Geneva, Switzerland
[c] Department of Pediatric Neuroradiology, G. Gaslini Children's Hospital, Largo G. Gaslini 5, I-16147 Genoa, Italy
* Corresponding author.
E-mail address: Jacques.schneider@ukbb.ch

Magn Reson Imaging Clin N Am 19 (2011) 761–775
doi:10.1016/j.mric.2011.08.013

staphylococci, and a decrease in incidence of early onset sepsis caused by group B streptococci (GBS).[3] In early onset sepsis, the neonate can acquire the organism from his or her GBS-colonized mother through vertical transmission from the lower genital tract or from acquisition during passage through the birth canal. Risk factors that predispose a neonate to become infected are prematurity,[4] lack of maternal anti-GBS IgG protection,[5] placental infections with septic emboli, prolonged rupture of the fetal membranes, and high inoculum of the organism in the maternal anogenital tract. In some cases, direct or iatrogenic contamination of the CNS may occur (eg, after ventricular shunting). Maternal antepartal antibiotics have dramatically reduced the risk of early onset GBS infection in newborns by more than 80%.[6] A corresponding change in *Escherichia coli* meningitis has not occurred and gram-negative bacillary meningitis still carries a worse prognosis than meningitis with a gram-positive organism.[7] Maternal antibiotics may also have increased antibiotic resistance in *E coli* isolates from early onset bloodstream infections.[8] Recent studies found no outcome difference between early onset GBS meningitis and gram-negative meningitis, but early onset GBS meningitis still has a worse outcome that late-onset GBS meningitis.[9,10]

Pathophysiology

Meningitis complicates 5% to 20% of the cases of early onset neonatal sepsis.[11] CNS damage is the result of a cascade of events, which begins with an extensive inflammatory vasculitis that may be followed by small or large vessel obstruction and infarctions. This vasculitis, which enables bacteria to cross the blood–brain barrier, takes place primarily at the level of the choroid plexus leading to plexitis and ventriculitis, with consecutive dissemination into the cerebrospinal fluid (CSF). Although in the strictest sense ventriculitis accompanies all cases of meningitis, it has been suggested that ventriculitis may occur as a primary process.[12] After CSF dissemination, bacteria gain access to the leptomeningeal space and induce arachnoiditis. Through this inflammatory-destructive process, bacteria eventually invade the brain parenchyma, followed by cerebral tissue liquefaction and encephalomalacia.[13] At the same time, inflammation of the arachnoid leads to adhesions and consecutive hydrocephalus development.[14] However, the major element that contributes to an increase in intracranial pressure during bacterial meningitis is the development of cerebral edema, which may be vasogenic, cytotoxic, or interstitial in origin.[15–17] Vasogenic cerebral edema is a consequence of increased blood–brain barrier permeability. Cytotoxic cerebral edema results from swelling of the cellular elements of the brain, most likely caused by the release of toxic factors in bacterial meningitis. Interstitial edema reflects obstruction of flow in normal CSF pathways, as in hydrocephalus. In neonates, cerebral edema is often the presenting clinical manifestation, because of rapid disease progression and higher vulnerability of the immature brain to the infectious agent. Nevertheless, distensibility of neonates' cranial vault reduces the risk of fatal complication in case of brain herniation, which occurs in approximately 6% of acute meningits.[17]

The pathophysiology of GBS meningitis varies according to age of onset. In early onset disease, autopsy studies demonstrate little or no evidence of leptomeningeal inflammation, despite the presence of abundant bacteria, vascular thrombosis, and parenchymal hemorrhage.[18] By contrast, infants with late-onset disease usually have diffuse purulent arachnoiditis with prominent involvement of the base of the brain.[13] These differences reflect the immaturity of the host immunologic response in the immediate neonatal period.[19] A prominent sign of leptomeningeal inflammation is fluid accumulation in the subarachnoid or subdural space. Subdural effusions, which are initially sterile and mainly caused by toxin-induced increased permeability of the capillaries and veins of the internal layer of the dura mater, are rare in neonates and sometimes not easy to distinguish from enlarged subarachnoid spaces. True subdural purulent effusion and empyema or intraventricular pus accumulation whether caused by ventriculitis or recirculation of subarachnoid purulent collections are very rare in neonates.[20]

After bacteria have gained access to brain parenchyma, focal purulent complications and brain abscesses may develop. Intracerebral abscesses complicating meningitis are most commonly related to *Citrobacter*, *Proteus*, *Pseudomonas*, *Serratia*, and *Staphylococcus aureus*.[21] Gram-negative organisms and especially members of the *Citrobacter* and *Proteus* genus were reported to be the causative organism in most of the children younger than 1 month, whereas various *Streptococcus* species were the most common isolates in children older that 1 month.[22,23] In this setting, hematogenous dissemination is the major source of origin in neonates, whereas contiguous infections (from sinusitis or otitis) and penetrating injuries are almost exclusively seen in older children. It must be emphasized that bacteria associated with brain abscess are those that cause meningitis and severe vasculitis,[20] with only rare exceptions.[24] Neonatal brain abscesses are characteristically large at the time of diagnosis, often multiple and typically lacking a complete capsule, which favors rapid enlargement.[25] In more than 80% of cases, they are located in the cerebral hemispheres, especially frontal and parietal lobes, usually originating in the periventricular white matter, whereas the subcortical white matter and basal ganglia are more common locations in older children.[26] Deeply located abscesses may rupture into the ventricular system.[27] There is a continuum from focal cerebritis to mature abscess, a process that takes place during a period of 2 to 3 weeks, although it may be as short as a few days in neonates. Early cerebritis is characterized by intensive vasculitis, local inflammation, petechial hemorrhages, and surrounding edema, followed by necrosis of the center with irregular peripheral inflammatory tissue in later cerebritis stage.[28] This host response builds the peripheral capsule of the abscess, which is initially poorly defined, thicker on the cortical side, and thinner on the medial or ventricular side, probably related to differences in vascularization.[27–29] This difference may explain why abscesses predominantly rupture into the ventricular system, a sometimes fatal complication responsible for sudden death. In the late-capsule stage, a five-layer structure is recognizable at histology, with a thick granulation circumferential reaction and extensive peripheral edematous changes.[29]

Long-term pathologic changes are mainly related to gliosis and encephalomalacia with variable amount of scarring and atrophy of the cortex and white matter, and hydrocephalus complications.

Neuroimaging

Imaging findings in acute neonatal bacterial meningitis vary greatly with the stage of infection. Extracerebral spaces and ventricular system may be normal, enlarged, or show evidence of protein or pus accumulation. Cerebral parenchyma alike may show normal signal intensity, evidence of edema, ischemia, infarction, hemorrhage, or necrosis with abscess and central purulent accumulation. Because of brain immaturity and poor immunologic response capabilities of the newborn in the immediate postnatal period, the physiopathologic cascade is not strictly timed and severe edema or abscess formation may be the most prominent or even the single presenting neuroimaging finding. Because of the lack of radiation, its higher sensitivity for ischemic lesions and infarctions, and its ability to easily detect purulent collections, MR imaging is the preferred imaging modality over

CT, even in an emergency situation. In all cases, MR imaging scans must include pre–contrast- and post–contrast-enhanced T1-weighted and T2-weighted images in at least two perpendicular planes. Fluid attenuated inversion recovery (FLAIR) sequence and DWI are both recommended in this situation because of their high sensitivity in detecting purulent collections.[30–32]

Choroid plexus infection and ventriculitis are often detected together, and show a characteristic triad consisting of choroid plexus engorgement, ependymal lining contrast enhancement, and intraventricular dependant debris and pus accumulation mainly in the occipital horns (**Fig. 1**). Periventricular edema may be related to bacteria-induced periventricular white matter necrosis or to unbalanced CSF circulation with development of hydrocephalus (**Fig. 2**).

Once inflammation has reached the CSF compartment, arachnoiditis is the natural next step in the cascade of events. Nevertheless, the initial signs of involvement of the meninges, such as enlargement of the subdural or subarachnoid space, are nonspecific and may go unrecognized (**Fig. 3**). However, contrast enhancement of the arachnoidea may be completely lacking in the natural history of GBS meningitis of the newborn. When present, contrast enhancement is seen as a pencil-shaped line covering the gyri and sometimes seen extending within the depth of the sulci (**Fig. 4**). Contrast enhancement of the dura,

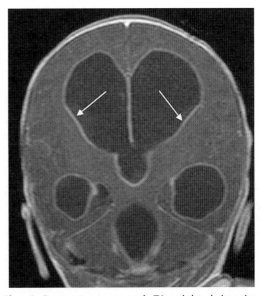

Fig. 1. Postcontrast coronal T1-weighted imaging shows dilatation of the ventricular system and ventriculitis with pencil-shaped contrast enhancement of the ependymal lining (*arrows*) in a case of *Serratia marcescens* infection.

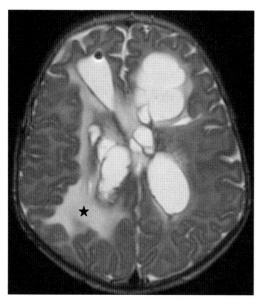

Fig. 2. Axial T2-weighted imaging shows ventricular dilatation and multiple intraventricular septae in a case of *Serratia marcescens* infection. Extensive T2-hyperintensity of the white matter of the right cerebral hemisphere (*asterisk*), most probably related to direct bacteria-induced white matter necrosis, and not to CSF resorption imbalance because almost no signal change on the contralateral side can be detected.

however, is seen as a thickened line underneath the calvarium opposite to the arachnoid membrane and separated from it by the subdural space, and may persist several months after complete clinical recovery (**Fig. 5**). Adhesions may occur everywhere within the CSF and consist of enhancing fibrin webs in the subarachnoid, subdural, and even intraventricular spaces (**Fig. 6**). Before true purulent accumulation occurs, the intense inflammatory reaction produces cellular debris from leuocytic infiltrates and fibrin or protein residues, which can be seen as high signal intensity change of the CSF-filled spaces on FLAIR imaging (**Fig. 7**), but may be difficult to recognize on T1-weighted, T2-weighted, or DWI (**Fig. 8**). DWI is best at demonstrating the presence of truly purulent accumulation, which shows very high signal intensity, because of the higher viscosity of these collections (**Fig. 9**). It must be emphasized that purulent collections may be completely missed on T1- or T2-weighted imaging (**Fig. 10**).

Large territorial or small lacunar peripheral infarctions result from either primary involvement of the vessels by way of blood-borne bacteria, or secondary caused by extension of the infection along the perivascular subpial spaces with inflammation of the walls of the arteries (arteritis). Vascular complications may also occur because of a breakdown of the blood–brain barrier. It may also induce cortical pseudolaminar necrosis, which appears as T1- and T2-hyperintensity and shows contrast enhancement (**Figs. 11** and **12**).

Venous involvement in meningitis is rare. It mainly expresses itself as thrombophlebitis and venous thrombosis, a complication usually seen in combination with dehydration.[27] On MR imaging, venous thrombosis displays itself as T1-isointensity to -hyperintensity of the thrombus within the vessel, depending on the age of the clot. Known complications of venous thrombosis are hemorrhagic transformations, which involve the matching venous drainage area.

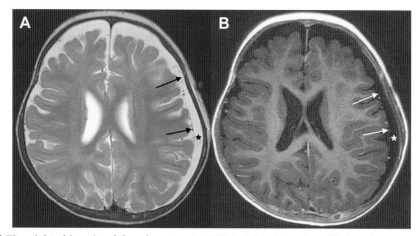

Fig. 3. Axial T2-weighted imaging (*A*) and postcontrast T1-weighted imaging (*B*) show in a case of late-onset pneumococcal meningitis in a 5-month-old boy enlargement of the subdural space on the left side (*asterisks*). Note the thin arachnoid membrane (*arrows*) demarcating the subarachnoid from the subdural space, which is void of vessels. There is no contrast enhancement in *B* and the subdural fluid has the same intensity as normal CSF in all sequences.

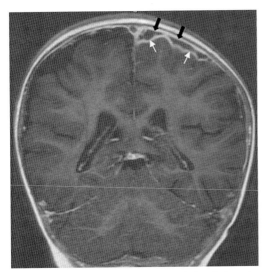

Fig. 4. Postcontrast coronal T1-weighted imaging demonstrates pencil-shaped contrast enhancement of the thickened dura (*black arrows*) and the arachnoid at the surface of the gyri (*white arrows*) in a case of pneumococcal meningitis.

Last in the chain of events in meningitis, brain parenchymal involvement leading to focal cerebritis produces an ill-defined area of T1-hypointensity and T2-hyperintensity on MR imaging. Mass effect is moderate and best identified through narrower sulci compared with the other side. Faint contrast enhancement may be detected within the edematous area. There is a continuum in MR imaging

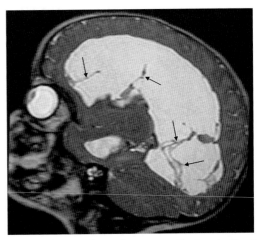

Fig. 6. Follow-up from the same patient as in Fig. 2. Sagittal T2-weighted imaging shows multiple residual intraventricular septations (*arrows*).

findings from early cerebritis to full-blown late-capsule stage abscess, with a continuously stronger demarcation of the purulent center against a peripheral initially incomplete, later complete inflammatory capsule. This last stage consists of a highly T1-hypointense and T2-hyperintense center, surrounded by a marked closed ring that consistently shows strong contrast enhancement. Peripheral edema is present to a variable amount in all stages (**Fig. 13**). The presence of hemorrhagic foci is revealed by focal T1-hyperintensity on pre–contrast-enhanced imaging. In analogy to the

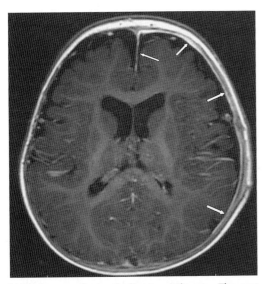

Fig. 5. Same patient as in Fig. 4 posttherapy. The postcontrast axial T1-weighted imaging shows a residual thickening and contrast enhancement of the dura over the left hemisphere (*arrows*).

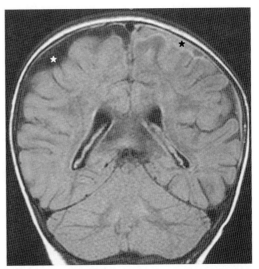

Fig. 7. Same patient as in Fig. 4. On coronal FLAIR, there is a clear signal hyperintensity of the CSF overlying the left cerebral convexity (*black asterisk*) compared with the opposite side (*white asterisk*), consistent with inflammatory exudate.

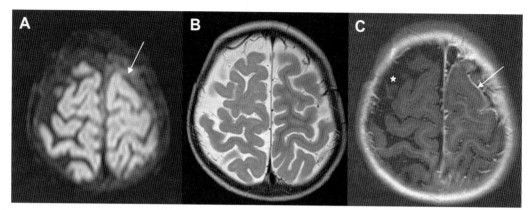

Fig. 8. Pneumococcal meningitis of the left cerebral hemisphere with moderate diffusion restriction of the CSF space. (*A*) Axial diffusion-weighted image (*arrow*). (*B*) No signal intensity change on axial T2-weighted imaging. (*C*) Strong contrast enhancement of the arachnoid in axial contrast-enhanced T1-weighted imaging (*arrow*), compared to the normal contralateral side (*asterisk*).

previously described extracerebral purulent fluid, DWI is highly sensitive in showing central pus accumulation in late-stage abscess, because of the high viscosity of the fluid (**Fig. 14**).[33–35] Markedly reduced diffusivity (bright on DWI and dark on apparent diffusion coefficient [ADC] maps) is characteristic and can be used as a surrogate marker of treatment response.[36] MR spectroscopy has been used to analyze the central components of abscesses, revealing first the absence of normal brain metabolites (*N*-acetylaspartate, choline, and creatine) and second the presence of residues from anaerobic glycolysis (lactate, lipids, acetate,

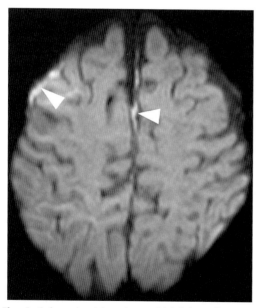

Fig. 9. Subarachnoid and parafalcial hyperintensity on axial diffusion-weighted image. Diffusion restriction is more pronounced than in **Fig. 8**, indicative of purulent coating (*arrowheads*).

and succinate) and proteolysis (aminoacids) (**Fig. 15**).[37,38]

VIRAL INFECTION
Epidemiology

Compared with bacteria-induced sepsis, the estimated incidence of neonatal viral infection, led by herpes simplex virus (HSV), is much lower and varies from 1.6 to 50 in 100,000 live births with a lower incidence in Europe compared with the United States. Newborns get contaminated through direct contact with infected maternal secretions in the birth canal in 85% of cases.[39] Vesicular lesions usually occur over the scalp and face in cephalic presentations, and over the buttocks in breech presentations.[40] Neonatal herpes can result from infection with HSV-1 or -2. In a study comparing the long-term outcome of treated neonatal herpes encephalitis, infants infected with HSV-2 have a higher morbidity.[41] The highest risk of transmission (50%) is present in pregnant women with a primary infection at the end of the third trimester. Nevertheless, in most cases, neonatal infection occurs in children of asymptomatic mothers, whose serologic status is a critical determinant of the risk of infectious transmission.[42] Isolated CNS disease occurs in 35% of HSV-infected infants and is probably the result of neuronal spread. Even under adequate therapy and good response, neurologic sequelae are present in 70% of surviving neonates and mortality is related to brainstem involvement.[43] With primary disseminated HSV disease, the brain becomes secondarily infected by the blood-borne route in 60% to 75% of infected neonates.[44] There is a high mortality (30%) rate and a 15% incidence of neurologic sequelae in the survivors.[45]

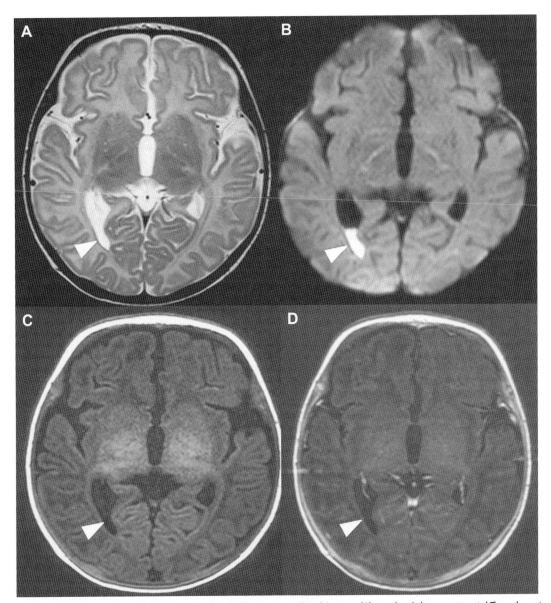

Fig. 10. Axial T2-weighted imaging (*A*), axial diffusion-weighted image (*B*), and axial precontrast (*C*) and post-contrast axial T1-weighted imaging (*D*). Staphylococcal meningitis with purulent accumulation with fluid–fluid level in the right occipital horn, only visible on diffusion imaging (*arrowheads*).

Beside HSV infection, there is a large entero-virus population (represented mainly by Coxsack-ie B virus and poliovirus) and echovirus, which can cause severe meningitis and meningoen-cephalitis in the neonatal period. A prevalence of 12 symptomatic cases per 100,000 infants younger than 2 months has been identified,[46] but this reported incidence is a gross underesti-mate of the real prevalence because of the large number of asymptomatic cases. As with HSV infection, clinically significant infection may occur by transplacental route (although exceptional before the third trimenon); during labor (about 4% of mothers excrete enterovirus near the time of delivery[47]); or after delivery, mainly caused by transmission from a mother to her infant. Most enteroviral nursery epidemics have involved Coxsackie B virus, but echovirus are well known as a major cause of febrile illness and aseptic meningitis in young infants. Echovirus meningo-encephalitis has been associated with severe neurodevelopmental disabilities.[48] In one review of neonatal echovirus infection, 26% exhibited evidence for meningitis or meningoencephalitis

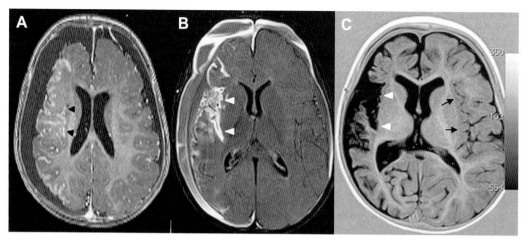

Fig. 11. A case of pneumococcal meningoencephalitis. (A) Postcontrast axial T1-weighted imaging shows enlargement of CSF spaces bilaterally and prominent contrast enhancement of the arachnoid on the right side (*arrowheads*) reaching deep within the sulci. (B) Precontrast axial FLAIR shows gray matter involvement on FLAIR imaging with thick hyperintensity mainly of the insular cortex on the right side (*arrowheads*). (C) Precontrast axial T1-weighted imaging. Long-term follow-up demonstrating cortical necrosis and atrophy on the right side (*white arrowheads*), compared to the normal insula on the contralateral side (*black arrowheads*).

and half of these cases were attributed to echovirus 11.[49]

Recently, a new virus genus, human parechovirus (HPeV) 1 to 6, has been identified that has been associated with severe meningoencephalitis, extensive white matter damage, and adverse neurologic sequelae (especially with HPeV 3).[50] In a recent study, in all patients with parechovirus

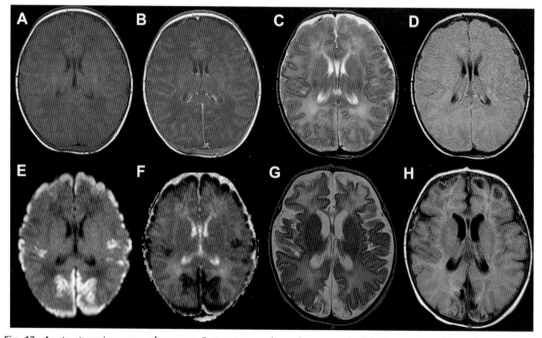

Fig. 12. Acute stage in a case of a group B streptococcal meningoencephalitis. Precontrast (A) and postcontrast (B) axial T1-weighted imaging. (C) Axial T2-weighted imaging. (D) FLAIR. (E) Axial diffusion-weighted image. (F) ADC map. Follow-up of same patient: axial T2-weighted imaging (G) and axial FLAIR (H). There is an extensive cortical involvement in the acute stage with cytotoxic edema (severe cortical hyperintensity in E). The cortical ribbon itself is blurred and even missing especially in the frontal and occipital lobes on A and C. Follow-up demonstrates cortical destruction, most severe in the frontal and occipital lobes, and diffuse atrophy of cerebral white matter, resulting in e vacuo dilatation of the ventricular system (G, H).

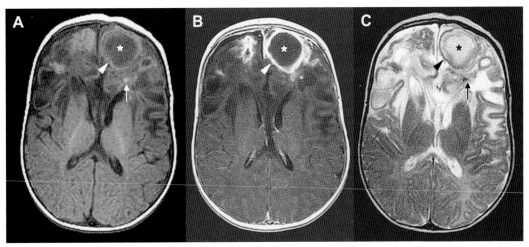

Fig. 13. Axial precontrast (*A*) and postcontrast (*B*) T1-weighted imaging, and axial T2-weighted imaging (*C*) in a case of *Citrobacter* meningoencephalitis with development of cerebral abscesses in both frontal lobes. Central pus accumulation (*asterisks*) and peripheral thick and multilayered capsule with intensive contrast enhancement (*arrowheads*). Within the extensive edematous changes in the frontal white matter, there are scattered foci of hemorrhage (*arrows in A and C*). (*Courtesy of* Ianina Scheer, MD, University Children's Hospital, Zürich, Switzerland.)

infection who developed clinical meningoencephalitis, white matter abnormalities found on cranial imaging were not distinguishable from those found in neonates with echovirus meningoencephalitis.[51]

Pathophysiology

Herpes simplex
Neonatal herpes simplex infections may result in a wide range of affection of the CNS, but neonates usually demonstrate significant brain involvement.

Meningoencephalitis is characterized by meningeal inflammation, perivascular cellular infiltration, and multifocal necrotic foci, followed by microglial and astrocytic proliferation. These findings are often accompanied by a variable degree of brain swelling and hemorrhagic foci within the necrotic areas.[52] Perinatal herpes simplex infection has a mostly devastating effect on neuronal development and later brain function. Severe atrophy and microcephaly are commonly seen. It must be emphasized that in a previously published study,

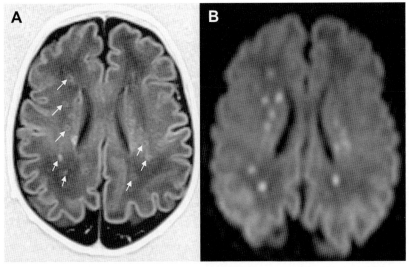

Fig. 14. Axial postcontrast T1-weighted imaging (*A*) and axial diffusion-weighted image (*B*) in a case of staphylococcal encephalitis with multiple small cerebral abscesses showing peripheral contrast enhancement (*arrows in A*) and central pus as demonstrated on diffusion imaging (*B*).

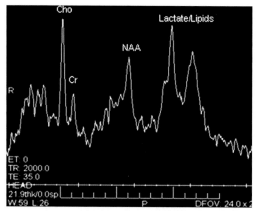

Fig. 15. MR spectroscopy of the abscess in Fig. 13. The short echo-time single-voxel spectrum at TE 35 ms demonstrates reduced peaks of N-acetylaspartate (NAA) and creatine (Cr), with high levels of choline (Cho), lactate, and lipids, indicating breakdown of cell membranes and anaerobic metabolism. (*Courtesy of* Ianina Scheer, MD, University Children's Hospital, Zürich, Switzerland.)

children infected with HSV-1 were neurologically normal on follow-up, whereas those with HSV-2 had increased rates of microcephaly, seizures, cerebral palsy, and mental retardation.[41]

Enterovirus

Perinatal enteroviral intracranial infection manifests itself most commonly as viral "aseptic" meningitis (by CSF criteria), caused by primary viral infection of the meninges and characterized by inflammatory infiltration of the pia-arachnoidea.[46] Much less common is primary viral encephalitis, caused by primary infection of brain parenchyma

and characterized by foci of parenchymal necrosis with glial proliferation. This characteristic has been documented only for prenatal Coxsackie B infection.[20,53] This encephalitis shows characteristically mononuclear and lymphocytic meningeal infiltration, perivascular inflammation, and multifocal neuronal necrosis coupled with isolation of virus from CNS parenchyma.[53]

Neuroimaging

Herpes virus

Although in older children the limbic and paralimbic cortex are predominantly involved and hemorrhagic necrosis are often seen,[54] neonatal CNS herpes infection is rarely hemorrhagic. Temporal and frontal lobes are spared and lesions can be demonstrated within the deep and periventricular white matter. MR imaging shows diffuse hypointensity on T1-weighted and hyperintensity on T2-weighted imaging, whereas DWI has been shown to be sensitive in the early course of the disease with restricted diffusion in the periventricular area (**Fig. 16**).[55,56] In these areas, MR spectroscopy may reveal a decrease in N-acetylaspartate, elevated glutamine and glutamate, and sometimes the presence of lactate.[27] Postcontrast images only rarely show enhancement of the leptomeninges. Later in the course of disease, cystic encephalomalacia and atrophy can develop in all supratentorial cortical and subcortical regions.[56–59]

Enterovirus and echovirus/parechovirus

Coxsackie B encephalitis has been shown to affect some specific regions: the anterior horn cells of the spinal cord, the medulla and pons, and the cerebellum. The most consistently

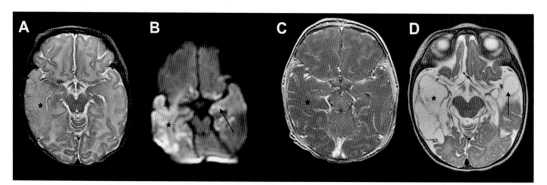

Fig. 16. Acute stage: axial T2-weighted imaging (*A*), axial diffusion-weighted image (*B*), and axial postcontrast T1-weighted imaging (*C*). Follow-up of the same patient: axial T2-weighted imaging (*D*) in a case of herpes encephalitis with diffuse white matter edema, diffusion restriction, and contrast enhancement of the right temporal lobe (*asterisk* in *A–C*). There is also cortical involvement of the left temporal lobe seen only as a diffusion restriction on diffusion imaging (*arrow* in *B*). On follow-up there is extensive encephalomalacia and cystic transformation of the involved temporal areas (*asterisk* and *arrow* in *D*). (*Courtesy of* Thierry A.G.M. Huisman, Johns Hopkins Hospital, Baltimore, MD.)

involved structure has been the inferior olivary nucleus.[20] This predilection for brainstem involvement has been confirmed in an outbreak of enterovirus infection in Taiwan in which the basal ganglia showed edematous and T2-hyperintensities in three patients and brainstem or spinal cord were involved in 15 patients. The cerebral hemispheres were less affected, presumably in correlation with the paucity of cerebral neuropathologic changes (**Fig. 17**).[60]

In echovirus and parechovirus infections, some reports have shown focal cerebral white matter necrosis, consecutive predominantly periventricular atrophy, in analogy to periventricular leucomalacia (**Fig. 18**).[61]

FUNGAL INFECTION
Epidemiology

Systemic fungal infections affect predominantly either extremely preterm neonates, because of the immaturity of their immune systems, their poor skin barrier to fungal invasion, and the use of corticosteroids to treat chronic lung disease, or neonates with congenital or acquired immunodeficiency.[62] The most commonly encountered organism is *Candida albicans*.[63] Invasive aspergillosis is rare; only 77 cases have been reported in children in the largest recent review[64] and only 35 neonatal cases have been published.[62] *Candida* has been shown to be the principal pathogen in only 15% of neonatal late-onset sepsis,[65] but at least one-third of cases are known to show signs of CNS involvement.[66] In an older series, a 29% mortality and hydrocephalus or developmental delay as common sequelae of *Candida* meningitis in infants has been reported.[67] In the last two decades, perhaps because of earlier recognition or improved therapy, outcomes have been more favorable, and mortality rates for neonates and infants were much lower than in older children.[64] The brain is a common site of invasive aspergillosis with an incidence of 10% to 15% and is infected by hematogenous dissemination from an extracranial focus that is commonly the lung.[68] Brain aspergillosis in immunocompromised patients has a poor prognosis with a mortality rate approaching 85% to 100%, and death usually occurs within 1 week of neurologic onset.[69] Nevertheless, recent

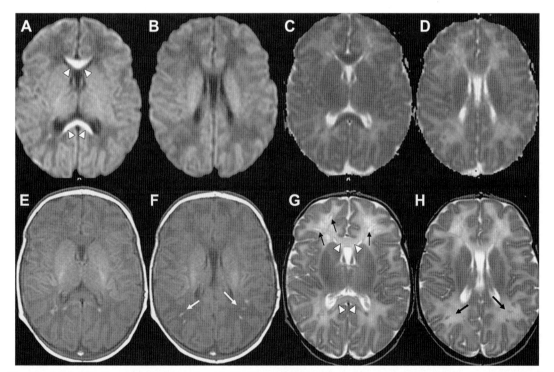

Fig. 17. Axial diffusion-weighted imaging (*A, B*), ADC maps (*C, D*), precontrast axial T1-weighted imaging (*E, F*), and axial T2-weighted imaging (*G, H*) in a case of enteroviral encephalitis demonstrating acute injury to the corpus callosum with severe diffusion restriction (*arrowheads* in *A*) and edema in the T2-weighted imaging (*arrowheads* in *G*). Multifocal white matter injury with punctuate hemorrhagic foci seen as T1-hyperintensity and T2-hypointensity (*arrows* in *F* and *H*) but also cystic lesions in the frontal deep white matter bilaterally (*arrows* in *G*).

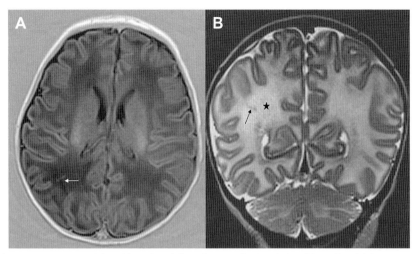

Fig. 18. Axial precontrast T1-weighted imaging (*A*) and coronal T2-weighted imaging (*B*) in a case of parechovirus encephalitis. Discrete white matter edema parietooccipital right (*asterisk* in *B*) and central hemorrhagic focus (*arrows* in *A* and *B*).

aggressive antifungal therapies have provided effective methods of treatment.

Physiopathology

The most common pathologic types of CNS aspergillosis and candidiasis alike were single or multiple brain abscesses. Vasculitis and meningoencephalitis or encephalitis have also been found in a few cases of CSN aspergillosis. In the disseminated form of brain aspergillosis, aspergillus hyphae thrombose arteries and cause brain infarction that is commonly hemorrhagic.[64] These sterile infarcts are readily converted to cerebritis or abscess by erosion of the arterial wall resulting in mycotic vasculitis and aneurysm.[70] This vasculitis-related septic infarction has an anatomic predilection for the corticomedullary junction, because of the hematogenous route of dissemination of aspergillus hyphae and of the vascular anatomy of this interface. The involvement of the basal nuclei and thalami is also characteristic and indicates the involvement of the lenticulostriate and thalamoperforator arteries. In addition, the corpus callosum is also a common site, which again reflects the predisposition of perforating arteries to aspergillosis.

Neuroimaging

Imaging changes are not expected in the first days of candidemia, but become apparent in all cases after 1 week into the course of disease.[71] MR imaging shows numerous parenchymal foci throughout the supratentorial and infratentorial brain, sometimes even within the ventricular system (**Fig. 19**).[71] Contrast enhancement seems

to depend on host immunologic response and variates from nodular enhancement, in cases of small foci, up to ring enhancement in larger abscesses. Under therapy, repeat imaging shows slow resolution of parenchymal lesions and disappearance at 6 months.[71]

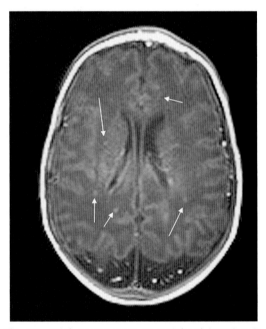

Fig. 19. Axial postcontrast T1-weighted imaging in a case of candida meningoencephalitis. Numerous small contrast-enhancing fungal nodules (*arrows*) disseminated through cerebral hemispheres. (*Courtesy of* Catherine Christophe, MD, University Children's Hospital of Queen Fabiola, Brussels, Belgium.)

In the disseminated form of brain aspergillosis, cortical vessels may show dilatation and sometimes do grossly enhance.[72] Microscopic examination has revealed numerous aspergillus hyphae within the vessel walls, along with vessel thrombosis.[73] At the corticomedullary junction, focal T2-hypointensity may represent aspergillus hyphae, fresh thrombus in the vessel, or small foci of hemorrhage around the vessel.[73]

SUMMARY

MR imaging is an invaluable tool for early and accurate detection of pathologic findings in neonatal brain infections. It allows to differentiate infections from others entities, which may share the same and mostly nonspecific neonatal neurologic symptoms, such as hemorrhages, infarctions, tumors, or metabolic diseases. It easily demonstrates involvement of ependymal lining, meninges, and parenchyma early in the course of the disease. DWI not only enables detection of ischemic foci but also of purulent accumulations not readily evident on conventional imaging. MR imaging allows not only early identification of complications, but is the best modality to monitor treatment and predict outcome. Even if ultrasound or even CT are valuable first-line imaging tools, MR imaging is the modality of choice for early and comprehensive identification of infections, and has been shown to improve clinical outcome because of earlier therapy initiation.

REFERENCES

1. Stoll BJ, Hansen NI, Higgins RD, et al. Very low birth weight preterm infants with early onset neonatal sepsis: the predominance of gram-negative infections continues in the National Institute of Child Health and Human Development Neonatal Research Network, 2002–2003. Pediatr Infect Dis J 2005; 24(7):635–9.
2. Klein JO. Bacterial sepsis and meningitis. In: Remington JS, Klein JO, editors. Infectious diseases of the fetus and newborn infant. Philadelphia: WB Saunders; 2000. p. 943–98.
3. Schuchat A. Group B streptococcus. Lancet 1999; 353(9146):51–6.
4. Anderson DC, Hughes BJ, Edwards MS, et al. Impaired chemotaxigenesis by type III group B streptococci in neonatal sera: relationship to diminished concentration of specific anticapsular antibody and abnormalities of serum complement. Pediatr Res 1983;17(6):496–502.
5. Baker CJ, Kasper DL. Correlation of maternal antibody deficiency with susceptibility to neonatal group B streptococcal infection. N Engl J Med 1976; 294(14):753–6.
6. Lukacs SL, Schoendorf KC, Schuchat A. Trends in sepsis-related neonatal mortality in the United States, 1985–1998. Pediatr Infect Dis J 2004;23(7): 599–603.
7. May M, Daley AJ, Donath S, et al. Early onset neonatal meningitis in Australia and New Zealand, 1992–2002. Arch Dis Child Fetal Neonatal Ed 2005;90(4):F324–7.
8. Cordero L, Rau R, Taylor D, et al. Enteric gram-negative bacilli bloodstream infections: 17 years' experience in a neonatal intensive care unit. Am J Infect Control 2004;32(4):189–95.
9. Edwards MS, Rench MA, Haffar AA, et al. Long-term sequelae of group B streptococcal meningitis in infants. J Pediatr 1985;106(5):717–22.
10. Franco SM, Cornelius VE, Andrews BF. Long-term outcome of neonatal meningitis. Am J Dis Child 1992;146(5):567–71.
11. Isaacs D, Barfield CP, Grimwood K, et al. Systemic bacterial and fungal infections in infants in Australian neonatal units. Australian Study Group for Neonatal Infections. Med J Aust 1995;162(4):198–201.
12. Miyairi I, Causey KT, DeVincenzo JP, et al. Group B streptococcal ventriculitis: a report of three cases and literature review. Pediatr Neurol 2006;34(5): 395–9.
13. Berman PH, Banker BQ. Neonatal meningitis. A clinical and pathological study of 29 cases. Pediatrics 1966;38(1):6–24.
14. Hristeva L, Booy R, Bowler I, et al. Prospective surveillance of neonatal meningitis. Arch Dis Child 1993;69(Spec No 1):14–8.
15. Chan PH, Fishman RA. Brain edema: induction in cortical slices by polyunsaturated fatty acids. Science 1978;201(4353):358–60.
16. Fishman RA. Brain edema. N Engl J Med 1975; 293(14):706–11.
17. Horwitz SJ, Boxerbaum B, O'Bell J. Cerebral herniation in bacterial meningitis in childhood. Ann Neurol 1980;7(6):524–8.
18. Quirante J, Ceballos R, Cassady G. Group B beta-hemolytic streptococcal infection in the newborn. I. Early onset infection. Am J Dis Child 1974;128(5): 659–65.
19. Maisey HC, Doran KS, Nizet V. Recent advances in understanding the molecular basis of group B Streptococcus virulence. Expert Rev Mol Med 2008; 10:e27.
20. Volpe JJ. Neurology of the newborn. 4th edition. Philadelphia: WB Saunders; 2001.
21. Fitz CR. Inflammatory diseases of the brain in childhood. AJNR Am J Neuroradiol 1992;13(2):551–67.
22. Renier D, Flandin C, Hirsch E, et al. Brain abscesses in neonates. A study of 30 cases. J Neurosurg 1988; 69(6):877–82.

23. Goodkin HP, Harper MB, Pomeroy SL. Intracerebral abscess in children: historical trends at Children's Hospital Boston. Pediatrics 2004;113(6): 1765–70.

24. Sundaram V, Agrawal S, Chacham S, et al. *Klebsiella pneumoniae* brain abscess in neonates: a report of 2 cases. J Child Neurol 2009;25(3):379–82.

25. Krajewski R, Stelmasiak Z. Brain abscess in infants. Childs Nerv Syst 1992;8(5):279–80.

26. Raybaud C, Girard N, Sévely A, et al. Neuroradiologie pédiatrique (I). In: Raybaud C, Girard N, Sévely A, et al, editors. Radiodiagnostic - neuroradiologie - appareil locomoteur. Paris (France): Elsevier; 1996. p. 26.

27. Barkovich A. Pediatric neuroimaging. 3rd edition. Philadelphia: Lippincott Williams & Williams; 2000.

28. Gray F, Nordmann P. Bacterial infections. In: Graham D, Lantos P, editors. Greenfield's neuropathology. 6th edition. London: Arnold; 1997. p. 113–52.

29. Falcone S, Post MJ. Encephalitis, cerebritis, and brain abscess: pathophysiology and imaging findings. Neuroimaging Clin N Am 2000;10(2):333–53.

30. Fujikawa A, Tsuchiya K, Honya K, et al. Comparison of MRI sequences to detect ventriculitis. AJR Am J Roentgenol 2006;187(4):1048–53.

31. Fukui MB, Williams RL, Mudigonda S. CT and MR imaging features of pyogenic ventriculitis. AJNR Am J Neuroradiol 2001;22(8):1510–6.

32. Han KT, Choi DS, Ryoo JW, et al. Diffusion-weighted MR imaging of pyogenic intraventricular empyema. Neuroradiology 2007;49(10):813–8.

33. Ebisu T, Tanaka C, Umeda M, et al. Discrimination of brain abscess from necrotic or cystic tumors by diffusion-weighted echo planar imaging. Magn Reson Imaging 1996;14(9):1113–6.

34. Kim YJ, Chang KH, Song IC, et al. Brain abscess and necrotic or cystic brain tumor: discrimination with signal intensity on diffusion-weighted MR imaging. AJR Am J Roentgenol 1998;171(6):1487–90.

35. Desprechins B, Stadnik T, Koerts G, et al. Use of diffusion-weighted MR imaging in differential diagnosis between intracerebral necrotic tumors and cerebral abscesses. AJNR Am J Neuroradiol 1999; 20(7):1252–7.

36. Fanning NF, Laffan EE, Shroff MM. Serial diffusion-weighted MRI correlates with clinical course and treatment response in children with intracranial pus collections. Pediatr Radiol 2006;36(1):26–37.

37. Remy C, Grand S, Lai ES, et al. 1H MRS of human brain abscesses in vivo and in vitro. Magn Reson Med 1995;34(4):508–14.

38. Grand S, Passaro G, Ziegler A, et al. Necrotic tumor versus brain abscess: importance of amino acids detected at 1H MR spectroscopy—initial results. Radiology 1999;213(3):785–93.

39. Whitley RJ. Herpes simplex virus infections of women and their offspring: implications for a developed society. Proc Natl Acad Sci U S A 1994;91(7):2441–7.

40. Whitley RJ, Nahmias AJ, Visintine AM, et al. The natural history of herpes simplex virus infection of mother and newborn. Pediatrics 1980;66(4):489–94.

41. Corey L, Whitley RJ, Stone EF, et al. Difference between herpes simplex virus type 1 and type 2 neonatal encephalitis in neurological outcome. Lancet 1988;1(8575-6):1–4.

42. Brown ZA, Benedetti J, Ashley R, et al. Neonatal herpes simplex virus infection in relation to asymptomatic maternal infection at the time of labor. N Engl J Med 1991;324(18):1247–52.

43. Whitley RJ, Corey L, Arvin A, et al. Changing presentation of herpes simplex virus infection in neonates. J Infect Dis 1988;158(1):109–16.

44. Whitley RJ. Herpes simplex virus infections. In: Klein JO, editor. Infectious diseases of the fetus and newborn infants. 3rd edition. Philadelphia: W.B. Saunders Company; 1990. p. 282–305.

45. Kimberlin DW, Lin CY, Jacobs RF, et al. Safety and efficacy of high-dose intravenous acyclovir in the management of neonatal herpes simplex virus infections. Pediatrics 2001;108(2):230–8.

46. Morens DM. Enteroviral disease in early infancy. J Pediatr 1978;92(3):374–7.

47. Brightman VJ, Scott TF, Westphal M, et al. An outbreak of coxsackie B-5 virus infection in a newborn nursery. J Pediatr 1966;69(2):179–92.

48. Verboon-Maciolek MA, Groenendaal F, Cowan F, et al. White matter damage in neonatal enterovirus meningoencephalitis. Neurology 2006;66(8):1267–9.

49. Modlin JF. Perinatal echovirus infection: insights from a literature review of 61 cases of serious infection and 16 outbreaks in nurseries. Rev Infect Dis 1986;8(6):918–26.

50. Verboon-Maciolek MA, Groenendaal F, Hahn CD, et al. Human parechovirus causes encephalitis with white matter injury in neonates. Ann Neurol 2008;64(3):266–73.

51. Verboon-Maciolek MA, Krediet TG, Gerards LJ, et al. Severe neonatal parechovirus infection and similarity with enterovirus infection. Pediatr Infect Dis J 2008;27(3):241–5.

52. Friede RL. Developmental neuropathology. New York: Springer Verlag; 1989.

53. Fechner RE, Smith MG, Middlekamp JN. Coxsackie B virus infection of the newborn. Am J Pathol 1963; 42:493–505.

54. Barnes DW, Whitley RJ. CNS diseases associated with varicella zoster virus and herpes simplex virus infection. Pathogenesis and current therapy. Neurol Clin 1986;4(1):265–83.

55. Dhawan A, Kecskes Z, Jyoti R, et al. Early diffusion-weighted magnetic resonance imaging findings in neonatal herpes encephalitis. J Paediatr Child Health 2006;42(12):824–6.

56. Kubota T, Ito M, Maruyama K, et al. Serial diffusion-weighted imaging of neonatal herpes encephalitis: a case report. Brain Dev 2007;29(3):171–3.

57. Kuker W, Nagele T, Schmidt F, et al. Diffusion-weighted MRI in herpes simplex encephalitis: a report of three cases. Neuroradiology 2004; 46(2):122–5.

58. McCabe K, Tyler K, Tanabe J. Diffusion-weighted MRI abnormalities as a clue to the diagnosis of herpes simplex encephalitis. Neurology 2003; 61(7):1015–6.

59. Enzmann D, Chang Y, Augustyn G. MR findings in neonatal herpes simplex encephalitis type II. J Comput Assist Tomogr 1990;14(3):453–7.

60. Shen WC, Chiu HH, Chow KC, et al. MR imaging findings of enteroviral encephalomyelitis: an outbreak in Taiwan. AJNR Am J Neuroradiol 1999; 20(10):1889–95.

61. Haddad J, Messer J, Gut JP, et al. Neonatal echovirus encephalitis with white matter necrosis. Neuropediatrics 1990;21(4):215–7.

62. Groll AH, Jaeger G, Allendorf A, et al. Invasive pulmonary aspergillosis in a critically ill neonate: case report and review of invasive aspergillosis during the first 3 months of life. Clin Infect Dis 1998;27(3):437–52.

63. Miller MJ. Fungal infections. In: Remington JS, Klein JO, editors. Infectious diseases of the fetus and newborn infant. Philadelphia: WB Saunders; 1995. p. 704.

64. Dotis J, Iosifidis E, Roilides E. Central nervous system aspergillosis in children: a systematic review of reported cases. Int J Infect Dis 2007;11(5): 381–93.

65. Wu JH, Chen CY, Tsao PN, et al. Neonatal sepsis: a 6-year analysis in a neonatal care unit in Taiwan. Pediatr Neonatol 2009;50(3):88–95.

66. Faix RG. Systemic Candida infections in infants in intensive care nurseries: high incidence of central nervous system involvement. J Pediatr 1984; 105(4):616–22.

67. Chesney PJ, Justman RA, Bogdanowicz WM. Candida meningitis in newborn infants: a review and report of combined amphotericin B–flucytosine therapy. Johns Hopkins Med J 1978;142(5):155–60.

68. Torre-Cisneros J, Lopez OL, Kusne S, et al. CNS aspergillosis in organ transplantation: a clinicopathological study. J Neurol Neurosurg Psychiatry 1993; 56(2):188–93.

69. Harris DE, Enterline DS. Neuroimaging of AIDS. I. Fungal infections of the central nervous system. Neuroimaging Clin N Am 1997;7(2):187–98.

70. Cox J, Murtagh FR, Wilfong A, et al. Cerebral aspergillosis: MR imaging and histopathologic correlation. AJNR Am J Neuroradiol 1992;13(5):1489–92.

71. Pahud BA, Greenhow TL, Piecuch B, et al. Preterm neonates with candidal brain microabscesses: a case series. J Perinatol 2009;29(4):323–6.

72. van der Knaap MS, Valk J, Jansen GH, et al. Mycotic encephalitis: predilection for grey matter. Neuroradiology 1993;35(8):567–72.

73. Okafuji T, Yabuuchi H, Nagatoshi Y, et al. CT and MR findings of brain aspergillosis. Comput Med Imaging Graph 2003;27(6):489–92.

Birth-Related Injury to the Head and Cervical Spine in Neonates

Aylin Tekes, MD[a],*, Pedro S. Pinto, MD[a],
Thierry A.G.M. Huisman, MD, EQNR, FICIS[b]

KEYWORDS

• Neonate • Mechanical birth injury • Head and cervical spine

Birth-related injury is defined as any traumatic/ischemic event sustained during the process of delivery. In this article the authors focus on perinatally acquired disease processes secondary to birth-related injury, either traumatic or ischemic in nature. Other diseases of the perinatal time period, including germinal matrix hemorrhages and hypoxic-ischemic encephalopathy (HIE), are beyond the objective of this review.

ETIOLOGY

Birth-related injury may affect any organ system; however, because the head is the presenting body part in the majority of deliveries, and is one of the largest anatomic structures to pass through the birth canal, and does not tolerate too much molding during delivery, traumatic head injury is the most frequently encountered type of birth-related trauma. In addition, during the delivery hyperextension and shear forces at the craniocervical junction may result in additional cervical spinal cord injury. Although many traumatic head and spine injuries are benign and do not require therapy, some may require rapid diagnosis and treatment to avoid progression, permanent disability, or even death. In addition, hypoxic-ischemic injuries may be superimposed on "purely" mechanical types of injury, which may worsen functional and neurologic outcome.

Advancements in obstetric management in the last few decades have significantly decreased the incidence of birth-related deaths. Birth-related injury accounts for fewer than 2% of neonatal deaths.[1] From 1970 to 1985, rates of newborn mortality due to birth-related trauma fell from 64.2 to 7.5 deaths per 100,000 live births, a remarkable decline of 88%. This decrease reflects, in part, the technologic advancements that allow today's obstetrician to recognize perinatal risk factors using prenatal ultrasonography (US) and fetal monitoring prior to vaginal delivery. The use of potentially injurious instrumentation, such as forceps or vacuum delivery, has also declined.[2]

Instrumental delivery (forceps, vacuum extraction) may be performed for fetal or maternal indications. The most common indication is a prolonged second stage of labor with fetal distress or presumed fetal compromise whereby any additional delay may result in hypoxic-ischemic neonatal brain injury or fetal death. Maternal indications include severe heart disease or cerebral vascular malformations.[3]

Birth trauma should be suspected in cases with difficult delivery, or in the presence of predisposing maternal or neonatal risk factors. Newborn risk factors include macrosomia (>4500 g), perinatal decelerations/depression, shoulder dystocia, abnormal presentation of the fetus such as breech position, and the use of instruments during delivery. Maternal risk factors include diabetes mellitus, obesity, small pelvis, induced labor, or previous history of a macrosomic neonate. Placental abruption predisposes a significant risk for hypoxic-ischemic injury in newborns.[4] Although many injuries are believed to occur secondary to birth-related

[a] Division of Pediatric Radiology, Department of Radiology and Radiological Science, Johns Hopkins Hospital, Baltimore, MD, USA
[b] Division of Pediatric Radiology, Department of Radiology and Radiological Science, Johns Hopkins Hospital, 600 North Wolfe Street, Nelson, B-173, Baltimore, MD 21287–0842, USA
* Corresponding author. Division of Pediatric Radiology, Department of Radiology and Radiological Science, Johns Hopkins Hospital, 600 North Wolfe Street, Nelson Basement, B-172, Baltimore, MD 21287-0842.
E-mail address: atekes1@jhmi.edu

Magn Reson Imaging Clin N Am 19 (2011) 777–790
doi:10.1016/j.mric.2011.08.004

complications, injuries in the absence of identifiable risk factors are well described, which makes their occurrence unpredictable and difficult to "catch" early.[5]

Consequently, the true incidence of birth-related head and cervical spine injury is not well known. In asymptomatic newborns, unless they are imaged for other reasons, it is impossible to know the incidence of intracranial injuries. Increasing use of imaging modalities in asymptomatic newborns shows that even spontaneous vaginal deliveries are associated with intracranial hemorrhages (**Fig. 1**).

Birth-related injury to the head and cervical spine may result in:

1. Extracranial injuries: skin abrasions and hemorrhage between the various layers of the scalp; caput succedaneum; cephalohematoma; subgaleal hemorrhage
2. Intracranial, extra-axial hemorrhage: epidural, subdural, or subarachnoid hemorrhage
3. Intracranial, intra-axial hemorrhage
   a. Cortical contusions, shear force, diffuse axonal injury, or intraparenchymal hemorrhage

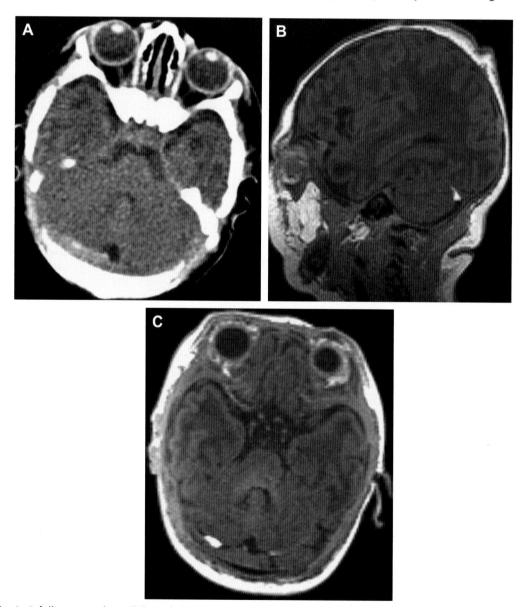

Fig. 1. A full-term newborn delivered via spontaneous vaginal delivery. (*A*) Axial computed tomography (CT) of the head shows curvilinear increased density along the right tentorial leaflet. (*B*) Sagittal and (*C*) axial T1-weighted magnetic resonance imaging shows T1 bright signal along the right tentorial leaflet, confirming that this is a small subdural hemorrhage, not a dural venous sinus thrombosis.

b. Cerebral injury secondary to perinatal hypoxia-ischemia
4. Skull injury: diasthesis of the sutures, and calvarial or facial fracture
5. Peripheral nerve injury in the face (facial nerve palsy), and injury to the cervical spinal cord, including the brachial plexus and phrenic nerve.

The authors discuss each category separately to provide general information. In the second half of the article imaging modalities used to diagnose each pathologic condition are discussed.

Extracranial Injuries

Most newborns delivered by instrumentation, particularly after vacuum extraction, exhibit scalp injury, most of which are transient and are of no clinical significance. The incidence of scalp abrasions and lacerations after vacuum extraction is estimated at 10%. The majority are superficial and of a minor degree.[6] The more significant injuries are related to incorrect placement of the vacuum cup, inability to achieve a correct application, excessive or poorly directed traction, cephalopelvic disproportion, or fetal coagulation defects.

Scalp lesions are classified according to the involved spaces. A proper knowledge is essential for correct characterization of the lesions. The scalp is composed of 5 layers: skin, subcutaneous fibrofatty tissue, galea aponeurotica, loose areolar connective tissue, and the periosteum of the calvarial bones. The temporalis muscle arises from the periosteum of the temporal fossa, and therefore lies beneath the galea and subgaleal space.[7]

Caput succedaneum is a serosanguinous, extraperiosteal collection within the subcutaneous fibrofatty space between the skin and the adjacent galea aponeurotica. It presents as a soft tissue swelling with purpura/ecchymosis over the affected part of the scalp. It is caused by the mechanical trauma of the presenting part of the fetal cranium pushing through the dilating cervix.[5] Due to its location, caput succedaneum typically extends across suture lines and usually resolves within the first few days of life. No treatment is necessary.

Subgaleal hemorrhages are located in the space between the galea aponeurosis of the scalp and the calvarial periosteum. This space extends from the orbital margins anteriorly, to the nuchal ridge posteriorly, and the temporal fascia laterally.[8] Subgaleal hematoma presents as a firm/fluctuant mass that crosses the suture lines. Unlike cephalohematoma, subgaleal hemorrhage is superficial to the temporal muscle. The subgaleal space is composed of loose connective tissue and contains small blood vessels. Subgaleal hemorrhage is most often associated with vacuum extraction

and forceps delivery in which the traction forces pull the aponeurosis from the calvarium. Typically it is clinically noted within a few hours after birth. The loose connective tissue in this space allows massive bleeding, which may result in hemorrhagic shock. Treatment is largely supportive.[8,9]

Cephalohematoma is a subperiosteal bleed that accumulates between the calvarial periosteum and the adjacent outer table of the skull. It is located beneath the temporalis muscle. Cephalohematoma presents typically as a firm swelling overlying the parietal or occipital bone confined by the sutures. It occurs in approximately 2.5% of newborns, being the most common extracranial scalp injury after abrasion/lacerations. Cephalohematoma is commonly associated with forceps and breech deliveries.[10] Often it is unilateral and is not associated with discoloration. The subperiosteal bleeding may grow slowly over a couple of days, thus may present with a few days of delay after birth. In the majority of cases, cephalohematomas resolve within a few weeks. Rarely complications may occur, such as significant blood loss or infection. Coexisting skull fractures may be present in up to 5% of the cases. Cephalohematomas occasionally may calcify and present as a "bony swelling."[5]

Intracranial Extra-Axial Injury

The incidence or prevalence of birth-related intracranial, extra-axial hemorrhage (subdural, epidural, or subarachnoid hemorrhage) is not well known or prospectively studied. A percentage of term newborns with intracranial hemorrhage present with clinical or neurologic symptoms such as apnea, bradycardia, and seizures that may initiate diagnostic workup. In addition, imaging studies indicate that intracranial, extra-axial hemorrhage may be found in asymptomatic newborns.[11-13] The reported incidence of asymptomatic and symptomatic intracranial extra-axial hemorrhage varies from study to study, probably due to differences in the studied newborn populations and the sensitivity and timing of the used diagnostic tests.

While intracranial extra-axial injury can be observed with spontaneous vaginal delivery,[14,15] additional maternal and fetal risk factors may increase the susceptibility of the neonate for perinatal intracranial injuries. Risk factors include forceps delivery, vacuum extraction, prolonged second stage (>2 hours), or fetal macrosomia.[16-18] In addition, factors such as birth asphyxia, prematurity, hemorrhagic diathesis, infection, and vascular anomalies have a significant impact.

Subdural hemorrhage (SDH) is the most common intracranial extra-axial hemorrhage related to birth trauma. Pollina and colleagues[17] reported that it accounts for 73% of intracranial birth injuries in term newborns. Although frequently related to birth trauma, SDH have been diagnosed in utero before the start of the birth process,[5,14,15] in newborns who were delivered by caesarean section,[17] and in asymptomatic newborns after uncomplicated vaginal deliveries.[12,13,19] In a study by Whitby and colleagues,[19] SDH were noted in 6.1% of uncomplicated deliveries, and follow-up magnetic resonance (MR) imaging showed resolution in all newborns by 4 weeks. All children showed normal neurologic development by 2 years of age.

In the newborns, the majority of birth-related SDH are found in the posterior fossa, along the tentorium or over the occipital-parietal lobes of the supratentorial brain (see **Fig. 1**). Isolated supratentorial SDH are quite rare. The location and extension suggests that these SDH result from nontraumatic vascular insults affecting the tributaries of the dural sinuses within the dural folds of the posterior fossa, as discussed by Volpe and others.[20,21] Formerly it was believed that subdural hemorrhages resulted from a tentorial tear, from damage to the occipital sinus accompanying occipital osteodiastasis, or to a rupture of bridging superficial cerebral convexity veins.[22] Most common clinical symptoms include apnea and seizures, focal neurologic deficits, lethargy, and hypotonia.

Many neonates with SDH are treated conservatively. Occasionally surgical intervention may be required, depending on the size and clinical symptoms such as compression of vital structures. Finally, in neonates and young babies, SDH may occur as part of the lesions encountered in nonaccidental trauma (NAI) (shaken baby). NAI is the leading cause of death and lifelong disability for neonates; half of which occur before 4 months of age.[23]

Epidural hematomas (EDH) are venous or arterial hemorrhages located between the internal tabula and the adjacent internal periosteum of the calvarium. EDH is typically limited by the sutures. The prevalence of EDH is rare in the newborn. Tagaki and colleagues[24] reported that EDH occurs in 2.2% of autopsies of newborns who had intracranial hemorrhage. The rarity can be explained by the absence of a middle meningeal artery groove in the neonate, which makes the artery less susceptible to skull fracture–related injury. EDH is frequently associated with skull fracture and cephalohematoma.[25] Presenting symptoms may include increased intracranial pressure, bulging fontanel, or focal neurologic symptoms including seizures. Surgical intervention may be necessary, although Negishi and colleagues[25] reported that outcome may be favorable without surgical treatment.

Subarachnoid hemorrhages (SAH) are located in the space between the arachnoid membrane and pia mater (**Fig. 2**). The prevalence of symptomatic SAH has been reported to range from 1.3 per 10,000 live births in spontaneous vaginal deliveries to 2 to 3 per 10,000 live births in vacuum and forceps deliveries.[17] Fenichel and colleagues[7,26,27] reported primary SAH as the most common type of intracranial

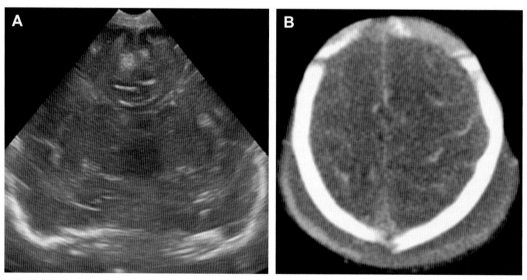

Fig. 2. A 35 gestational weeks newborn delivered via cesarean section due to failure to progress. (*A*) Coronal ultrasonography (US) of the head shows generalized increased echogenicity of the white matter with pronounced gray-white matter differentiation and effacement of the lateral ventricles representing edema. In addition, note the lobular increased densities in the sulci, representing subarachnoid hemorrhage. (*B*) Axial head CT confirms the brain edema and subarachnoid hemorrhage.

hemorrhage over a 5-year period among "symptomatic" term newborns (n = 22) in a neonatal intensive care unit.[26] SAH occur more frequently as a result of prematurity and postperinatal asphyxia.[28] In newborns, SAH is believed to result from a rupture of the fragile veins that cross the subarachnoid space, or from injury to small leptomeningeal vessels.[26] Although a SAH may be asymptomatic, the most common presentation is seizures that often occur on the second day of life.[26] Neurologic examination often may be normal during interictal periods; however, irritability or depressed level of consciousness may be present. An adjacent/combined cortical contusion may cause focal neurologic signs. In patients with ischemic encephalopathy, clinical deterioration may be rapid and progressive. Usually there are no long-term sequelae of minor SAH if underlying cortical injury and hypoxic injury are not present.[5,26,29]

Intracranial Intra-Axial Injuries

Intracerebral hemorrhage (ICH) is less frequent than SDH and SAH in term newborns. Sandberg and colleagues[27] published a large series, in which they reviewed a neurosurgical computerized database spanning more than 40 years, and identified 11 cases of intracerebral, lobar hemorrhage. Of these 11 neonates, 8 were delivered by spontaneous vaginal delivery, 2 by vacuum extraction, and 1 by cesarean section. Other than large ICH, newborns may suffer from smaller parenchymal injuries, small cortical contusions, and shear or diffuse axonal injuries. In contrast to the rarity of cases reported in the literature, ICH is not uncommon in clinical practice. The discrepancy in the reported number of cases and clinical experience can be explained by the imaging techniques that have been used in the published series. The increasing use of MR imaging sequences more sensitive to blood products such as susceptibility-weighted imaging may increase detection of birth-related intracranial injuries in the newborn (**Fig. 3**).

Cerebral injury secondary to intrapartum hypoxia-ischemia

Hypoxic-ischemic injury is one of the most commonly recognized causes of severe, long-term neurologic deficits in children. Initial ischemic episode is followed by a "reperfusion state." During this reperfusion state interventional procedures such as "hypothermia" can be beneficial for the neurologic outcome. Details of this topic are covered in an article by Izbudak and Grant elsewhere in this issue.

Skull Injury

Overlapping of the calvarial bones especially of the parietal bones is a normal physiologic pheno-

menon during delivery, allowing the neonatal head to pass the narrow birth canal (**Fig. 4**). Postnatal residual overlap may be palpated in some newborns, which usually resolves spontaneously. Skull fractures are rarely seen after spontaneous birth. Skull fractures may occur in assisted deliveries, for example, by compression of the forceps, or from the skull pushing against the maternal symphysis or ischial spines. Skull fractures can be linear, affecting the parietal bones, or may be depressed, forming the so-called ping-pong ball type fracture.[30] Occipital osteodiastasis is a special type of skull injury of the newborn resulting from separation of the squamous and lateral parts of the occipital bone. This injury is commonly observed in breech delivery, with anterior displacement and upward rotation of the squamous bone[31]; this may result in posterior fossa SDH, cerebellar contusion, or even cervicomedullary compression.[30] Presence of cephalohematoma or SAH should raise the suspicion for skull fracture, and cross-sectional imaging should be performed.

Peripheral Nerve and Spinal Cord Injuries

Brachial plexus injury, facial nerve injury, phrenic nerve injury, or spinal cord injuries can be seen as a complication of birth.

The prevalence of brachial plexus injury is rare, and ranges from 0.1% to 0.2% of births.[32–36] Risk factors include macrosomia, shoulder dystocia, instrumented deliveries, and malpresentation.[34] The pathogenesis of injury often involves stretch injury when shoulder dystocia requires extreme lateral flexion and traction of the head. However, there are increasing reports of injury that occurs when lateral flexion and traction of the head has not been applied, such as during precipitous deliveries or when there is injury to the posterior shoulder. These findings indicate that intrauterine maladaptation may also play a role in the development of the injury.[37,38] Brachial plexus injury has also been reported during the intrauterine period.[39] Hematomas of the sternocleidomastoid muscle and fractures of the clavicle and humerus can be observed in children with brachial plexus injuries, and should be used as a lead sign to rule out brachial plexus lesions (**Fig. 5**).

There are 3 types of injuries to the brachial plexus:

1. Injury to the upper plexus—Erb palsy—involves nerve roots C5 to C7, and accounts for approximately 90% of cases. The biceps reflex is not present and the Moro reflex is asymmetric. The involved arm is held in the "waiter's tip" position, with adduction and internal rotation of the shoulder, extension of the elbow,

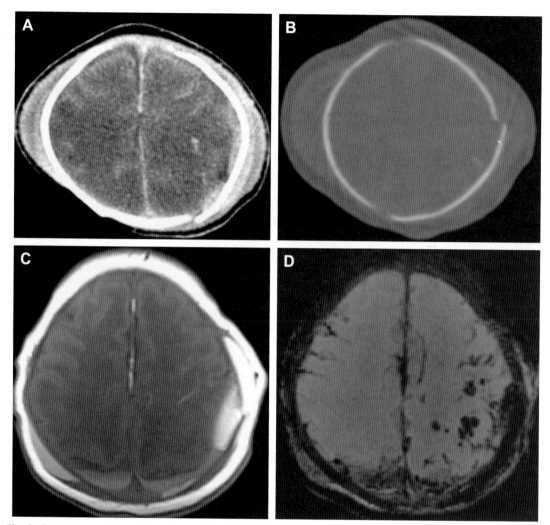

Fig. 3. Premature rupture of membranes in a 33-week newborn delivered via cesarean section, after failure to progress and failed vacuum extraction. Multiple bilateral extensive intracranial and extracranial injuries are seen. (*A*) Axial CT of the brain shows bilateral cephalohematomas, diffuse brain edema, subarachnoid hemorrhage, and punctuate parenchymal hemorrhage. Note the left epidural hemorrhage and irregularity in the left parietal bone. (*B*) Bone algorithm at the same level demonstrates the left parietal bone fracture. (*C*) Axial T1-weighted image shows presence of bilateral subdural hemorrhages, in addition to the cephalohematomas, and left epidural hemorrhage. (*D*) Susceptibility-weighted imaging demonstrates multiple foci of decreased signal in the left parietal parenchyma, indicating diffuse axonal injury.

pronation of the forearm, and flexion of the wrist and fingers. Erb palsy can be associated with phrenic nerve injury, which is innervated by nerve fibers from C3 to C5.[40]

2. Klumpke palsy is rare, and accounts for 1% of all brachial plexus injuries. It involves the nerve roots C8 and T1, and results in weakness of the intrinsic hand muscles and long flexors of the wrist and fingers. The grasp reflex is typically absent while the biceps reflex is present. Klumpke palsy is associated with ipsilateral Horner syndrome (ptosis, miosis, anhydrosis) if an accompanying injury to the sympathetic fibers of T1 exists.[5,41]

3. Involvement of the entire plexus is seen in about 10% of the cases, which results in a flaccid upper extremity with absent reflexes.

Diagnosis is usually made by physical examination. Radiographs of the shoulder and upper arm should be obtained to exclude bony injury, namely clavicle fracture. Cerebral injury often can be excluded by the lack of other accompanying neurologic findings. The presence of respiratory

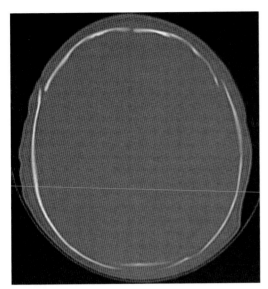

Fig. 4. A full-term newborn delivered via cesarean section after failed attempted vaginal delivery presenting with seizure. Axial head CT with bone algorithm shows normal mild override of the coronal and lambdoid sutures.

distress may indicate an accompanying phrenic nerve injury.[5] Approximately 90% of brachial plexus injuries recover spontaneously.[42] Patients with injury of the C5 and C6 nerve roots have a better prognosis than neonates with a lower or total brachial plexus involvement. Initial treatment is conservative (supportive physiotherapy,

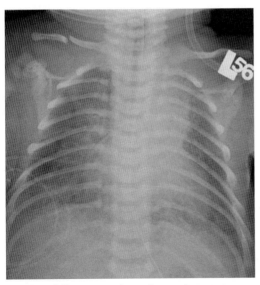

Fig. 5. A full-term newborn born via spontaneous vaginal delivery. Note the right clavicle fracture in the distal one-third in this newborn with meconium aspiration.

preferential positioning); selected cases may benefit from surgical repair of the brachial plexus, although controversy remains concerning the timing and final benefit of surgical exploration.[43]

Facial nerve injury and resulting palsy occurs in 1.8 to 7.5 per 1000 live births.[44] Next to the motor deficit, focal facial nerve twitching or oblique seizing may be observed. Forceps delivery with direct injury to the facial nerve partially explains the facial nerve injury. The posterior blade of the forceps is believed to exert pressure on the stylomastoid foramen, or compresses the bone overlying the vertical segment of the facial nerve.[45] However, 33% of cases occur in spontaneous delivery, indicating that other causes should be considered. Acquired facial nerve palsy by birth trauma must be differentiated from developmental facial nerve palsy. The prognosis of acquired facial palsy by birth trauma is good, with spontaneous recovery in a matter of hours to weeks. Electromyography is recommended, as well as auditory brainstem response to rule out additional cochlear or vestibular nerve involvement. Some investigators recommend surgical intervention within 1 to 3 months[45]; however, most reports favor observation for a year or even up to 2 years if repeat electromyography findings improve over time.

The majority of neonatal phrenic nerve injury cases (75%) are associated with brachial plexus palsy (namely Erb palsy, because phrenic nerve arises from C3–C5 nerve roots). Phrenic nerve injury usually is unilateral. The etiology involves traction injury of the neck and arm during delivery.[44] Clinical symptoms include respiratory distress (paralysis of the ipsilateral hemidiaphragm), with diminished breath sounds on the affected side. Treatment is supportive. Spontaneous recovery can be observed in up to 30% of cases in the first month. Surgical diaphragmatic plication may be performed when no recovery is seen within the first month.[46]

Birth-related spinal cord injuries are rare, and are traumatic/ischemic in nature. The prevalence is 0.14 per 10,000 live births. Lesions of the upper cervical cord are more common than cervicothoracic and thoracolumbar lesions. High cervical lesions are most often associated with forceps rotation during vertex delivery. Lower cervical and thoracic lesions usually occur during vaginal breech delivery, when the head is hyperextended or the head is trapped secondary to cephalopelvic disproportion.[47,48] Spinal cord injury has rarely been reported following cesarean section delivery.[49]

The newborn is more susceptible to longitudinal traction and rotation forces of the spine, given that the craniocervical junction ligaments are lax, the neck muscles are weak, and the vertebral column is predominantly cartilage with premature/ongoing mineralization.

Clinically, spinal cord injury should be suspected in cases of decreased or absent spontaneous movement, absent deep tendon reflexes, absent or periodic breathing, and lack of response to painful stimuli below the level of the lesion. Lesions above C4 almost always are associated with apnea.[47] Lesions between C4 and T4 may have respiratory distress secondary to varying degrees of involvement of the phrenic nerve and impaired innervation to the intercostal muscles. Paralysis of the abdominal musculature leads to the presence of a soft, distended abdomen. The anal sphincter is atonic and the bladder is distended. The diagnosis may be delayed initially, because spinal cord injury is often associated with hypoxic-ischemic encephalopathy, which may challenge the clinical presentation.[50] The differential diagnosis includes intracranial injury, neuromuscular disease, and congenital abnormalities of the spinal cord. If cord injury is suspected in the delivery room, head, neck, and spine should be immobilized. Therapy is in general supportive.

IMAGING

Accurate diagnosis of birth-related injuries to the head and neck region should start with a complete and detailed birth history including the mode of delivery, duration of labor, pharmaceutic augmentation, gestational age at birth, observed complications during delivery, and identification of other maternal and fetal risk factors such as preeclampsia, diabetes, maternal drug use, or fetal macrosomia. In addition the Apgar score, umbilical cord pH, base excess, and hematocrit are valuable parameters for accurate imaging and image interpretation. The more clinical information is conveyed to the radiologist, the more accurate the diagnosis will be.

The increasing use of advanced cross-sectional imaging techniques (eg, diffusion-weighted MR imaging, MR spectroscopy) enhances the early and sensitive recognition of birth-related head and spinal cord injuries.[51]

Plain Radiography

Plain radiography of the skull and cervical spine was the choice of imaging before the advent and common use of cross-sectional imaging modalities. Although skull radiographs can demonstrate fracture or suture separation/override, the sensitivity is low. Negative skull radiography does not exclude intracranial injury, and by the same token a skull fracture does not necessarily indicate an intracranial injury. In newborns with suspected phrenic nerve palsy, chest radiographs can show elevation of the affected diaphragm, with mediastinal shift to the contralateral side. These radiographic findings may not be evident in newborns who receive positive pressure ventilation. Real-time fluoroscopic examination of the hemidiaphragms during inspiration and expiration can confirm the diagnosis by showing paradoxic movement of the affected hemidiaphragm.

Ultrasonography

US imaging of the head is commonly used in neonates; with the advantage that US can be performed bedside, does not use ionizing radiation, and can consequently be repeated as frequently as necessary. In addition, US allows anatomic evaluation of the brain with the additional functional analysis provided by color-coded duplex sonography through measurements of the resistive index in the arterial circulation. Newborns with birth-related head injuries can have bradycardia, apnea, or hemodynamic instability, whereby transportation can be challenging and may dispose added risk to the newborn. Extracranial soft-tissue injuries in the scalp can be easily evaluated with US. High-frequency linear transducers are preferred to delineate the layers of scalp. Fluid collection/hemorrhage underneath the subcutaneous fat would represent caput succedaneum. Cephalohematoma is subperiosteal in location, and subgaleal hemorrhage lies in the subgaleal aponeurosis. Identification of temporalis muscle is very useful in differentiating the latter two. Cephalohematoma is the scalp injury most commonly associated with fractures. Given the subperiosteal nature, cephalohematoma tends to be limited by the sutures whereas subgaleal hemorrhages are more infiltrative, and if large enough may extend from the orbital ridges to neck.

In the evaluation of intracranial injuries, head US is routinely performed through the anterior fontanel in coronal and sagittal planes. Gray-scale images should be combined with resistive index measurements of the intracranial circulation and sampling of the superior sagittal sinus.

Parenchymal diffuse/focal ischemic and/or hemorrhagic insult can be demonstrated by US. Pronounced gray-white matter differentiation, hyperechogenicity of the white matter, effacement of the sulci and lateral ventricles, and increased echogenicity of the basal ganglia can be observed in newborns with diffuse ischemic brain injury in the acute phase. In addition, decrease in resistive index of the anterior arterial circulation (<0.60) supports the other described findings of ischemia (**Fig. 6**).[52]

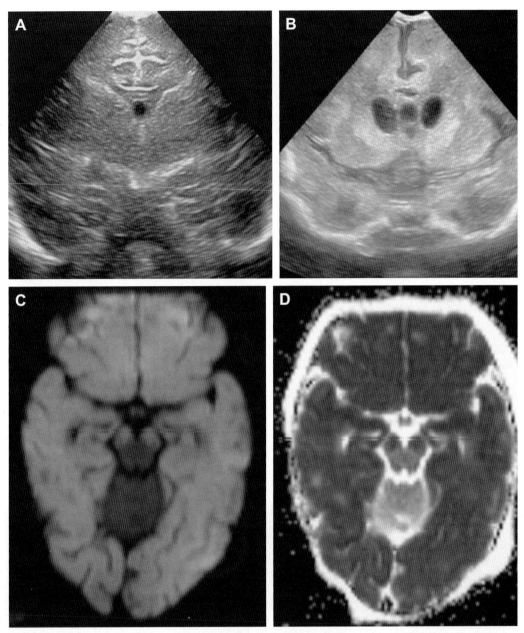

Fig. 6. A full-term newborn with history of placental abruption. Head US gives comparably good diagnostic quality with CT. (*A*) Head US at day of life 1 shows pronounced gray-white matter differentiation, increased echogenicity of the white matter, and effacement of the sulci, secondary to diffuse ischemic changes, (*B*) Head US at day of life 6 shows significantly increased signal of the gray matter, white matter, and basal ganglia, and diffuse global volume loss. (*C, D*) Corresponding diffusion-weighted imaging and analog-to-digital converter map obtained at day of life 6 shows restricted diffusion in the entire supratentorial brain.

Parenchymal hemorrhages can present as focal areas of hyperechogenicity, with a variable degree of mass effect depending on the size and location of the hemorrhage. Typical intracranial hemorrhage of prematurity is rarely seen in relation to birth trauma. US is limited in detection of subarachnoid hemorrhages, peripherally located lesions such as subdural hemorrhages, and imaging of cerebellum and brainstem, due to the fact that these areas are less accessible to the ultrasound probe. Secondary signs of mass effect such as unilateral effacement of the lateral ventricle and midline shift may, however, be alarming for peripheral hemorrhages in either the parenchyma or subdural/epidural space, and should initiate further imaging. US should serve as the first modality in imaging of the head in newborns with birth-related trauma.

US is also useful in diagnosing focal calvarial fractures: linear probes have demonstrated that they can differentiate between sutures and fracture lines in the calvarium.[53] In addition, US should be considered in brachial plexus lesions and phrenic nerve palsies. Soft-tissue hematoma secondary to a clavicle fracture may result in significant compression of the neurovascular structures (see **Fig. 5**). A hematoma within the sternocleidomastoid muscle may also be seen by US. Follow-up examination may be helpful in distinguishing between an acute hematoma and fibromatosis colli. Finally, US enables evaluation of patency of the major arteries and veins along the upper thoracic inlet as well as along the clavicle.

Computed Tomography

Cross-sectional imaging with computed tomography (CT) should be considered when the clinical findings do not correlate well, or cannot be explained by the US findings or clinical history. CT has the advantage that it can display simultaneously the soft tissues as well as the bony structures in high detail. Consequently, CT has a high accuracy in detecting cranial fractures. In addition, CT is superior to US for the evaluation of posterior fossa abnormalities, especially retrocerebellar and tentorial subdural hemorrhages in the setting of birth-related injuries.

Thin-slice axial images of the head and cervical spine are performed with soft-tissue and bone algorithms, which enables the radiologist to perform 2-dimensional (2D) coronal and sagittal and 3-dimensional (3D) reconstructions. 2D reformats of the skull can show overriding sutures, which is a frequent normal finding in neonates (see **Fig. 4**). 3D surface reconstructions of the skull are very helpful in the interpretation of skull fractures, especially in differentiating fractures from Wormian bones in the neonate (**Fig. 7**).

In the developing brain the white matter is incompletely myelinated, and consequently appears relatively hypodense (**Fig. 8**), which may present a challenge, especially if ischemic injury has to be ruled out (see **Fig. 2**).

CT is frequently preferred over MR imaging if the newborn has respiratory and/or hemodynamic instability. The ultrafast CT scanners allow imaging in a couple of seconds, rendering motion-free images even when the neonate is not sedated. The major disadvantage, however, is that CT uses high doses of radiation in this very vulnerable patient group. Not only is the myelinating brain radiated, but also the radiation-sensitive lens may be injured, especially if multiple repeat examinations are considered.

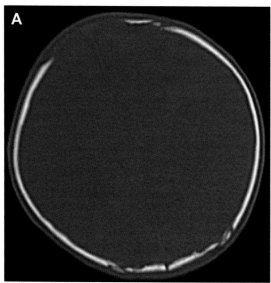
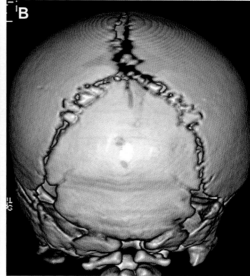

Fig. 7. A full-term newborn delivered via cesarean section with vacuum assistance after failure to progress and prolonged labor. (*A*) Fragmented appearance of the bones at the lambdoid sutures can be misleading for fractures on the axial CT. (*B*) 3D surface reconstruction of the skull confirms that this represents the Wormian bones in the neonate.

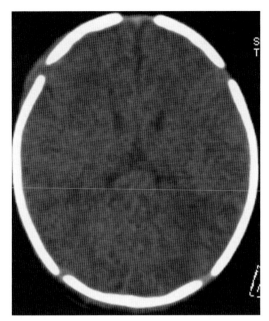

Fig. 8. A full-term infant born via vacuum-assisted vaginal delivery. Note bilateral symmetric normal hypodense appearance of the white matter.

Magnetic Resonance Imaging

MR imaging really revolutionized the high-end sensitive and specific imaging of the developing neonatal brain. Multiplanar sequences that render multiple image contrasts depending on the chosen sequence parameter and the large toolbox of functional sequences, including diffusion-weighted MR imaging, perfusion-weighted MR imaging, MR spectroscopy, and functional MR imaging, allow the study of the neonatal brain in high detail without the use of ionizing radiation. In addition, MR imaging does not suffer from beam-hardening artifacts (as in CT), which allows one to study the brainstem and cerebellum in high anatomic detail. The major disadvantage is that the neonates are in a so-called hostile environment in which the neonate is less accessible and has usually to be transported outside of the safe environment of the neonatal intensive care unit. MR-compatible incubators have partially solved these problems. However, the duration of imaging is still significantly longer compared with CT and, consequently, imaging is more susceptible to motion artifacts. However, if the clinical and MR imaging team are well prepared, many neonates can be studied without the need for sedation by taking advantage of "natural sleep" in which the neonate is fed immediately before the MR imaging examination, is nicely swaddled, and all sequences are optimized for fast imaging.[54]

In newborns, especially those with birth-related injuries to the head and cervical spine, MR imaging is valuable in mapping the full extent and quality of injury, and may better guide treatment, predict outcome, and consequently help in counseling the parents.

Neonatal MR imaging not only sheds light on sick newborns but also helps clinicians to understand that physiologic processes such as spontaneous vaginal delivery can cause subdural hemorrhages in up to almost 50% of asymptomatic newborns.[55] MR can easily demonstrate the full depth of soft-tissue birth-related injuries, from scalp injuries to intracranial hemorrhagic/ischemic lesions (see **Fig. 3**). Subdural hematomas are the most common intracranial hemorrhage, and are seen along the tentorium or cranial convexities, the infratentorial location being more common than supratentorial ones. Birth-related tentorial SDH should be differentiated from transverse sinus thrombosis. Birth-related SDH accumulate along the tentorial leaflets, sometimes with extension along the midline (see **Fig. 1**). These SDH are generally of the same age and resolve spontaneously within 1 to 3 months after birth.[19,51,55] The pattern of SDH related to birth trauma appears to be different to that of nonaccidental trauma. Nonaccidental injuries generally cause SDH overlying the cerebral convexities or interhemispheric fissure; these hematomas are often, but not always, of differing ages.[56] Medicolegal cases with suspected nonaccidental head trauma during the first weeks of life stand as a challenge for the child life protection team. In general, radiologists are the first to see the intracranial manifestations of the inflicted trauma, and have the responsibility of informing the emergency department physicians. Cranial MR imaging is superior to CT in identification of hemorrhages, especially of the extracerebral hemorrhages, and posterior fossa subdural hemorrhages in neonates.[57–59] Conventional MR imaging sequences such as T1-weighted, T2-weighted, and fluid-attenuated inversion recovery are more sensitive than CT in demonstrating different ages of blood products.

Differential diagnosis of intracranial hemorrhage and ischemia in the newborn is not limited to nonaccidental injuries. Deep venous sinus thrombosis, neonatal encephalitis, glutaric aciduria type I, and vascular anomalies should be considered in the right clinical setting if an unusual pattern of imaging findings is encountered.

MR angiography and venography can be performed when deep venous sinus thrombosis is suspected. In cases with deep intracranial hemorrhage, that is, involvement of the basal ganglia and intraventricular hemorrhage, coagulopathy should be actively investigated.

Imaging of peripheral nerve injuries has been revolutionized with the use of MR imaging. In the past, indirect imaging findings such as a clavicle fracture or shoulder dislocation sett the clue for possible nerve injury. The use of heavily T2-weighted imaging enables one to visualize the nerve roots and brachial plexus directly, and thus to diagnose possible nerve root avulsion with identification of pseudomeningocele at the exact level of nerve injury.

Spinal cord injuries are rare but devastating injuries. Early on in postnatal life, the respiratory difficulty and electromyography findings can be misleading and diagnoses can be delayed. Birth-related cord injury most commonly compromises the cervical spinal cord. The spinal cord is best evaluated with MR imaging. In the acute phase, increased caliber and T2 hyperintense signal are seen at the level of insult, evolving into progressive thinning of the cord in the later subacute and chronic phases. Use of diffusion-weighted imaging of the brainstem and cervical spinal cord is very helpful in demonstrating the early changes of ischemia, when it is not yet evident using the conventional imaging techniques.

In conclusion, birth-related head and cervical spine injuries are various. The great majority of these injuries resolve spontaneously in newborns; however, when significant they may result in devastating neurologic injuries and may be fatal. Appropriate use of imaging techniques and timely diagnosis plays an important role in the management of the newborn with birth-related trauma, providing appropriate counseling to the parents and guidance for the best possible neurologic outcome. Imaging findings, combined with detailed clinical history and physical examination, is crucial in differential diagnosis of birth-related injuries, and requires teamwork between obstetrics, the neonatal intensive care unit, and pediatric radiology.

REFERENCES

1. Leestma J. Forensic neuropathology. In: Duckett S, editor: In: Pediatric neuropathology. Williams; 1995. p. 243–83.
2. Laroia N. 2008. Available at: http://emedicine.medscape.com/article/980112-overview. Accessed February 1, 2010.
3. Society of Obstetricians and Gynaecologists of Canada. SOGC clinical practice guidelines. Guidelines for vaginal birth after previous caesarean birth. Number 155 (replaces guideline Number 147), February 2005. Int J Gynaecol Obstet 2005;89(3):319–31.
4. Wen SW, Liu S, Kramer MS, et al. Comparison of maternal and infant outcomes between vacuum extraction and forceps deliveries. Am J Epidemiol 2001;153(2):103–7.
5. Uhing MR. Management of birth injuries. Clin Perinatol 2005;32(1):19–38, v.
6. McQuivey RW. Vacuum-assisted delivery: a review. J Matern Fetal Neonatal Med 2004;16(3):171–80.
7. Gean AD, editor. Imaging of head trauma. 1st edition. New York: Raven Press; 1995.
8. Plauche WC. Subgaleal hematoma. A complication of instrumental delivery. JAMA 1980;244(14):1597–8.
9. Ng PC, Siu YK, Lewindon PJ. Subaponeurotic haemorrhage in the 1990s: a 3-year surveillance. Acta Paediatr 1995;84(9):1065–9.
10. Thacker KE, Lim T, Drew JH. Cephalhaematoma: a 10-year review. Aust N Z J Obstet Gynaecol 1987;27(3):210–2.
11. Heibel M, Heber R, Bechinger D, et al. Early diagnosis of perinatal cerebral lesions in apparently normal full-term newborns by ultrasound of the brain. Neuroradiology 1993;35(2):85–91.
12. Holden KR, Titus MO, Van Tassel P. Cranial magnetic resonance imaging examination of normal term neonates: a pilot study. J Child Neurol 1999;14(11):708–10.
13. Tavani F, Zimmerman RA, Clancy RR, et al. Incidental intracranial hemorrhage after uncomplicated birth: MRI before and after neonatal heart surgery. Neuroradiology 2003;45(4):253–8.
14. Mateos F, Esteban J, Ramos JT, et al. Fetal subdural hematoma: diagnosis in utero. Case report. Pediatr Neurosci 1987;13(3):125–8.
15. Hanigan WC, Ali MB, Cusack TJ, et al. Diagnosis of subdural hemorrhage in utero. Case report. J Neurosurg 1985;63(6):977–9.
16. Jhawar BS, Ranger A, Steven D, et al. Risk factors for intracranial hemorrhage among full-term infants: a case-control study. Neurosurgery 2003;52(3):581–90 [discussion: 588–90].
17. Pollina J, Dias MS, Li V, et al. Cranial birth injuries in term newborn infants. Pediatr Neurosurg 2001;35(3):113–9.
18. Sachs BP, Acker D, Tuomala R, et al. The incidence of symptomatic intracranial hemorrhage in term appropriate-for-gestation-age infants. Clin Pediatr (Phila) 1987;26(7):355–8.
19. Whitby EH, Griffiths PD, Rutter S, et al. Frequency and natural history of subdural haemorrhages in babies and relation to obstetric factors. Lancet 2004;363(9412):846–51.
20. Volpe JJ. Intracranial haemorrhage. In: Volpe JJ, editor. Neurology of the newborn. Philadelphia: W.B. Saunders; 1995. p. 377–8.
21. Squier W, Mack J. The neuropathology of infant subdural haemorrhage. Forensic Sci Int 2009;187(1–3):6–13.
22. Steinbok P, Haw CS, Cochrane DD, et al. Acute subdural hematoma associated with cerebral

infarction in the full-term neonate. Pediatr Neurosurg 1995;23(4):206–15.

23. Overpeck MD, Brenner RA, Trumble AC, et al. Risk factors for infant homicide in the United States. N Engl J Med 1998;339(17):1211–6.

24. Takagi T, Fukuoka H, Wakabayashi S, et al. Posterior fossa subdural hemorrhage in the newborn as a result of birth trauma. Childs Brain 1982;9(2):102–13.

25. Negishi H, Lee Y, Itoh K, et al. Nonsurgical management of epidural hematoma in neonates. Pediatr Neurol 1989;5(4):253–6.

26. Fenichel GM, Webster DL, Wong WK. Intracranial hemorrhage in the term newborn. Arch Neurol 1984;41(1):30–4.

27. Sandberg DI, Lamberti-Pasculli M, Drake JM, et al. Spontaneous intraparenchymal hemorrhage in full-term neonates. Neurosurgery 2001;48(5):1042–8 [discussion: 1048–9].

28. Abroms IF, Rosen BA. Neurologic trauma in newborn infants. Semin Neurol 1993;13(1):100–5.

29. Harpold TL, McComb JG, Levy ML. Neonatal neurosurgical trauma. Neurosurg Clin N Am 1998;9(1):141–54.

30. Volpe JJ. Neonatal intracranial hemorrhage. Pathophysiology, neuropathology, and clinical features. Clin Perinatol 1977;4(1):77–102.

31. Reichard R. Birth injury of the cranium and central nervous system. Brain Pathol 2008;18(4):565–70.

32. Bryant DR, Leonardi MR, Landwehr JB, et al. Limited usefulness of fetal weight in predicting neonatal brachial plexus injury. Am J Obstet Gynecol 1998;179(3 Pt 1):686–9.

33. Gonen R, Spiegel D, Abend M. Is macrosomia predictable, and are shoulder dystocia and birth trauma preventable? Obstet Gynecol 1996;88(4 Pt 1):526–9.

34. Gilbert WM, Nesbitt TS, Danielsen B. Associated factors in 1611 cases of brachial plexus injury. Obstet Gynecol 1999;93(4):536–40.

35. Walle T, Hartikainen-Sorri AL. Obstetric shoulder injury. Associated risk factors, prediction and prognosis. Acta Obstet Gynecol Scand 1993;72(6):450–4.

36. Bennet GC, Harrold AJ. Prognosis and early management of birth injuries to the brachial plexus. Br Med J 1976;1(6024):1520–1.

37. Hankins GD, Clark SL. Brachial plexus palsy involving the posterior shoulder at spontaneous vaginal delivery. Am J Perinatol 1995;12(1):44–5.

38. Sandmire HF, DeMott RK. Erb's palsy: concepts of causation. Obstet Gynecol 2000;95(6 Pt 1):941–2.

39. Dunn DW, Engle WA. Brachial plexus palsy: intrauterine onset. Pediatr Neurol 1985;1(6):367–9.

40. al-Qattan MM, el-Sayed AA, al-Kharfy TM, et al. Obstetrical brachial plexus injury in newborn babies delivered by caesarean section. J Hand Surg Br 1996;21(2):263–5.

41. Amar AP, Aryan HE, Meltzer HS, et al. Neonatal subgaleal hematoma causing brain compression: report of two cases and review of the literature. Neurosurgery 2003;52(6):1470–4 [discussion: 1474].

42. Michelow BJ, Clarke HM, Curtis CG, et al. The natural history of obstetrical brachial plexus palsy. Plast Reconstr Surg 1994;93(4):675–80 [discussion: 681].

43. McNeely PD, Drake JM. A systematic review of brachial plexus surgery for birth-related brachial plexus injury. Pediatr Neurosurg 2003;38(2):57–62.

44. Hughes CA, Harley EH, Milmoe G, et al. Birth trauma in the head and neck. Arch Otolaryngol Head Neck Surg 1999;125(2):193–9.

45. Manning JJ, Adour KK. Facial paralysis in children. Pediatrics 1972;49(1):102–9.

46. de Vries TS, Koens BL, Vos A. Surgical treatment of diaphragmatic eventration caused by phrenic nerve injury in the newborn. J Pediatr Surg 1998;33(4):602–5.

47. Menticoglou SM, Perlman M, Manning FA. High cervical spinal cord injury in neonates delivered with forceps: report of 15 cases. Obstet Gynecol 1995;86(4 Pt 1):589–94.

48. MacKinnon JA, Perlman M, Kirpalani H, et al. Spinal cord injury at birth: diagnostic and prognostic data in twenty-two patients. J Pediatr 1993;122(3):431–7.

49. Morgan C, Newell SJ. Cervical spinal cord injury following cephalic presentation and delivery by Caesarean section. Dev Med Child Neurol 2001;43(4):274–6.

50. Rossitch E Jr, Oakes WJ. Perinatal spinal cord injury: clinical, radiographic and pathologic features. Pediatr Neurosurg 1992;18(3):149–52.

51. Looney CB, Smith JK, Merck LH, et al. Intracranial hemorrhage in asymptomatic neonates: prevalence on MR images and relationship to obstetric and neonatal risk factors. Radiology 2007;242(2):535–41.

52. Daneman A, Epelman M, Blaser S, et al. Imaging of the brain in full-term neonates: does sonography still play a role? Pediatr Radiol 2006;36(7):636–46.

53. Sorantin E, Brader P, Thimary F. Neonatal trauma. Eur J Radiol 2006;60(2):199–207.

54. Huisman TA, Tekes A. Advanced MR brain imaging. Why? Pediatr Radiol 2008;38(Suppl 3):S415–432.

55. Rooks VJ, Eaton JP, Ruess L, et al. Prevalence and evolution of intracranial hemorrhage in asymptomatic term infants. AJNR Am J Neuroradiol 2008;29(6):1082–9.

56. Lonergan GJ, Baker AM, Morey MK, et al. From the archives of the AFIP. Child abuse: radiologic-pathologic correlation. Radiographics 2003;23(4):811–45.

57. Keeney SE, Adcock EW, McArdle CB. Prospective observations of 100 high-risk neonates by high-field (1.5 Tesla) magnetic resonance imaging of

the central nervous system. II. Lesions associated with hypoxic-ischemic encephalopathy. Pediatrics 1991;87(4):431–8.

58. McArdle CB, Richardson CJ, Hayden CK, et al. Abnormalities of the neonatal brain: MR imaging.

Part II. Hypoxic-ischemic brain injury. Radiology 1987;163(2):395–403.

59. Kidwell CS, Chalela JA, Saver JL, et al. Comparison of MRI and CT for detection of acute intracerebral hemorrhage. JAMA 2004;292(15):1823–30.

Imaging of Neonatal Child Abuse with an Emphasis on Abusive Head Trauma

Rick R. van Rijn, MD, PhD[a,b,*], Melissa R. Spevak, MD[c]

KEYWORDS

• Imaging • Neonatal child abuse • Abusive head trauma

Child abuse is defined by the World Health Organization as "Child abuse, sometimes referred to as child abuse and neglect, includes all forms of physical and emotional ill-treatment, sexual abuse, neglect, and exploitation that results in actual or potential harm to the child's health, development or dignity. Within this broad definition, 5 subtypes can be distinguished – physical abuse; sexual abuse; neglect and negligent treatment; emotional abuse; and exploitation."[1] Although radiologists can potentially be confronted with all 5 forms of child abuse and neglect (CAN), this article deals exclusively with physical abuse.

The exact incidence and prevalence of CAN are unknown, because researchers use their own definitions of such abuse, which makes comparison between studies difficult. Among such studies are the National Incidence Study of Child Abuse and Neglect in the United States, the Canadian Incidence Study of Reported CAN, and the Dutch Prevalence Study of Maltreatment of Youth.[2–4] In these 3 studies the incidence was reported to range from 17.2 to 30.0 per 1000 children. Another way of looking at the magnitude of this problem is presented by Lord Laming, who in his report on the tragic death of Victoria Climbié, stated "I have no difficulty in accepting the proposition that this problem (deliberate harm to children) is greater than that of what are generally recognized as common health problems in children, such as diabetes or asthma."[5]

Besides an immediate impact on the child's health status, which can be severe or even lethal, there are serious social and medical long-term consequences of CAN. In the Adverse Childhood Experiences study, Felitti and colleagues[6] found a graded relationship between the number of categories of adverse childhood exposures and adult health risk behaviors and diseases. Although beyond the scope of this publication it is of general interest to address the potential economic cost of CAN. In a 2010 publication Corso and Fertig[7] presented corrected data for the United States, reporting that the annual cost, both direct and indirect, of CAN is a staggering $65,139,889,962. This figure does not even take into account the costs associated with mortality or reduced life expectancy.

In evaluating child abuse, a multidisciplinary approach is essential. Ideally, a team, which may be called the child advocacy team (CAT), consisting of all involved specialties including pediatric radiology should be involved. The CAT should support the attending physician and, if necessary, ask for help from a pediatric forensic physician. It interesting to note that the Royal College of

[a] Department of Radiology, Academic Medical Centre/Emma Children's Hospital Amsterdam, Meibergdreef 9, 1105 AZ Amsterdam Zuid-Oost, The Netherlands
[b] Section of Pediatric Forensics, Department of Forensic Medicine, Netherlands Forensic Institute, The Hague, The Netherlands
[c] Division of Pediatric Radiology, The Russell H. Morgan Department of Radiology and Radiological Science, Johns Hopkins University, 600 North Wolfe Street, Baltimore, MD 21287, USA
* Corresponding author. Department of Radiology, Academic Medical Centre Amsterdam, Meibergdreef 9, 1105 AZ Amsterdam Zuid-Oost, The Netherlands.
E-mail address: r.r.vanrijn@amc.uva.nl

Magn Reson Imaging Clin N Am 19 (2011) 791–812
doi:10.1016/j.mric.2011.08.006

Pathologists (RCP), at a meeting specifically aimed at the discussion on the cause of abusive head trauma (AHT), agreed that "in the current state of knowledge the presence of 'the triad' [see later discussion], even in its 'characteristic' form, should not be regarded as absolute proof of traumatic head injury in the absence of any other corroborative evidence."[8] The evaluation of child abuse is often challenging; the combined opinion of many specialists in the CAT lends credibility and certainty to the diagnosis.

Because this edition of *Radiological Clinics of North America* is devoted to imaging of the neonate, we focus on the most prevalent finding in physical abuse at the age: AHT. Given the importance of secondary findings in AHT, imaging of fractures is also discussed. Although the neonatal period is only the first month of life, most of the material discussed in this article can also be applied to the infant.

AHT

AHT is one of the most devastating forms of child abuse, and in children less than 2 years it is the leading cause of death in CAN.[9] In 1946, the pediatric radiologist, J. Caffey reported on the unusual association of long bone fractures and subdural hematomas (SDHs) and suggested these 2 injuries may be secondary to child abuse, a radical idea at the time.[10] Later, in 1962, Silverman, a radiologist, and Kempe, a pediatrician, and others described the battered child syndrome in a study that described the results of direct trauma on the child, renewing general interest in the problem of child abuse.[11] In 1972, the shaken baby syndrome term was introduced in another study by J. Caffey.[12] In his seminal paper, the classic triad consisting of encephalopathy, subdural hemorrhages, and retinal hemorrhages was first presented. However, the term shaken baby syndrome is not just a description of radiological findings but also implies an underlying mechanism (ie, shaking). In recent years, there has been much debate about the cause of AHT; in particular, whether shaking alone could lead to the findings seen on imaging.[12–20] It was therefore deemed inappropriate to continue the use of shaken baby syndrome, and in 2009, the American Academy of Pediatrics (AAP) proposed the use of AHT instead.[21] Other terms that are used besides AHT are nonaccidental head injury and inflicted traumatic brain injury.

In Great Britain the Crown Prosecution Service issued this statement on the diagnosis of AHT: "Each case will clearly turn on its own facts but it would appear unlikely that a charge of murder can be justified where the only evidence available is the triad of injuries" (the triad of injuries referred to is the so-called classic triad in AHT). Furthermore, it specifically states that "Cases of alleged non-accidental head injury are fact specific and will be determined on their individual facts. All the circumstances, including the clinical picture, must be taken into account." This statement means, as stated in the introduction, that the diagnosis of AHT should be made only in close collaboration with a CAT. In each case of suspected AHT a complete clinical history and thorough physical examination are mandatory.[22] Mcguire and colleagues[23] performed a systematic literature analysis in which 8151 publications were identified and 14 of 320 reviewed publications were included. In total the study population consisted of 1655 children with neurotrauma (799 with AHT). From their data these investigators concluded that apnea (positive predictive value [PPV] 93%, odds ratio [OR] 17.06, $P<.001$), retinal hemorrhages (PPV 71%, OR 3.504, $P = .03$) and rib fractures (PPV 73%, OR 3.03, $P = .13$) were significant positive predictors for AHT. Although the presence of retinal hemorrhages is strongly related to AHT, the discussion of this topic falls outside the scope of this article and the interested reader is therefore referred to relevant publications.[24,25]

CLINICAL PRESENTATION

The clinical presentation of children with AHT can be variable, rendering it difficult to make an accurate diagnosis in many cases. Jenny and colleagues[26] have shown in a series of 173 abused children with head injuries, 54 (31.2%) cases were initially misdiagnosed. More important than these statistical findings is these investigators' finding that 4 of 5 deaths might have been prevented by a timely recognition of CAN. This finding is in keeping with other publications on the diagnosis of CAN.[27–29]

According to Minns and Busuttil,[30] 4 main presenting patterns of AHT are seen:

1. Hyperacute encephalopathy:

Approximately 6% of all children present with hyperacute encephalopathy, otherwise known as a cervicomedullary syndrome. These are mostly young children with acute brainstem conditions (ie, apnea and cerebral edema). In many, if not most cases, these children are dead on arrival in the hospital.

2. Acute encephalopathy:

Most AHT cases, approximately 53%, are cases of acute encephalopathy. At presentation, these children have a low level of consciousness, increased cranial pressure, convulsions, apnea, hypotonia, anemia, or shock. Often additional injuries, such as rib fractures, are found. This pattern of AHT was originally described by J. Caffey[10] as the shaken baby syndrome.

3. Subacute nonencephalopathy:

This group of patients, approximately 19% of all cases, present with similar but less severe symptoms as seen in acute encephalopathy.

4. Chronic extracerebral presentation:

Approximately 22% of all patients with AHT present with growing head circumference and mild symptoms of raised intracranial pressure (eg, failure to thrive and behavioral problems).

IMAGING
Conventional Radiography

Historically, conventional radiographs of the skull were an important diagnostic tool. However, with the advent of computed tomography (CT), the use of skull radiographs in the trauma setting has been abolished. Several studies have shown that the sensitivity of skull radiographs for intracranial conditions is poor. The Children's Head injury Algorithm for the prediction of Important Clinical Events (CHALICE) study, a prospective diagnostic cohort study of 22,772 children, assessed the value of the conventional skull radiograph.[31] In this study, a total of 5318 skull radiographs were obtained, and in 259 cases the radiological report stated the presence of a fracture. Of these fractures, 44 (17%) were missed by emergency physicians. In 59 cases (1% of normal radiographs) a fracture was diagnosed by emergency physicians but read as normal by the radiologist. A subpopulation of 98 children with abnormalities (not otherwise specified) on CT also had a skull radiograph. In these patients, radiography had a sensitivity of 77% (95% confidence interval [CI] 67%–85%, 75 fractures in 98 patients) for a positive condition on CT. In a series of 47 children who sustained AHT, studied by Rao and colleagues,[32] 31 (65.9%) did not have a skull fracture. In a study by Merten and colleagues[33] among children with AHT, a skull fracture was seen in 45% of cases and intracranial conditions were seen in 56% of children with a skull fracture. Based on these and other publications, it can be concluded that the continued use of skull radiographs for children with acute head injury is not warranted. This finding is in keeping with previous studies.[34–37] The AAP states in their position paper on the

management of minor closed head injury that the skull radiograph has only a limited role in the evaluation of these children.[38]

In child abuse, skeletal radiography is used to show the presence of occult trauma and clinical evident conditions and aid in the diagnosis of underlying disease (Fig. 1). In rare cases, a skull fracture in the plane of scanning can be missed on CT.[39] In these cases, the fracture may be visible on the skull radiographs. The reporting radiologist should be aware of sutural anatomy (ie, not only the normally seen sutures but also the normal variants, because these can resemble fractures).[40] In a significant proportion of cases of AHT, skull fractures are seen.

Most skull fractures, whether from accidental trauma or CAN, are linear fractures; this finding is not discriminating. It has been reported that when there are bilateral fractures, multiple fractures with depression and diastases greater than 3 mm, depression fractures, fractures with diastases of the fracture lines, or occipital fractures, child abuse should be considered in the differential diagnosis (Fig. 2A and B).[41–43] No single skull fracture is pathognomonic for child abuse.

In the most recent guidelines of the American College of Radiology (ACR) and the joint guideline from the Royal College of Paediatrics and Child Health (RCPCH) and Royal College of Radiologists (RCR), the skull radiograph is a mandatory part of the skeletal survey.[44–46] This statement implies that even when a CT of the head has been performed, a skull radiograph should be obtained in all cases.

Ultrasonography

Cranial ultrasonography, which is widely adopted by pediatric radiologists because of its clear benefit to patient care, has no role in the primary

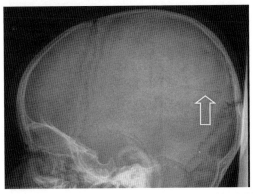

Fig. 1. Skull radiograph of a 15-month-old child shows a skull fracture (arrow). Further workup of CAT ruled out child abuse.

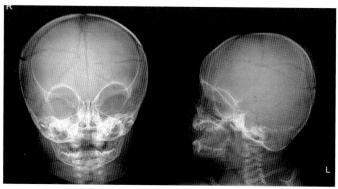

Fig. 2. Anteroposterior and lateral skull radiograph of a 6-month-old girl shows complex skull fractures as a result of an impact trauma in AHT.

detection of child abuse. Because of the convexity of the skull, SDH can be missed and detection of subarachnoid hemorrhage (SAH) is virtually impossible.

However, there are instances when the pediatric radiologist is asked to perform a cranial ultra-sonographic study. This request may be in a situation when the patient is unstable and an urgent bedside examination is necessary. Change in status such as enlarging head circumference, at which time an SDH may be seen, may be the indication for the ultrasonographic examination. Using color Doppler imaging it is possible to discern between an SDH and benign enlargement of the subarach-noid space, a common finding in children who are referred for large cranial circumference (**Fig. 3** and **Fig. 4**A, B).[47–50] Jaspan and colleagues[51] presented 6 children in whom contusional tears of subcortical white matter were detected using high-resolution ultrasonography, a finding that indicates AHT in these investigators' opinion. Another use of cranial ultrasound, using a high-resolution probe, is for

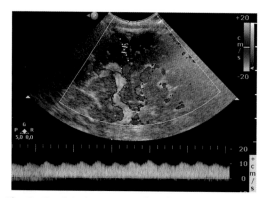

Fig. 3. Cranial ultrasonography of a 6-month-old girl with large cranial circumference shows benign enlarge-ment of the subarachnoid space. Color Doppler ultraso-nography clearly shows the presence of bridging veins.

follow-up of SDH. When properly used this tech-nique can obviate repeat CT or magnetic resonance (MR) imaging scanning.[52]

CT

CT is the first-line imaging tool in the setting of traumatic brain injury, irrespective of the cause of trauma. With its wide availability and short scan times, it can readily identify acute conditions needing neurosurgical intervention. Images should be acquired using thin collimation, necessary for three-dimensional (3D) reconstruction. The images should be reconstructed with a maximum slice thickness of 5 mm in both a soft tissue algorithm (with, eg, window width (WW)/window level (WL) 80/25) and a bone algorithm (with, eg, WW/WL 3000/300). Standard 3D reconstructions, which should be obtained in all cases of AHT, are useful for showing radiological findings, especially (but not exclusively) to nonmedical personnel (**Fig. 5**). The use of more advanced 3D techniques has been described in the literature but has not been validated in large samples.[53]

Noncontrast-enhanced CT has good sensitivity for acute hemorrhage and midline shift (**Figs. 6** and **7**). However, it is less sensitive, especially in the acute stage, for nonhemorrhagic intracranial conditions such as shear injury and perfusion disorders. In adults, the use of perfusion CT has been described in the evaluation of mild head injury. Metting and colleagues[54] reported that disturbed cerebral perfusion, in patients with nor-mal noncontrast-enhanced CT scans, was related to the severity of injury and outcome. This condi-tion has not been studied in children and, given the lack of evidence, perfusion CT should not be performed in children with neurotrauma. In gen-eral, there is no indication for contrast-enhanced CT scanning. If a vascular lesion is considered,

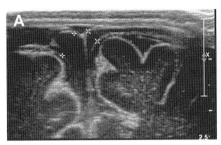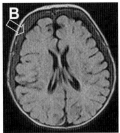

Fig. 4. (A) Cranial ultrasonography of an 8-week-old girl shows bilateral SDH (*calipers*). The study was requested because of failure to thrive. (B) T2 fluid-attenuated inversion recovery weighted MR imaging of the same patient obtained 4 days after the initial ultrasound study confirms the presence of bilateral SDHs (*arrow*).

MR imaging angiography should be the modality of choice.

Subdural hemorrhage is seen in a significant proportion of children with AHT. Subdural hemorrhage is found in up to 90% of autopsied cases of AHT.[55] In most instances it consists of a thin film of blood, over the cerebral convexities, often bilaterally. In young children, unlike adults, the subdural hemorrhage often extends into the posterior interhemispheric fissure (**Fig. 8**). On a CT scan, a small amount of interhemispheric subdural hemorrhage can be visualized that might be missed at autopsy because of its location. However, compared with autopsy, CT is less sensitive in detecting small convexity subdural hemorrhages, a result of both beam hardening artifacts and partial volume effects of the inner table of the skull.

SAH is seen in most autopsy cases of AHT. However, because it can also be found after accidental trauma it cannot be used as a discriminating factor. Epidural hemorrhage is seen after impact trauma, in accidental as well as AHT cases. Like SAH, it cannot be seen as a discriminating factor.

CT of the head is indicated in all children who present with signs of physical abuse in combination with neurologic deficits or retinal hemorrhages. There is much debate about routine cranial CT in all physically abused children less than a certain age, irrespective of their neurologic status.[56–60] There have been publications both supporting and rejecting routine CT in all children with suspected or proven physical child abuse. In a prospective study by Rubin and colleagues[56]

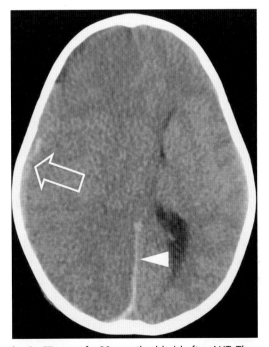

Fig. 6. CT scan of a 29-month-old girl after AHT. There is an SDH along the right convexity (*arrow*) extending into the posterior interhemispheric fissure (*arrowhead*). There is a significant shift of the midline because of the SDH and right-sided brain edema.

Fig. 5. 3D reconstruction of the skull of a 6-week-old boy. A diastatic parietal skull fracture, the result of impact trauma in AHT, is clearly visible.

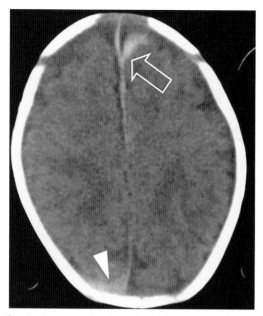

Fig. 7. CT scan of a 6-week-old boy after admitted AHT. CT shows a left frontal SDH extending into the anterior interhemispheric fissure (*arrow*) and a smaller right-sided occipital SDH (*arrowhead*).

involving 65 patients, 51 patients met the inclusion criteria for their study, of which 19 patients (37.3%, 95% CI 24.2–50.4%) had occult head injury. Based on the skeletal survey alone 26% (5/19) patients would have been missed. All children with occult head injury were less than the age of 1 year. In

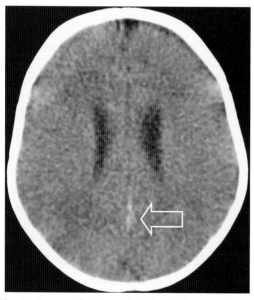

Fig. 8. CT scan of a 2-month-old girl after AHT. There is blood in the posterior interhemispheric fissure (*arrow*).

contrast to this finding, Mogbo and colleagues[57] published a study in which only 19% of children had evidence of acute intracranial injury. Based on their findings these investigators concluded that CT scans neither changed clinical management nor altered clinical or legal outcome. However, this study is limited: only children with radiologically apparent skull fractures were included. The current guidelines of the RCPCH and RCR state that CT is indicated in "any child under the age of one where there is evidence of abuse" (in this context, abuse means physical abuse).[46] In contrast, the ACR states its revised appropriateness criteria that for any child less than the age of 2 years without focal neurologic signs or symptoms CT is usually indicated, particularly for those patients who are high risk (eg, who have rib fractures, multiple fractures, or facial injury or who are less than 6 months of age).[61]

Guidelines reflect the growing concern of the long-term effects of ionizing radiation (eg, radiation-induced tumors) related to CT scanning, an issue emphasized by the 2001 publications of Paterson and Brenner in the *American Journal of Roentgenology*.[62,63] As a result of these publications and ensuing international discussions, the Society for Pediatric Radiology started the Image Gently Campaign, aiming to increase radiation awareness and decrease radiation dose to the pediatric population. Recently a study from Canada has shown that in adults who underwent angiocardiography, a 3% increase in cancer rate was seen for every 10 mSv radiation exposure. However, as in all clinical situations, there should be a risk-benefit assessment, and tumor induction risk should be weighed against the clinical benefits of a CT scan. Clearly, a missed case of child abuse can lead to a serious, even lethal, outcome. Thus, the radiation issue alone should not preclude the CT scan.

MR Imaging

MR imaging is not the imaging method of first choice in cases of AHT. First and foremost, the sensitivity for acute hemorrhage is less compared with CT. Second, MR imaging is more difficult to perform because the examination takes a relatively long time (even with modern sequences), and in many cases sedation or general anesthesia, requiring MR-compatible anesthesia equipment, is mandatory. It also requires that a sometimes critically ill and instable patient be transferred from the safety of a pediatric intensive care environment to the relative insecurity of the radiology department for a considerable time. This situation limits the application of MR imaging in the acute phase of patient treatment. In the subacute phase of injury,

MR imaging becomes superior to CT in delineating an evolving SDH and parenchymal condition. At that stage, MR imaging can be used to assess the true extent of damage and the potential clinical outcome.

There are no international guidelines for MR imaging protocols. In the United Kingdom, the RCR and the RCPCH have published a standard for cranial MR imaging in children with suspected nonaccidental injury (**Table 1**).[46] The protocol consists of standard sequences (T1-weighted and T2-weighted imaging) to delineate the anatomy and presence of pathologic conditions (**Fig. 9**; **Fig. 10A, B** and **Fig. 11**), as well as advanced imaging sequences (ie, susceptibility-weighted imaging [SWI] and diffusion-weighted imaging [DWI]).

SWI, a relatively new technique, makes use of a high-spatial-resolution 3D gradient-recalled-echo sequence that is sensitive for paramagnetic blood breakdown products such as deoxyhemoglobin, intracellular methemoglobin, and hemosiderin (**Figs. 12 and 13**). Research has shown that the use of SWI is superior to other sequences in detecting microhemorrhage in patients with head trauma (**Fig. 14**).[64] In children, a correlation between the number of microhemorrhages, as a parameter of diffuse axonal injury (DAI), and

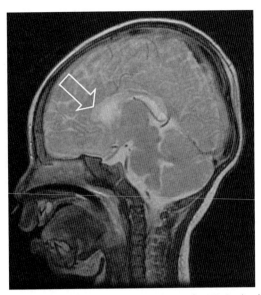

Fig. 9. 4-month-old boy, after admitted AHT. Sagittal T2-weighted MR imaging shows increased signal intensity of the anterior part of the corpus callosum (*arrow*). This is a clear sign of diffuse axonal injury.

Table 1 RCR and RCPCH MR imaging protocol for brain imaging in AHT	
Early	
Plane	**Sequence**
Axial	Dual-echo SE (<1 y of age)
	Dual-echo FSE (>1 y of age)
	T2* gradient (or EPI susceptibility sequence)
	DWI
Coronal	T1 SE and FLAIR or T2 FSE
Sagittal	T1 SE
Late	
Axial	Dual-echo SE (less than 1 year of age)
	Dual-echo FSE (more than 1 year of age)
Coronal	T1 SE
	T2 FSE
Sagittal	T1 SE

Abbreviations: DWI, diffusion-weighted imaging; EPI, echoplanar imaging; FLAIR, fluid-attenuated inversion recovery; FSE, fast spin echo; SE, spin echo.
Data from The Royal College of Radiologists and the Royal College of Paediatrics and Child Health. Standards for radiological investigations of suspected non-accidental injury. London: RCR and RCPCH; 2008. p. 37.

neurologic outcome has been described.[65–67] In a study of 101 children (62 boys, mean age 8.4 months, and 39 girls, mean age, 7.4 months), with forensic pediatric specialist-confirmed AHT, microhemorrhages seen on SWI correlated with significantly poor long-term neurologic outcome.[67]

DWI is a technique in which MR imaging displays the characteristics of water diffusion and each voxel represents the rate of diffusion in that specific voxel. In DWI, 2 images are obtained: the DWI scan and the calculated apparent diffusion coefficients (ADC). This technique was initially used in adults for stroke imaging but has also found an important application in pediatric radiology. In areas of restricted diffusion (cytotoxic edema), the DWI image, which is T2-weighted, shows high signal intensity in the affected area of the brain. If the same area on the ADC map has low signal intensity, the presence of cytotoxicity is confirmed (**Fig. 15A–C** and **Fig. 16A–C**). However, if the same area also has high signal intensity on the ADC map, then this is called T2 shine-through and the DWI should be reported as negative. A literature analysis by the Welsh Child Protection Systematic Review Group showed that DWI reveals more conditions than routine MR sequences.[68] Clinical studies in neonates find DWI to be a good predictor of long-term neurologic outcome.[69–72]

Besides these sequences, MR angiography can be used, with or without intravenous contrast administration. Although its use has been reported

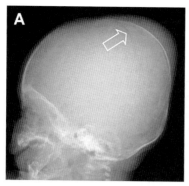
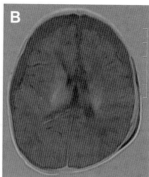

Fig. 10. (A) Postmortem radiograph of the skull of a 2-month-old boy shows a parietal skull fracture (arrow). (B) Postmortem T1-weighted MR imaging, obtained several hours after demise, of the same patient shows a normal development of the brain. A bilateral SDH is present.

in the evaluation of AHT, there is no evidence that MR angiography has additional diagnostic value.[73]

If there is an indication for imaging of the spine, sagittal T1-weighted and T2-weighted series (slice thickness 3 mm) should be obtained. If any abnormalities are seen on sagittal imaging, axial imaging (T1-weighted and T2-weighted series) can then be performed through these areas.

Young children less than the age of approximately 3 months, or older if they are small for age, can be scanned using a knee coil, which has superior signal-to-noise ratio to the adult head coil.

CT or MR imaging or both, and when?
As discussed in the previous 2 sections, CT and MR imaging should not be seen as opposing but as complementary techniques. Each has a specific role to play in the diagnosis of AHT and its differential diagnosis. The question remains as to what is the ideal order of these examinations. No studies are available comparing different imaging strategies, related to timing, using CT and MR imaging. The RCR and the RCPCH have published in their guidelines a flowchart on this subject (Fig. 17)[46] that can easily be implemented in clinical practice. Because it is the only available guideline, it should be followed in all cases of suspected AHT. MR imaging is especially useful in the follow-up of AHT and is preferred over CT (Fig. 18A, B).

Dating subdural hemorrhage
A question arises in many court cases concerning the potential timing of the events leading to the

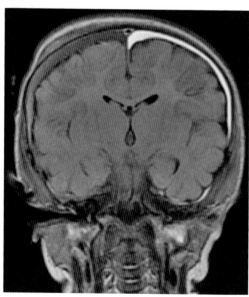

Fig. 11. Coronal fluid-attenuated inversion recovery MR imaging of a 10-week-old boy showing bilateral SDHs with different signal intensities.

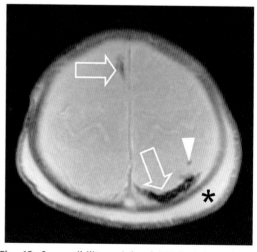

Fig. 12. Susceptibility-weighted MR imaging of a 4-month-old boy shows a large hematoma along the scalp (asterisk), SDHs (arrows), and a focal hemorrhagic lesion, as a sign of diffuse axonal injury (arrowhead).

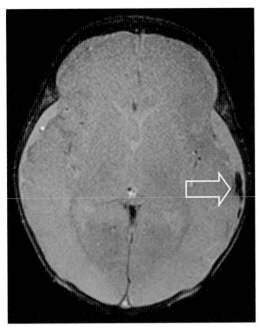

Fig. 13. Susceptibility-weighted MR imaging of a 2-month-old girl shows a left-sided SDH (*arrow*).

intracranial condition. This question can be important in including or excluding possible perpetrators. In most clinical CT examinations, we assume that a hyperdense SDH is acute and a hypodense

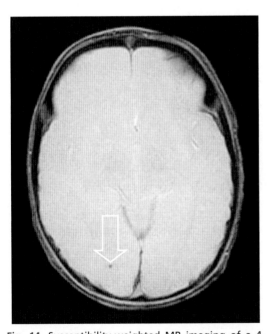

Fig. 14. Susceptibility-weighted MR imaging of a 4-month-old boy shows, as the only finding on the initial MR imaging, a small focal hemorrhagic lesion (*arrow*). This boy later developed severe multicystic encephalopathy and subsequently died.

SDH is older. For MR imaging changes in T1 and T2 signal intensity over time are reported in literature. This finding is sufficient for day-to-day clinical evaluation. Response to the question of timing for AHT, with all its legal implications, is different.

In both CT and MR imaging, there can be exceptions to the rule (eg, in an anemic patient an acute SDH on CT can be isodense compared with normal brain tissue [**Fig. 19**]).[74] An SDH showing both hyperdense and hypodense components on CT, which could be seen as a chronic SDH with re-bleed, has been reported in hyperacute SDH.[75] Admixture of cerebrospinal fluid into the SDH can make interpretation even more difficult.

Because there is no solid evidence for dating SDHs this should not be attempted on imaging. Close collaboration with the involved pediatric specialists (CAT) is essential.

Differential Diagnosis

In case of suspected CAN, as is the case for all other medical diagnoses, a differential diagnosis should be considered.[21,23,76–80] Some of the most important differential diagnoses are discussed briefly.

In the last few years several studies have shown that birth trauma can cause SDH.[80–82] SDH after vaginal delivery has, in a prospective study, been shown to be present in up to 26% of asymptomatic neonates.[81] Another study looking at the natural history of neonatal SDH showed that in asymptomatic patients rescanned at 4 weeks of age, spontaneous resolution occurred in all cases.[81]

Several genetic and metabolic disorders (eg, osteogenesis imperfecta, glutaric aciduria type 1) should be considered in the differential diagnosis and tested for if appropriate. Most of these disorders are rare, but the presence of such a disorder does not rule out CAN.

It is rare for common childhood bleeding disorders to cause intracranial hemorrhage (**Fig. 20**). However, a well-known cause of intracranial hemorrhage in neonates is coagulopathy because of vitamin K deficiency (**Fig. 21**).[83,84] In most cases vitamin K deficiency is seen in breastfed neonates who have not received vitamin K prophylaxis at birth; however, in rare cases an underlying liver disease is present.[85–88]

A final consideration to be discussed is an accidental fall. Two different scenarios exist: a fall from standing and a fall from a height. Falls from standing in young children, especially when they are just becoming ambulatory, are common accidents and should be regarded as part of this specific stage in life. There are no reports of children sustaining a significant head trauma after

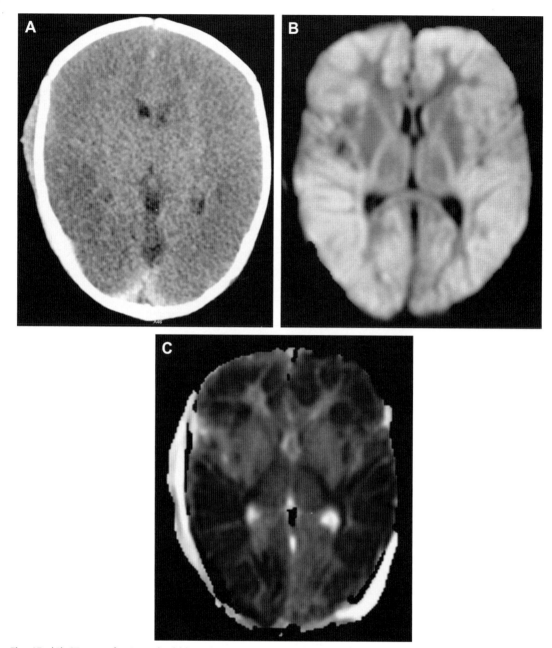

Fig. 15. (*A*) CT scan of a 6-week-old boy shows bilateral hypodense areas located occipitally. (*B*) DWI-weighted MR imaging performed 1 day later shows extensive restricted diffusion in keeping with cytotoxic edema. (*C*) The corresponding ADC map shows a low attenuation corresponding with the abnormalities seen on DWI, thus confirming the diagnosis of cytotoxic edema.

a fall from standing. In contrast, falls from a height can cause an intracranial condition if from a substantial height with a subsequent impact force. There is much debate whether a fall from a short height (eg, from a couch or out of the arms of a caretaker) can cause serious cranial conditions.[89,90] In most studies, a discrepancy has been found between witnessed and nonwitnessed short distance falls, in which the latter lead to severe trauma.

Falls from a great height, such as out of a second-floor window, can lead to serious intracranial conditions, but in these cases the clinical information is usually consistent with this trauma.

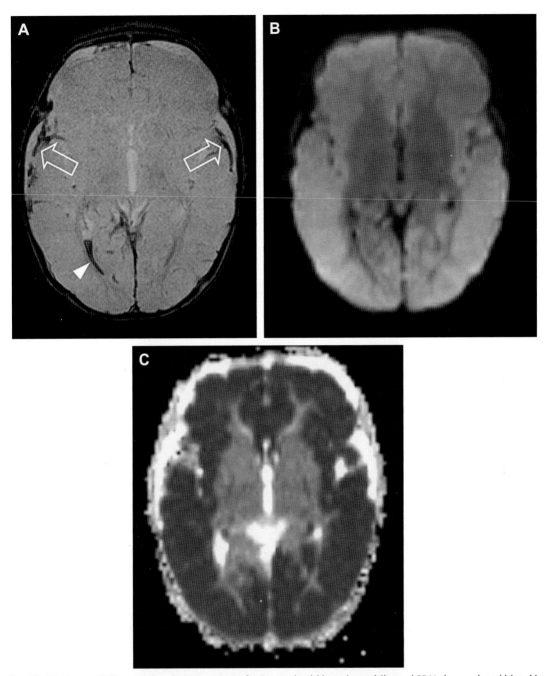

Fig. 16. (*A*) Susceptibility-weighted MR imaging of a 5-month-old boy shows bilateral SDHs (*arrows*) and blood in the posterior right ventricle (*arrowhead*). (*B*) DWI-weighted MR imaging performed during the same session shows extensive restricted diffusion in keeping with cytotoxic edema. (*C*) The corresponding ADC map shows a low attenuation corresponding with the abnormalities seen on DWI, thus confirming the diagnosis of cytotoxic edema.

Skeletal survey

The second most common finding in child abuse, after skin lesions such as bruises and contusions, is fractures.[91,92] In case of CAN, fractures are most likely to occur in younger children, are often multiple, and may show diverse stages of healing.[41,93–95] In

contrast to popular belief, a significant proportion of these children with fractures, especially neonates and infants, show no external physical findings (eg, bruises or hematomas) of the injury.[96,97]

Given the current discussion on the cause of AHT and the legal value of the classic triad

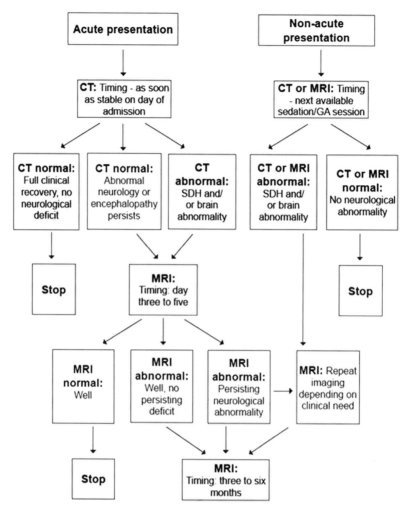

Acute presentation

Non-acute presentation

CT: Timing - as soon as stable on day of admission

CT or MRI: Timing - next available sedation/GA session

CT normal: Full clinical recovery, no neurological deficit

CT normal: Abnormal neurology or encephalopathy persists

CT abnormal: SDH and/or brain abnormality

CT or MRI abnormal: SDH and/or brain abnormality

CT or MRI normal: No neurological abnormality

Stop

MRI: Timing: day three to five

Stop

MRI normal: Well

MRI abnormal: Well, no persisting deficit

MRI abnormal: Persisting neurological abnormality

MRI: Repeat imaging depending on clinical need

Stop

MRI: Timing: three to six months

Fig. 17. Imaging algorithm for suspected AHT as proposed by the RCR and the RCPCH. (*From* The Royal College of Radiologists and the Royal College of Paediatrics and Child Health. Standards for radiological investigations of suspected non-accidental injury. London: RCR and RCPCH; 2008. p. 35; with permission.)

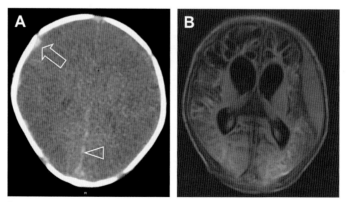

Fig. 18. (*A*) CT scan of a 1-month-old boy showing a right-sided SDH (*arrow*) and an SDH in the posterior inter-hemispheric fissure (*arrowhead*). (*B*) MR imaging obtained 1 month later shows severe multicystic encephalopathy and a large left-sided subdural effusion.

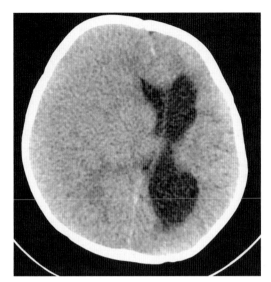

Fig. 19. CT scan of a 4-month-old boy with anemia (hemoglobin level 3.5) shows shift of the midline. The surgically proven SDH is isodense compared with brain tissue and therefore not visible.

(subdural hemorrhages, encephalopathy, and retinal hemorrhages), extracranial findings of CAN may be important in medicolegal proceedings.[98–102]

Imaging

Conventional radiology

The cornerstone of imaging the skeleton in suspected CAN is, and will most likely remain, conventional radiography. The ACR as well as the RCR and RCPCH have published guidelines for the skeletal survey (**Table 2**).[44,46] The difference between them is the addition of oblique chest radiographs in the RCR and RCPCH guideline. Implementation of oblique chest radiographs increases the sensitivity for the detection of rib fractures by 17% (95% CI 2%–36%) and the specificity by 7% (95% CI 2%–13%).[103] Several studies have also shown that adherence to these guidelines is poor, resulting in nondiagnostic examinations (**Fig. 22**).[104–106]

A repeat skeletal survey after 14 days increases sensitivity and specificity in cases with equivocal findings. The skull should be excluded from the follow-up survey, because fractures of the skull do not heal with callus formation. In 2 studies additional information was found, respectively, in 46% and 66% of cases.[107,108]

Other imaging techniques

In children less than the age of 2 to 3 years, the skeletal survey is the radiological gold standard for detecting fractures and is usually the only evaluation of the skeletal system necessary. Other techniques may have a place in the workup of suspected CAN in older children and in special situations.

Bone scintigraphy can be used in cases of suspected child abuse. Its use is declining, partly because of the marginal sensitivity and specificity and partly because of the radiation dose involved. Its strength lies in the detection of occult fractures in more anatomically complex and rarely involved locations such as the ribs, pelvis, and feet, although it is less sensitive for detection of metaphyseal fractures now known as classic

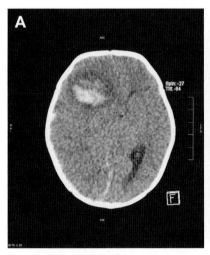
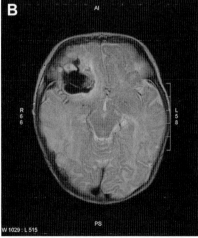

Fig. 20. (A) CT scan of a 4-week-old girl with an intracranial parenchymal hemorrhage. Layering, as a result of sedimentation, is visible in the hemorrhage. (B) MR imaging of the same patient was performed to rule out an underlying vascular malformation. T2-weighted imaging clearly delineates the parenchymal location of the hemorrhage. Laboratory investigation showed that this patient suffered from α_1-antitrypsin deficiency.

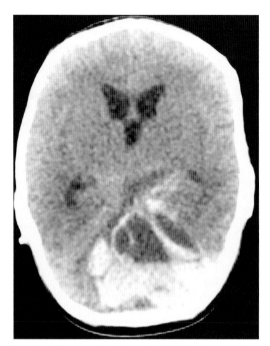

Fig. 21. CT scan of a 6-week-old girl shows a large hematoma in the posterior fossa. The child was exclusively breastfed and had not received vitamin K, resulting in a bleeding diathesis.

metaphyseal lesions (CMLs), a distinctive finding in CAN.[42,109–113]

In the trauma setting, there is an increasing use of CT of the skeleton. This practice might lead to the conclusion that CT, if performed at admission, could replace the skeletal survey.[114,115] In a retrospective study of 45 pediatric trauma patients, 18 of 45 (40%) patients had findings only at CT, including 2 patients with rib fractures.[116] A recent postmortem study showed a higher sensitivity of CT over radiography in 56 children.[117] Fractures were seen on radiography in 7 of 12 patients and on CT in 11 of 12 patients. However, the sensitivity and specificity for the detection of middle cranial fossa (MCF) fracture is unknown and expected to be low; this makes CT an invalid technique for the workup of suspected CAN.

In many institutions worldwide, bone scintigraphy is being replaced by whole-body short tau inverse recovery MR imaging (WB-STIR).[118] Because MR imaging has no radiation exposure, it could potentially be a replacement for the skeletal survey. However, in a study in 16 children (age range 1.5–37 months) with positive findings on conventional skeletal survey, WB-STIR had a sensitivity of 75% (33/44) for rib fractures and 67% (2/3) for MCF fracture.[119] In a recent study by Perez-Rossello and colleagues,[120] WB-STIR had a low sensitivity for MCF (31%) and rib fractures (57%). In light of these findings, the use of WB-STIR is not advised.

However, MR imaging has proved useful in specific skeletal injuries, especially those involving the growth plates. Injuries of the growth plate of the shoulder, hip, and elbow, in the abused child,

Table 2
Skeletal survey guidelines in suspected CAN

ACR	RCR and RCPCH
Thorax (AP and lateral), to include ribs[a] and thoracic and upper lumbar spine	AP thorax, **right and left oblique**[b] views of the ribs
Pelvis (AP), to include the midlumbar spine	Pelvis (AP)
Lumbosacral spine (lateral)	Lumbosacral spine (lateral)
Cervical spine (AP and lateral)	Cervical spine (**lateral**)
Skull (frontal and lateral), additional views if needed: oblique or Towne view	Skull (frontal and lateral), Towne view if occipital injury suspected
Humeri (AP)	Humeri (AP)[c]
Forearms (AP)	Forearms (AP)
Hands (PA)	Hands (PA)
Femora (AP)	Femora (AP)
Lower legs (AP)	Lower legs (AP)
Feet (PA) or (AP)	Feet (AP)

Abbreviations: AP, anteroposterior; PA, posteroanterior.
 [a] Oblique views recommended.
 [b] The difference between guidelines are shown in bold type.
 [c] Coned views are at the discretion of the attending radiologist.
 Data from ACR. ACR practice guideline for skeletal surveys in children. 2006. 17-6-0008; and the RCR and the RCPCH. Standards for radiological investigations of suspected non-accidental injury. 2008.

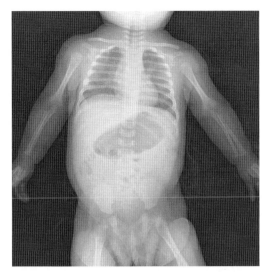

Fig. 22. A poor, and therefore often nondiagnostic, skeletal survey in a 2-month-old girl.

are not uncommon. These injuries are also known as epiphyseal separations and are difficult to detect if they involve only the growth plate and have no displacement (Salter-Harris I type). Although soft tissue swelling may be present, the acute fracture may not be apparent on radiographs especially when only 1 view is obtained

with a skeletal survey. This type of fracture may be detected with whole-body MR imaging examination or, if clinically suspected, site-specific MR imaging is useful for delineation and further characterization (**Fig. 23**).

Fractures

As stated earlier, fractures resulting from CAN may be found anywhere in the skeleton. Moreover, they may be multiple and can show diverse states of healing.[41,93–95]

An older study in the United States showed that, in children younger than 5 years, CAN accounts for approximately 10% of visits to the emergency department (ED).[121] In a study of 258 patients with fractures resulting from abuse, 20.9% had at least 1 medical contact at which signs of abuse were missed.[29] A retrospective case-based analysis of 435 child abuse victims by Carthy and Pierce[122] found 51 children (11.7%) in whom the diagnosis of child abuse could have been made at their first presentation to the hospital. Of these 51 children, 6 (12%) died and 10 (20%) survived with handicaps. A study of deceased children found that 55% had been seen by a physician with the complaint of physical trauma in the month before their demise.[123] These studies highlight the importance of timely detection and correct interpretation of CAN-related fractures.

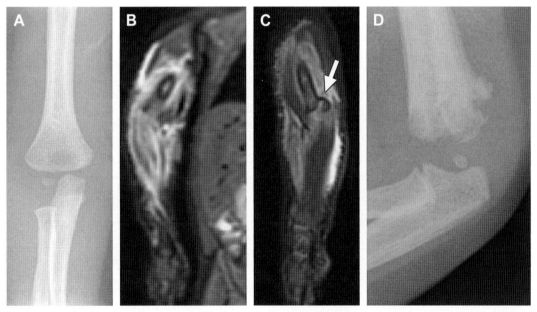

Fig. 23. 8-month-old abused boy brought to emergency department for not using right arm. Infant had multiple fractures. (*A*) Initial anteroposterior radiograph of the right elbow shows no fracture. (*B*) and (*C*) Coronal (*B*) and sagittal (*C*) STIR images of right upper extremity show Salter II-epiphyseal separation injury (*arrow, C*) with extensive hyperintensity in the muscles and subcutaneous tissues. (*D*) Lateral radiograph at 2-week follow-up confirms healing fracture. (*From* Perez-Rossello JM, Connolly SA, Newton AW, et al. Whole-Body MRI in suspected infant abuse. AJR 2010;195:748; with permission.)

Rib fractures

Rib fractures are the hallmark radiological findings of CAN, especially in cases of AHT. The most common mechanism is anterior-posterior compression of the chest.[124,125] In this situation excessive leverage of the ribs over the transverse processes of the vertebrae can lead to posterior rib fractures. These fractures can be clinically silent and found incidentally (**Fig. 24**).[126,127] Barsness and colleagues,[128] in a retrospective study, assessed the PPV of rib fractures in relation to CAN. Based on their findings in children less than 3 years of age, the PPV for abuse was 95%.

Metaphyseal fractures

Metaphyseal fracture or CML, first described by the pediatric radiologist John Caffey in 1957 and further elucidated in a landmark study by Kleinman and colleagues published in 1985, is also a highly specific finding for abuse.[129,130] CML is found mostly in the distal femur, proximal and distal tibia/fibula, and proximal humerus (**Fig. 25**).[129]

Dating fractures

As in the case of CT and MR imaging of AHT, dating of fractures in the context of child protection is often requested. Most often radiologists use the table published by Connor and Cohen in Kleinman's book on child abuse imaging (**Table 3**).[131] However, the scientific support for dating is poor. In a systematic review of 1556 papers by Prosser and colleagues,[132] only 3 studies, with combined data on 189 children, could be included. Based on this meta-analysis, the investigators concluded that fracture dating in children is an inexact science,

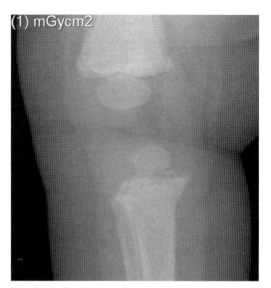

Fig. 25. Radiograph of the right knee of a 4-month-old boy shows CMLs of the distal femur and proximal tibia. Periosteal reaction, generally indicating a more severe injury, is also visible.

but that radiologists should be able to differentiate recent from old fractures.

Differential Diagnosis

In every fracture, a differential diagnosis should always be kept in mind, including CAN. Besides accidental trauma, the attending physician should think of disorders related to collagen production and bone mineralization, as well as other diseases leading to an increased risk in bone fragility. There are diseases that may mimic fractures, such as skeletal dysplasias, but also more common entities such as osteomyelitis or sickle cell disease. Normal variants such as metaphyseal step-off, metaphyseal spur, and physiologic subperiosteal

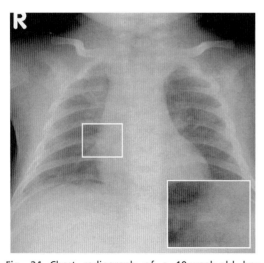

Fig. 24. Chest radiograph of a 10-week-old boy admitted to the hospital after AHT. A posterior rib fracture, showing callus formation, is seen (*inset*).

Table 3
Radiological fracture dating

Radiological Finding	Timing	Comment
Periosteal reaction	Minimum 1 wk	
Hard callus	Minimum 2–3 wk, peak 3–6 wk	Long time-distribution tail after 6 wk
Signs of remodeling	Minimum 8 wk	

Data from Refs.[146–149]

new bone formation may present as diagnostic dilemmas, especially for radiologists with a limited experience in pediatric radiology. The interested reader is referred to textbooks for an in-depth discussion on the differential diagnosis of pediatric fractures.[133]

REPORTING RADIOLOGICAL STUDIES IN CAN

When a radiological interpretation is written in a case of suspected or proven child abuse, the radiologist should be aware that the document can be critical in the decision to report the abuse to the authorities.[134,135] Moreover, the report can, and in most severe cases of child abuse most likely does, become part of legal proceedings.

The radiology report should specifically state the quality of the study and, in the case of a skeletal survey, adherence to international guidelines.[136] Every abnormality found on the radiological studies should be specifically documented and the radiologist should state the level of certainty. If the presence of a lesion is uncertain, it is advised that arrangements, in cooperation with the attending pediatrician, are made for follow-up studies and that this process is monitored. Although it has been shown that repeat skeletal survey can have a significant impact on patient care, this is performed only in some children.[107,108] The report should contain a detailed discussion of the relevant differential diagnosis and should have a clear and concise conclusion.[45] The findings should be discussed with the attending pediatrician and preferably the hospital's CAT, because the diagnosis of CAN depends on clinical, diagnostic, and social findings.

It is essential that the radiology report is as factual and objective as possible and that it reflects the level of uncertainty as it is reported in medical literature.[137] The radiologist should have expertise in pediatric radiology or at least be experienced in cases of child abuse and its differential diagnosis. If such a consultant is not available, then a local or national expert should be sought. It is important that the written report reflects medical and scientific state-of-the-art knowledge. It is also imperative to keep in mind that the report is, in general, read by nonmedically trained people. This factor makes it essential that difficult medical terminology, including Latin nomenclature, is explained.

The radiologist may be asked to testify as a result of primary clinical involvement, because of rendering a second opinion in a case, or as an expert witness. Before accepting an invitation to act as an expert witness, it is important to confirm that there is no conflict of interest and that they have the experience, knowledge, and expertise to act as an expert witness. In court, it is important that the radiologist's testimony states facts and that these facts are within the radiologist's field of knowledge and expertise.[137] The use of a diagram of the skeleton indicating the location of the lesions is something to be considered. The expert also should keep in mind that judges are not trained in statistical sciences. For example, it has been shown that they have difficulty with error rate, with only 4% showing a clear understanding of this principle.[138,139]

The position of an expert in a court case is exceptional; in contrast to other witnesses, they may give an opinion and not just state facts. However, this special position entails a moral obligation on the part of the expert that the opinions expressed are objective and well justified. In this respect, the RCP and the RCPCH in a joint statement specifically said that "the courtroom is not a place used by Doctors to fly their personal kites or push a theory from the far end of the medical spectrum."[140] In the United States, the Supreme Court has ruled (Frye v United States, 293 F 1013 (DC Cir 1923)) that testimony is admissible if it has achieved "general acceptance in the relevant scientific committee." The reporting radiologist should be aware of who has access to the report. In some cases the report can be kept confidential and accessible only to the requesting party; in other cases the report is made available to all parties involved.

There have been several publications on the role of the radiologist as expert witness. Although most of these publications are focused on malpractice cases, they make interesting reading for the radiologist involved in criminal prosecutions.[141–145]

SUMMARY

Radiological imaging plays a crucial role in the detection of physical child abuse. The result and interpretation of radiological studies in suspected CAN may have a serious impact on the patient's welfare as well as their social environment. Radiologists involved in this field of expertise should be aware of the differential diagnosis. When radiological studies obtained in cases of suspected CAN are interpreted and reported, the radiologist should be aware that the report could become part of legal proceedings and that the report should be factual and without bias. From the perspective of optimal patient care in the evaluation of child abuse, it is imperative that the pediatric radiologist is part of the group of pediatric specialists, the so-called CAT.

REFERENCES

1. Prevention of child abuse and neglect: making the links between human rights and public health. Geneva: World Health Organization [WHO] Department of Injuries and Violence Prevention; 2001.
2. US Department of Health and Social Services–Administration for Children and Families. Abuse, neglect and foster care research; national incidence study of child abuse and neglect (NIS-4), 2009-2009. Available at: http://www.acf.hhs.gov/programs/opre/abuse_neglect/natl_incid/index.html. 2010. Accessed January 18, 2011.
3. Public Health Agency of Canada. Canadian Incidence Study of Reported Child Abuse and Neglect–Major Findings–2003. Available at: http://www.phac-aspc.gc.ca/cm-vee/csca-ecve/toc-eng.php. 2011. Accessed January 18, 2011.
4. van IJzendoorn MH, Prinzie P, Euser EM, et al. Kindermishandeling in Nederland Anno 2005: De Nationale Prevalentiestudie Mishandeling van Kinderen en Jeugdigen (NPM-2005). 2007.
5. Laming, H. The Victoria Climbié inquiry. Available at: http://www.victoria-climbie-inquiry.org.uk. 2006. Accessed January 10, 2007.
6. Felitti VJ, Anda RF, Nordenberg D, et al. Relationship of childhood abuse and household dysfunction to many of the leading causes of death in adults. The Adverse Childhood Experiences (ACE) Study. Am J Prev Med 1998;14(4):245–58.
7. Corso PS, Fertig AR. The economic impact of child maltreatment in the United States: are the estimates credible? Child Abuse Negl 2010;34(5):296–304.
8. The Royal College of Pathologists. Report of a meeting on the pathology of traumatic head injury in children. Available at: http://www.rcpath.org/resources/sbs_meeting_report_final.pdf. 2009. Accessed January 19, 2011.
9. Duhaime AC, Christian CW, Rorke LB, et al. Nonaccidental head injury in infants–the "shaken-baby syndrome". N Engl J Med 1998;338(25):1822–9.
10. Caffey J. Multiple fractures in the long bones of infants suffering from chronic subdural hematoma. Am J Roentgenol Radium Ther Nucl Med 1946;56:163–73.
11. Kempe CH, Silverman FN, Steele BF, et al. The battered-child syndrome. JAMA 1982;251:3288–94.
12. Caffey J. On the theory and practice of shaking infants. Its potential residual effects of permanent brain damage and mental retardation. Am J Dis Child 1972;124(2):161–9.
13. Bandak FA. Shaken baby syndrome: a biomechanics analysis of injury mechanisms. Forensic Sci Int 2005;151(1):71–9.
14. Barnes PD, Galaznik J, Gardner H, et al. Infant acute life-threatening event–dysphagic choking versus nonaccidental injury. Semin Pediatr Neurol 2010;17(1):7–11.
15. Coglan A. Doctor gagged for doubting shaken baby syndrome. New Scientist; 2010. 23-8-2010.
16. Dyer C. Diagnosis of "shaken baby syndrome" still valid, appeal court rules. BMJ 2005;331(7511):253.
17. Galaznik JG. Thin-films of subdural hemorrhage in the absence of mechanical trauma: the new challenge of an expanding differential. Pediatr Radiol 2009;39(8):882–3.
18. Geddes JF, Tasker RR, Hackshaw CD, et al. Dural haemorrhage in non-traumatic infant deaths: does it explain the bleeding in 'shaken baby syndrome'? Neuropathol Appl Neurobiol 2003;29:14–22.
19. Punt J. Inflicted head injury in infants: issues arising from the Geddes hypothesis. Arch Dis Child 2006;91(8):714–5.
20. Talbert DG. Shaken baby syndrome: does it exist? Med Hypotheses 2009;72(2):131–4.
21. Christian CW, Block R. Abusive head trauma in infants and children. Pediatrics 2009;123(5):1409–11.
22. Glick JC, Staley K. Inflicted traumatic brain injury: advances in evaluation and collaborative diagnosis. Pediatr Neurosurg 2007;43(5):436–41.
23. Maguire S, Pickerd N, Farewell D, et al. Which clinical features distinguish inflicted from non-inflicted brain injury? A systematic review. Arch Dis Child 2009;94(11):860–7.
24. Levin AV, Christian CW. The eye examination in the evaluation of child abuse. Pediatrics 2010;126(2):376–80.
25. Morad Y, Wygnansky-Jaffe T, Levin AV. Retinal haemorrhage in abusive head trauma. Clin Experiment Ophthalmol 2010;38(5):514–20.
26. Jenny C, Hymel KP, Ritzen A, et al. Analysis of missed cases of abusive head trauma. JAMA 1999;281(7):621–6.
27. Oral R, Yagmur F, Nashelsky M, et al. Fatal abusive head trauma cases: consequence of medical staff missing milder forms of physical abuse. Pediatr Emerg Care 2008;24(12):816–21.
28. Rao P, Carty H. Non-accidental injury: review of the radiology. Clin Radiol 1999;54(1):11–24.
29. Ravichandiran N, Schuh S, Bejuk M, et al. Delayed identification of pediatric abuse-related fractures. Pediatrics 2010;125(1):60–6.
30. Minns RA, Busutttil A. Patterns of presentation of the shaken baby syndrome–four types of inflicted brain injury predominate [letter]. BMJ 2004;328:766.
31. Dunning J, Daly JP, Lomas JP, et al. Derivation of the children's head injury algorithm for the prediction of important clinical events decision rule for head injury in children. Arch Dis Child 2006;91(11):885–91.

32. Rao P, Carty H, Pierce A. The acute reversal sign: comparison to medical and non-accidental injury patients. Clin Radiol 1999;54:494–501.

33. Merten DF, Osborne D, Radkowski MS, et al. Cranio-cerebral trauma in the child abuse syndrome: radio-logical observation. Pediatr Radiol 1984;14:272–7.

34. Lloyd DA, Carty H, Patterson M, et al. Predictive value of skull radiography for intracranial injury in children with blunt head injury. Lancet 1997; 349(9055):821–4.

35. Quayle KS, Jaffe DM, Kuppermann N, et al. Diagnostic testing for acute head injury in children: when are head computed tomography and skull radiographs indicated? Pediatrics 1997;99(5):E11.

36. Masters SJ. Evaluation of head trauma: efficacy of skull films. AJR Am J Roentgenol 1980;135(3): 539–47.

37. Hofman PA, Nelemans P, Kemerink GJ, et al. Value of radiological diagnosis of skull fracture in the management of mild head injury: meta-analysis. J Neurol Neurosurg Psychiatry 2000;68(4):416–22.

38. Committee on quality improvement, AAoP. The management of minor closed head injury in children. Pediatrics 1999;104(6):1407–15.

39. Fleece DM, Kochan PS. Skull fracture in an infant not visible with computed tomography. J Pediatr 2009;154(6):934.

40. Weir P, Suttner NJ, Flynn P, et al. Normal skull suture variant mimicking intentional injury. BMJ 2006;332(7548):1020–1.

41. Leventhal JM, Thomas SA, Rosenfield NS, et al. Fractures in young children. Distinguishing child abuse from unintentional injuries. Am J Dis Child 1993;14:787–92.

42. Merten DF, Radlowski MA, Leonidas JC. The abused child: a radiological reappraisal. Radiology 1983;146:377–81.

43. Meservy CJ, Towbin R, McLaurin RL, et al. Radiographic characteristics of skull fractures resulting from child abuse. AJR Am J Roentgenol 1987; 149(1):173–5.

44. American College of Radiology (ACR). Standards for skeletal surveys in children. American College of Radiology 1997;23:1–4.

45. ACR practice guideline for skeletal surveys in children. American College of Radiology (ACR); 2006. 17-6-0008. Available at: http://www.acr.org/secon darymainmenucategories/quality_safety/guidelines/ pediatric/skeletal_surveys.aspx. Accessed August 3, 2011.

46. Standards for radiological investigations of suspected non-accidental injury. London: The Royal College of Radiologists and the Royal College of Paediatrics and Child Health; 2008.

47. Amodio J, Spektor V, Pramanik B, et al. Spontaneous development of bilateral subdural hematomas in an infant with benign infantile hydrocephalus: color Doppler assessment of vessels traversing extra-axial spaces. Pediatr Radiol 2005;35(11):1113–7.

48. Chen CY, Chou TY, Zimmerman RA, et al. Pericerebral fluid collection: differentiation of enlarged subarachnoid spaces from subdural collections with color Doppler US. Radiology 1996;201(2): 389–92.

49. McNeely PD, Atkinson JD, Saigal G, et al. Subdural hematomas in infants with benign enlargement of the subarachnoid spaces are not pathognomonic for child abuse. AJNR Am J Neuroradiol 2006; 27(8):1725–8.

50. Zenger MN, Kabatas S, Zenger S, et al. The value of power Doppler ultrasonography in the differential diagnosis of intracranial extraaxial fluid collections. Diagn Interv Radiol 2007;13(2): 61–3.

51. Jaspan T, Narborough G, Punt JA, et al. Cerebral contusional tears as a marker of child abuse–detection by cranial sonography. Pediatr Radiol 1992;22(4):237–45.

52. Chen CY, Huang CC, Zimmerman RA, et al. High-resolution cranial ultrasound in the shaken-baby syndrome. Neuroradiology 2001;43(8):653–61.

53. Ringl H, Schernthaner RE, Schueller G, et al. The skull unfolded: a cranial CT visualization algorithm for fast and easy detection of skull fractures. Radiology 2010;255(2):553–62.

54. Metting Z, Rödiger LA, Stewart RE, et al. Perfusion computed tomography in the acute phase of mild head injury: regional dysfunction and prognostic value. Ann Neurol 2009;66(6):809–16.

55. Duhaime AC, Gennarelli TA, Thibault LE, et al. The shaken baby syndrome. A clinical, pathological, and biomechanical study. J Neurosurg 1987;66(3): 409–15.

56. Rubin DM, Christian CW, Bilaniuk LT, et al. Occult head injury in high-risk abused children. Pediatrics 2003;111(6 Pt 1):1382–6.

57. Mogbo KI, Slovis TL, Canady AI, et al. Appropriate imaging in children with skull fractures and suspicion of abuse. Radiology 1998;208(2):521–4.

58. Laskey AL, Holsti M, Runyan DK, et al. Occult head trauma in young suspected victims of physical abuse. J Pediatr 2004;144(6):719–22.

59. Fickenscher KA, Dean JS, Mena DC, et al. Occult cranial injuries found with neuroimaging in clinically asymptomatic young children due to abusive compared to accidental head trauma. South Med J 2010;103(2):121–5.

60. Hymel KP. Traumatic intracranial injuries can be clinically silent. J Pediatr 2004;144(6):701–2.

61. ACR appropriateness criteria–suspected physical abuse child. J Am Coll Radiol 2011;8(2):87–94.

62. Brenner DJ, Elliston CD, Hall EJ, et al. Estimated risks of radiation induced fatal cancer from pediatric CT. AJR Am J Roentgenol 2001;176:289–96.

63. Paterson A, Frush DP, Donnelly L. Helical CT of the body: are settings adjusted for pediatric patients? AJR Am J Roentgenol 2001;176:297–301.

64. Akiyama Y, Miyata K, Harada K, et al. Susceptibility-weighted magnetic resonance imaging for the detection of cerebral microhemorrhage in patients with traumatic brain injury. Neurol Med Chir (Tokyo) 2009;49(3):97–9.

65. Ashwal S, Babikian T, Gardner-Nichols J, et al. Susceptibility-weighted imaging and proton magnetic resonance spectroscopy in assessment of outcome after pediatric traumatic brain injury. Arch Phys Med Rehabil 2006;87(12 Suppl 2):S50–8.

66. Babikian T, Freier MC, Tong KA, et al. Susceptibility weighted imaging: neuropsychologic outcome and pediatric head injury. Pediatr Neurol 2005;33(3):184–94.

67. Colbert CA, Holshouser BA, Aaen GS, et al. Value of cerebral microhemorrhages detected with susceptibility-weighted MR imaging for prediction of long-term outcome in children with nonaccidental trauma. Radiology 2010;256(3):898–905.

68. Kemp AM, Butler A, Morris S, et al. Which radiological investigations should be performed to identify fractures in suspected child abuse? Clin Radiol 2006;61(9):723–36.

69. Twomey E, Twomey A, Ryan S, et al. MR imaging of term infants with hypoxic-ischaemic encephalopathy as a predictor of neurodevelopmental outcome and late MRI appearances. Pediatr Radiol 2010;40(9):1526–35.

70. Babikian T, Tong KA, Galloway NR, et al. Diffusion-weighted imaging predicts cognition in pediatric brain injury. Pediatr Neurol 2009;41(6):406–12.

71. Liauw L, van Wezel-Meijler G, Veen S, et al. Do apparent diffusion coefficient measurements predict outcome in children with neonatal hypoxic-ischemic encephalopathy? AJNR Am J Neuroradiol 2009;30(2):264–70.

72. Vermeulen RJ, van Schie PE, Hendrikx L, et al. Diffusion-weighted and conventional MR imaging in neonatal hypoxic ischemia: two-year follow-up study. Radiology 2008;249(2):631–9.

73. McKinney AM, Thompson LR, Truwit CL, et al. Unilateral hypoxic-ischemic injury in young children from abusive head trauma, lacking craniocervical vascular dissection or cord injury. Pediatr Radiol 2008;38(2):164–74.

74. Vincent FM. Acute subdural hematomas may appear isodense in anemia. Neurology 1985;35(1):140–1.

75. Barnes PD, Robson CD. CT findings in hyperacute nonaccidental brain injury. Pediatr Radiol 2000;30(2):74–81.

76. Margolin EA, Dev LS, Trobe JD. Prevalence of retinal hemorrhages in perpetrator-confessed cases of abusive head trauma. Arch Ophthalmol 2010;128(6):795.

77. Chiesa A, Duhaime AC. Abusive head trauma. Pediatr Clin North Am 2009;56(2):317–31.

78. Sirotnak AP. Medical disorders that mimic abusive head trauma. In: Frasier L, Rauth-Farley K, Alexander R, et al, editors. Abusive head trauma in infants and children: a medical, legal and forensic reference. 1st edition. St Louis (MO): GW Medical Publishing; 2006. p. 191–226.

79. Barnes PD, Krasnokutsky M. Imaging of the central nervous system in suspected or alleged nonaccidental injury, including the mimics. Top Magn Reson Imaging 2007;18(1):53–74.

80. Fernando S, Obaldo RE, Walsh IR, et al. Neuroimaging of nonaccidental head trauma: pitfalls and controversies. Pediatr Radiol 2008;38(8):827–38.

81. Whitby EH, Griffiths PD, Rutter S, et al. Frequency and natural history of subdural haemorrhages in babies and relation to obstetric factors. Lancet 2004;363(9412):846–51.

82. Looney CB, Smith JK, Merck LH, et al. Intracranial hemorrhage in asymptomatic neonates: prevalence on MR images and relationship to obstetric and neonatal risk factors. Radiology 2007;242(2):535–41.

83. Yilmaz C, Yuca SA, Yilmaz N, et al. Intracranial hemorrhage due to vitamin K deficiency in infants: a clinical study. Int J Neurosci 2009;119(12):2250–6.

84. Brousseau TJ, Kissoon N, McIntosh B. Vitamin K deficiency mimicking child abuse. J Emerg Med 2005;29(3):283–8.

85. Ertekin V, Selimoglu MA, Gursan N, et al. Image and diagnosis. Intracranial haemorrhage due to vitamin K deficiency, as the first symptom of extrahepatic biliary atresia. West Indian Med J 2005;54(6):392, 397.

86. van Hasselt PM, de Koning TJ, Kvist N, et al. Prevention of vitamin K deficiency bleeding in breastfed infants: lessons from the Dutch and Danish biliary atresia registries. Pediatrics 2008;121(4):e857–63.

87. Van WM, De BR, Van D, et al. Vitamin K, an update for the paediatrician. Eur J Pediatr 2009;168(2):127–34.

88. Puckett RM, Offringa M. Prophylactic vitamin K for vitamin K deficiency bleeding in neonates. Cochrane Database Syst Rev 2000;4:CD002776.

89. Lyons TJ, Oates RK. Falling out of bed: a relatively benign occurrence. Pediatrics 1993;92(1):125–7.

90. Nimityongskul P, Anderson LD. The likelihood of injuries when children fall out of bed. J Pediatr Orthop 1987;7(2):184–6.

91. McMahon P, Grossman W, Gaffney M, et al. Soft-tissue injury as an indication of child abuse. J Bone Joint Surg Am 1995;77(8):1179–83.

92. Maguire S, Mann MK, Sibert J, et al. Are there patterns of bruising in childhood which are diagnostic or suggestive of abuse? a systematic review. Arch Dis Child 2005;90(2):182–6.

93. Hobbs CJ, Hanks HGI, Wynne JM. Child abuse and neglect–a clinician's handbook. London and Edinburgh: Churchill Livingstone; 1993.

94. Pierce MC, Bertocci GE. Fractures resulting from inflicted trauma: assessing injury and history compatibility. Clin Pediatr Emerg Med 2006;71: 43–8.

95. Worlock P, Stower M, Barbor P. Patterns of fractures in accidental and non-accidental injury in children: a comparative study. BMJ 1986;293:100–2.

96. Mathew MO, Ramamohan N, Benet GC. Importance of bruising associated with paediatric fractures: prospective observational study. BMJ 1998; 317(7166):1117–8.

97. Valvano T, Binns H, Flaherty E, et al. The reliability of bruising in predicting which fractures are caused by child abuse. In: Pediatric Academic Societies' Abstract Archive 2000–2006, 3140.5.

98. Jaspan T. Current controversies in the interpretation of non-accidental head injury. Pediatr Radiol 2008;38(S3):378–87.

99. Geddes JF, Vowles GH, Hackshaw AK, et al. Neuropathology of inflicted head injury in children. II. Microscopic brain injury in infants. Brain 2001; 124(Pt 7):1299–306.

100. Geddes JF, Hackshaw AK, Vowles GH, et al. Neuropathology of inflicted head injury in children. I. Patterns of brain damage. Brain 2001;124(Pt 7): 1290–8.

101. Mack J, Squier W, Eastman JT. Anatomy and development of the meninges: implications for subdural collections and CSF circulation. Pediatr Radiol 2009;39(3):200–10.

102. Squier W. Shaken baby syndrome: the quest for evidence. Dev Med Child Neurol 2008;50(1):10–4.

103. Ingram JD, Connell J, Hay TC, et al. Oblique radiographs of the chest in nonaccidental trauma. Emerg Radiol 2000;7:42–6.

104. Kleinman PL, Kleinman PK, Savageau JA. Suspected infant abuse: radiographic skeletal survey practices in pediatric health care facilities. Radiology 2004;233(2):477–85.

105. Offiah AC, Hall CM. Observational study of skeletal surveys in suspected non-accidental injury. Clin Radiol 2003;58(9):702–5.

106. van Rijn RR, Kieviet N, Hoekstra R, et al. Radiology in suspected non accidental injury: theory and practice in the Netherlands. Eur J Radiol 2009; 71(1):147–51. [Epub ahead of print].

107. Zimmerman S, Makoroff K, Care M, et al. Utility of follow-up skeletal surveys in suspected child physical abuse evaluations. Child Abuse Negl 2005; 29(10):1075–83.

108. Kleinman PK, Nimkin K, Spevak MR, et al. Follow-up skeletal surveys in suspected child abuse. AJR Am J Roentgenol 1996;167(4):893–6.

109. Conway JJ, Collins M, Tanz RR. The role of bone scintigraphy in detecting child abuse. Semin Nucl Med 1993;23:321–33.

110. Haase GM, Ortiz VN, Sfanakis GN. The value of radionuclide bone scanning in the early recognition of deliberate child abuse. J Trauma 1980;208:73–5.

111. Jaudes PK. Comparison of radiography and radionuclide bone scanning in the detection of child abuse. Pediatrics 1984;73:166–8.

112. Sty JR, Starshak RJ. The role of bone scintigraphy in the evaluation of suspected child abuse. Radiology 1983;146:369–75.

113. Mandelstam SA, Cook D, Fitzgerald M, et al. Complementary use of radiological skeletal survey and bone scintigraphy in detection of bony injuries in suspected child abuse. Arch Dis Child 2003; 88(5):387–90.

114. Fung Kon Jin PH, Dijkgraaf MG, Alons CL, et al. Improving CT scan capabilities with a new trauma workflow concept: simulation of hospital logistics using different CT scanner scenarios. Eur J Radiol 2010. [Epub ahead of print].

115. Wurmb TE, Frühwald P, Hopfner W, et al. Whole-body multislice computed tomography as the first line diagnostic tool in patients with multiple injuries: the focus on time. J Trauma 2009;66(3): 658–65.

116. Renton J, Kincaid S, Ehrlich PF. Should helical CT scanning of the thoracic cavity replace the conventional chest x-ray as a primary assessment tool in pediatric trauma? An efficacy and cost analysis. J Pediatr Surg 2003;38(5):793–7.

117. Hong TS, Reyes JA, Moineddin R, et al. Value of postmortem thoracic CT over radiography in imaging of pediatric rib fractures. Pediatr Radiol 2011;41(6):736–48.

118. Kellenberger CJ, Epelman M, Miller SF, et al. Fast STIR whole-body MR imaging in children. Radiographics 2004;24(5):1317–30.

119. Evangelista P, Barron C, Goldberg A, et al. MRI STIR for the evaluation of nonaccidental trauma in children. In: Pediatric Academic Societies' Abstract Archive 2000–2006, 2912.433.

120. Perez-Rossello JM, Connolly SA, Newton AW, et al. Whole-body MRI in suspected infant abuse. AJR Am J Roentgenol 2010;195(3):744–50.

121. Holten JC, Friedman SB. Child abuse: early case finding in the emergency department. Pediatrics 1968;42(1):128–38.

122. Carty H, Pierce A. Non-accidental injury: a retrospective analysis of a large cohort. Eur Radiol 2002;12(12):2919–25.

123. Lucas DR, Wezner KC, Milner JS, et al. Victim, perpetrator, family, and incident characteristics of

infant and child homicide in the United States Air Force. Child AbuseNegl 2002;26(2):167–86.

124. Kleinman PK, Marks SC Jr, Nimkin K, et al. Rib fractures in 31 abused infants: postmortem radiologic-histopathologic study. Radiology 1996; 200(3):807–10.

125. Worn MJ, Jones MD. Rib fractures in infancy: establishing the mechanisms of cause from the injuries–a literature review. Med Sci Law 2007; 47(3):200–12.

126. Stover B. Diagnostic imaging in child abuse. Radiologe 2007;47(11):1037–48 [in German].

127. Chapman S. Radiological aspects of non-accidental injury. J R Soc Med 1990;83(2):67–71.

128. Barsness KA, Cha ES, Bensard DD, et al. The positive predictive value of rib fractures as an indicator of nonaccidental trauma in children. J Trauma 2003;54(6):1107–10.

129. Kleinman PK, Marks SC, Blackborn B. The metaphyseal lesion in abused infants: a radiologic-histopathologic study. AJR Am J Roentgenol 1985;146:895–905.

130. Caffey J. Some traumatic lesions in growing bones other than fractures and dislocations: clinical and radiological features: the Mackenzie Davidson Memorial Lecture. Br J Radiol 1957;30(353): 225–38.

131. O'Connor JF, Cohen J. Dating fractures. In: Kleinman PK, editor. Diagnostic imaging of child abuse. 2nd edition. St Louis (MO): Mosby; 1998. p. 168–77.

132. Prosser I, Maguire S, Harrison SK, et al. How old is this fracture? Radiologic dating of fractures in children: a systematic review. AJR Am J Roentgenol 2005;184(4):1282–6.

133. Bilo RA, Robben SG, van Rijn RR. Normal variants, congenital and acquired disorders. In: Bilo RA, Robben SG, van Rijn RR, editors. Forensic aspects of paediatric fractures; differentiating accidental trauma from child abuse. 1st edition. Berlin: Springer-Verlag; 2009. p. 133–70.

134. Dedouit F, Guilbeau-Frugier C, Capuani C, et al. Child abuse: practical application of autopsy, radiological, and microscopic studies. J Forensci Sci 2008;53(6):1424–9.

135. Jones R, Flaherty EG, Binns HJ, et al. Clinicians' description of factors influencing their reporting of suspected child abuse: report of the Child Abuse Reporting Experience Study Research Group. Pediatrics 2008;122(2):259–66.

136. Adamsbaum C, Méjean N, Merzoug V, et al. How to explore and report children with suspected non-accidental trauma. Pediatr Radiol 2010;40(6): 932–8.

137. Board of the Faculty of Clinical Radiology. TRCoR. Providing expert advice to the court: guidance for members and fellows. London: The Royal College of Radiologists; 2005.

138. Gatowski SI, Dobbin SA, Richardson JT, et al. Asking the gatekeepers: a national survey of judges on judging expert evidence in a post-Daubert world. Law Hum Behav 2001;25(5):433–58.

139. Moreno JA. Einstein on the bench? Exposing what judges do not know about science and using child abuse cases to improve how courts evaluate scientific evidence. Ohio State Law J 2003;64:531–85.

140. Sudden unexpected death in infancy: a multi-agency protocol for care and investigation. The Royal College of Pathologists and The Royal College of Paediatrics and Child Health; 2004. Available at: http://www.rcpath.org/resources/pdf/SUDI%20 report%20for%20web.pdf. Accessed August 3, 2011.

141. Muroff JA, Berlin L. Taming the expert: standards and implications of radiologist expert witness testimony. J Am Coll Radiol 2005;2(5):418–23.

142. Auxier JA. The role of the expert witness. Radiat Res 1989;117(2):178–80.

143. Berlin L, Hoffman TR, Shields WF, et al. When does expert witness testimony constitute a violation of the ACR code of ethics? The role of the ACR Committee on Ethics. J Am Coll Radiol 2006;3(4): 252–8.

144. Brenner RJ. The expert witness: understanding the rationale. J Am Coll Radiol 2007;4(9):612–6.

145. ACR practice guideline on the expert witness in radiology and radiation oncology. American College of Radiology (ACR); 2007. Available at: http://www.acr.org/SecondaryMainMenuCategories/quality_safety/guidelines/dx/expert_witness.aspx. Accessed August 3, 2011.

146. Cumming W. Fractures of the hands and feet in child abuse: imaging and pathologic features. J Can Assoc Radiol 1979;30(30):33.

147. Islam O, Soboleski D, Symons S, et al. Development and duration of radiographic signs of bone healing in children. AJR Am J Roentgenol 2000; 175(1):75–8.

148. Kleinman PK. Diagnostic imaging of child abuse. St Louis (MO): Mosby; 1998.

149. Yeo LI, Reed MH. Staging of healing of femoral fractures in children. Can Assoc Radiol J 1994; 45(1):16–9.

Congenital Cardiovascular Malformations: Noninvasive Imaging by MRI in Neonates

Rajesh Krishnamurthy, MD[a],*, Edward Lee, MD, MPH[b,c]

KEYWORDS

- Neonate • Cardiac • Imaging • MR imaging • Gadolinium
- Indications • Technique

Not too long ago, the perinatal period was fraught with peril for fetuses with severe congenital heart disease (CHD). Neonates presented in a critical condition at birth or in the first week of life, usually following ductal closure. Their survival was diminished by the lack of trained personnel and specialized infrastructure at the place of delivery, and by the emergent nature of the palliative intervention. Owing largely to advances in fetal echocardiography, in most developed countries the diagnosis of severe CHD is now made during gestation, and delivery is electively planned in hospitals that have the facilities and expertise to manage these patients. In the vast majority of cases, postnatal chest radiography and echocardiography (echo) are often the only diagnostic modalities needed for preoperative planning before initial palliation. When echo cannot provide a comprehensive picture of relevant cardiovascular anatomy, MR imaging performs an important complementary role,[1] with diagnostic catheterization being restricted to a small number of patients who need clarification of complex coronary anatomy, or measurement of chamber pressures and oxygen saturation. The role of MR imaging as a sole imaging modality for comprehensive presurgical evaluation is also increasingly being explored for conditions that have complex multisystem involvement, such as heterotaxy, or associated neurologic involvement that must be evaluated before surgery. This review focuses on the imaging of neonatal CHD by MR, followed by a brief discussion of the safety of gadolinium-based contrast agents in this age group.

NEONATAL CARDIAC MR IMAGING TECHNIQUE

Neonatal cardiovascular MR imaging is one of the most difficult imaging challenges in pediatrics, due to the adaptation needed for the complex structural changes in severe CHD, the small size of the structures of interest, rapid heart rate and breathing rate, altered hemodynamics, and the relatively high risk of sedating these sick neonates.[2] It is a dynamic user-dependent examination, with changes to the protocol being needed based on real-time evaluation of the initial sequences.

[a] Edward B. Singleton Department of Pediatric Radiology, Texas Children's Hospital, Baylor College of Medicine, 6701 Fannin Street, Suite 1280, Houston, TX 77030, USA
[b] Pulmonary Imaging, Department of Radiology, Children's Hospital Boston and Harvard Medical School, 300 Longwood Avenue, Boston, MA 02115, USA
[c] Pulmonary Division, Department of Medicine, Children's Hospital Boston and Harvard Medical School, 300 Longwood Avenue, Boston, MA 02115, USA
* Corresponding author.
E-mail address: rxkrishn@texaschildrenshospital.org

Magn Reson Imaging Clin N Am 19 (2011) 813–822
doi:10.1016/j.mric.2011.08.002

Patient Preparation

Before the start of an MR examination in a neonate with CHD, review of the chest radiograph helps to confirm position of the heart in the thorax, which will determine positioning of the electrocardiography (ECG) electrodes. Robust synchronization with the ECG signal using vectorcardiogram triggering as well as the use of respiratory bellows for pulse sequences needing respiratory triggering are part of the standard preparation.

Intravenous Access

Because the first-pass MR angiography is the gold standard for evaluation of the extracardiac vasculature, selecting an appropriate route of contrast administration is critical to the success of the study. In the immediate postnatal period, intravenous access in the arm or leg is preferred to an umbilical venous catheter, which could potentially terminate in an occluded ductus venosus. A 22-gauge or 24-gauge needle is used for intravenous access, with injection rates of 1 to 2 mL per second.

Sedation

Breath-holding will reduce motion blurring, and yield sharper and potentially more diagnostic images. However, breath-holding requires general endotracheal anesthesia (GETA) with controlled ventilation. In the authors' experience, most pulse sequences can be performed in sedated and freely breathing patients to yield diagnostic images, with GETA being restricted to evaluation of very small vascular structures such as aortopulmonary collaterals.

Coil Selection

Phased-array coils are preferred because they allow for the use of parallel imaging techniques, which significantly reduce scan time. A phased-array receive coil that provides adequate coverage should be used. The coverage should extend from the middle of the neck to the level of the renal vessels in all patients, so that important findings outside the thorax such as infradiaphragmatic total anomalous pulmonary venous return (TAPVR) or unusual branching patterns of the head and neck vessels can be identified. Ideal anatomic coverage is provided by the head or shoulder coil in neonates. Newer multipurpose coils such as the head and neck coil or the neurovascular coil are good choices if combined evaluation of the head and cardiovascular system is desired. Dedicated neonatal phased-array cardiac and body coils are becoming increasingly available,

providing an excellent signal with high spatial resolution. MR imaging–compatible incubator/coil combinations have also been introduced, which regulate temperature, humidity, and oxygen concentration while providing monitoring capabilities during transport and scanning for these critical neonates with tenuous hemodynamic and metabolic status.[3]

Pulse Sequences

All sequences have benefited from the advent of parallel imaging, which uses information from multiple coil elements to speed up acquisition or increase temporal resolution. The following is a summary of pulse sequences used for neonatal imaging.

Black-blood sequences

The most commonly used sequences are fast spin echo double-inversion recovery sequence, performed with ECG gating and breath-holding, or a spin echo echoplanar imaging sequence, performed with ECG gating and free breathing. In the free-breathing sequences, respiratory motion is compensated by multiple signal averages with or without respiratory triggering. Black-blood sequences provide multislice static images, with excellent spatial resolution even in neonates. These sequences provide an overview of vascular anatomy, spatial chamber relationships, airway morphology, and abdominal visceral anatomy.

Bright-blood sequences

The most commonly used cine sequence is segmented k-space steady-state free precession (SSFP). It has excellent temporal resolution, allowing for multiphase evaluation across the cardiac cycle, and optimal myocardial and blood pool contrast. However, cine SSFP is limited by out-of-plane flow-related phase incoherence artifact, especially in small patients with rapid flow. In addition, the spatial resolution achievable in cine SSFP is limited. Therefore, the old "workhorse" sequence, cine fast gradient echo (cine GRE) with segmented k-space sequence, is preferred to the SSFP sequence when thin slices with high resolution are required in neonates. Cine GRE can be acquired with free breathing and multiple signal averaging. It is more sensitive to in-plane intravoxel dephasing signal loss from flow turbulence, which can be used as an important diagnostic clue to the presence of shunts, stenosis, and regurgitation. In the neonatal period, the cine GRE sequence is frequently performed in the axial plane with overlapping thin slices, to track the course of the extracardiac vasculature and to determine venoatrial connections.

Alternatively, isotropic whole heart coverage using a 3-dimensional (3D) SSFP sequence with respiratory navigator gating has been used to provide comprehensive static, high-resolution morphologic bright-blood evaluation of intracardiac morphology, coronary anatomy, and extracardiac vascular anatomy in one sequence. It can serve as an alternative (or backup) angiographic data set, and is not subject to the vagaries of distribution of intravenous contrast. However, this technique is not available on all magnet platforms, and is not as robust in small children or in those with high heart rates. Tips to increase the quality of 3D SSFP imaging in neonates with high heart rates include using high spatial resolution (<1 mm isotropic), small respiratory navigator window (2–3 mm), small shot duration (50–70 milliseconds), timing the acquisition to end-systole, low parallel imaging factor, and dedicated phased-array coils with a larger number of elements.

Flow velocity mapping is accomplished by a gradient echo–based pulse sequence known as phase contrast (PC). PC imaging can be used to quantify stroke volume, valvular regurgitation, Qp:Qs, differential pulmonary artery flow, venous return, coronary flow, and pressure gradients across stenoses using the modified Bernoulli equation. There is usually little role for PC imaging in the preoperative setting in neonates.

MR angiography

The most common sequence used is contrast-enhanced MR angiography (CEMRA) performed in dynamic fashion following bolus injection of gadolinium using a 3D T1-weighted fast gradient echo sequence. CEMRA provides a high-resolution 3D data set, with its main application being evaluation of the extracardiac thoracic vasculature, including the pulmonary arteries, pulmonary veins, aorta, systemic veins, and collateral blood supply to the lungs.[4] CEMRA may be performed in a time-resolved fashion even in neonates with high heart rates by incorporating k-space undersampling techniques such as keyhole, with parallel imaging techniques such as SENSE (sensitivity encoding) and centric encoding of k-space to achieve highly accelerated dynamic times of up to 1 to 2 seconds while preserving spatial resolution (**Fig. 1**).[5] When used as a time-resolved technique, MR angiography also provides the added advantage of reliable first-pass imaging, which is independent of timing of contrast injection or acquisition, and dynamic information, which provides insights into the hemodynamics of the disease process. Techniques of postprocessing include multiplanar reformatting, maximum-intensity projection, volume rendering, and virtual endoscopy.

Imaging planes

Black-blood imaging is performed in the axial, oblique sagittal, or coronal planes, with the latter being aligned along the trachea and proximal bronchi. Bright-blood imaging is most commonly performed in the axial plane to track the course of the extracardiac vasculature. Vertical long-axis, 4-chamber, and short-axis planes are also routinely used, with right ventricular and left ventricular outflow tract views, aortic root short-axis views, with customized planes to image the aortic arch or pulmonary arteries being used whenever necessary. 3D MR angiograms are performed in the sagittal or coronal planes.

PROTOCOLS AND INDICATIONS FOR NEONATAL CARDIAC MR IMAGING

Initial palliation stands for first-stage surgical procedures that are typically done immediately after birth to stabilize the patient, including relieving pulmonary vein, pulmonary artery, or aortic outflow obstruction, augmentation of pulmonary blood flow with a modified Blalock-Taussig (BT) shunt, or reducing pulmonary blood flow with a pulmonary artery band. Echocardiography is an excellent tool in expert hands, providing most of the information required for planning initial palliation. However, it may be limited in some situations because of a narrow field of view, lack of acoustic windows, and inability to delineate complex spatial relationships and the extracardiac vascular anatomy, especially pulmonary veins, systemic veins, aortic arch, and arterial collaterals. MR imaging is complementary in this setting, providing a high-resolution 3D data set, with excellent delineation of complex spatial relationships and the extracardiac vascular anatomy with a high degree of diagnostic confidence. In a study comparing MR imaging with echocardiography and cardiac catheterization in presurgical planning of heterotaxy, accurate delineation of pulmonary venous connections was not achieved by echocardiography in 42% of patients, and by catheterization in 25% of patients. The interobserver agreement was also better on MR imaging relative to echocardiography or catheterization.[6]

A short and efficient MR imaging study is paramount in neonatal patients because neonatal patients with severe CHD are potentially unstable. A comprehensive evaluation is neither desirable nor feasible. The imaging question for MR imaging is discrete, frequently pertaining to the status of the pulmonary and systemic vasculature.

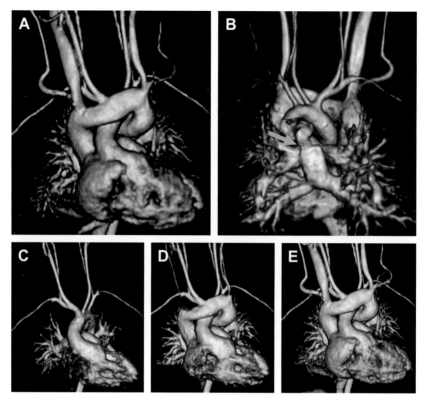

Fig. 1. Time-resolved MR angiography in a neonate. A newborn with functional single ventricle, and supracardiac total anomalous pulmonary venous return with suspicion of pulmonary venous obstruction on echo. (*A, B*) Anterior and posterior views of a 3-dimensional (3D) volume-rendered MR angiography using keyhole, SENSE (sensitivity encoding), and CENTRA (contrast-enhanced timing robust angiography), showing the anomalous vertical vein draining into the left innominate vein, with associated obstruction caused by mass effect from the left mainstem bronchus (*arrow* in *B*). (*C–E*) Anterior projections from successive dynamics of the time-resolved MR angiography showing successive filling of the aorta and pulmonary artery, pulmonary veins, and the systemic veins on (*C*), (*D*), and (*E*), respectively, following a lower-extremity intravenous injection of contrast.

Therefore, the MR imaging protocol is usually limited to axial and oblique cine GRE sequence performed with 3- to 4-mm slice thickness with overlap to diminish errors related to volume averaging, thin-section black-blood images in the axial and/or oblique planes through the chest, and a high-resolution gadolinium-enhanced 3D MR angiogram. Functional/flow/myocardial evaluation is not routinely performed unless it provides important diagnostic or prognostic information that is not available on echo.

A discussion of common indications for neonatal cardiac MR imaging follows, with suggestions on protocol modifications based on indication:

Evaluation of Cardiac Morphology

Echo is quite successful in delineating intracardiac morphology and function in this age group, including atrial, ventricular, and great arterial relationships, valvular status, and ventricular function,

and is aided by the liberal acoustic windows and the ability to use high-resolution transducers. There are only a few indications for MR imaging or computed tomography (CT) for determining intracardiac morphology, and they involve rare entities with complex segmental anatomy, alterations of the chest wall that affect acoustic windows, or entities that require rigorous quantitation of morphologic and functional parameters for decision making regarding management. Examples include:

- Clarification of unusual or complex segmental cardiac anatomy, as in some types of single ventricle (**Fig. 2**), criss-cross atrioventricular relationships, ectopia cordis, and conjoined twins with thoracopagus
- In the setting of cardiac tumors, to determine relationship to inflow and outflow pathways, and for tissue characterization
- For decision making regarding single-ventricle or two-ventricle therapy in patients

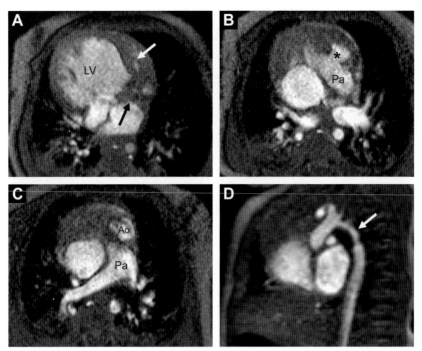

Fig. 2. MR imaging for evaluation of cardiac morphology. A newborn with {S,L,L} transposition of great arteries and tricuspid atresia. MR imaging was performed to assess the status of the aortic arch. (*A*) Four-chamber view of a cine fast gradient echo (cine GRE) sequence showing L-looped ventricles, hypoplastic right ventricle (*white arrow*), and tricuspid atresia (*black arrow*). LV, left ventricle. (*B*) Cranial to *A*, showing restrictive bulboventricular foramen (*asterisk*), leading to a hypoplastic infundibular outlet chamber, and pulmonary artery (Pa) arising from the left ventricle. (*C*) Cranial to *B*, showing L-malposed aorta (Ao) arising from the infundibular outlet chamber. (*D*) Oblique sagittal cine GRE image showing diffuse hypoplasia of the aortic arch (*arrow*) caused by proximal obstruction at the level of the bulboventricular foramen.

with borderline left ventricular hypoplasia,[7] or double-outlet right ventricle
- Assessment of myocardial perfusion and viability in patients with anomalous origin of the coronary artery from the pulmonary artery.[8]

Systemic Evaluation in the Setting of Cardiovascular Disease

There is growing recognition of the fact that CHD is a systemic disease, with cardiovascular, neurologic, and visceral involvement and/or sequelae. Therefore, MR imaging has been used as a "one-stop shop" for neonates with severe CHD to evaluate systemic involvement. MR offers several advantages in this setting, including large field of view, 3D data set with unlimited planes of evaluation, excellent soft-tissue contrast, ability to screen for acute changes like intracranial ischemia and hemorrhage, and screening for stigmata of associated syndromes (**Fig. 3**).

- MR imaging has been used to evaluate the entire spectrum of visceral, cardiac, and vascular abnormalities in heterotaxy in an efficient and accurate manner in comparison with echo.[9] The protocol comprises black-blood imaging performed in the coronal plane, aligned along the trachea and proximal bronchi, a rapid single-shot fast spin echo T2-weighted axial sequence through the abdomen to evaluate the abdominal manifestations of heterotaxy, an axial cine GRE bright-blood sequence with thin, overlapping slices to track the course of the systemic and pulmonary vessels, and gadolinium-enhanced MR angiography (**Fig. 4**).
- MR angiography is also being used for whole-body evaluation in the setting of infantile Marfan syndrome, Loeys-Dietz syndrome, and Kawasaki disease to determine extent of involvement that will determine prognosis and/or intensity of the treatment regimen.
- There is a growing number of large centers that routinely perform MR imaging of the brain of neonates with severe CHD before

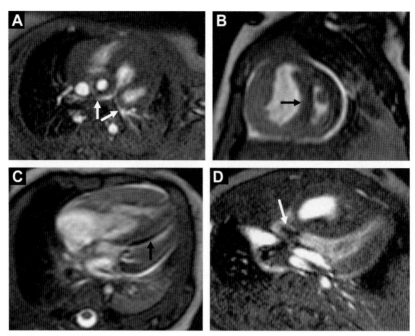

Fig. 3. A 20-day-old male with William syndrome. (*A*) Axial cine GRE image showing diffuse hypoplasia of the main pulmonary artery and bilateral branch pulmonary arteries (*white arrows*). (*B*) Short-axis cine steady-state free precession (SSFP) image showing severe right ventricular hypertrophy with convex bowing of the interventricular septum into the left ventricle (*black arrow*), consistent with pulmonary arterial hypertension and supra-systemic right ventricular pressures. (*C*) Cine SSFP 4-chamber view showing intracavitary flow acceleration within the left ventricle (*arrow*), caused by a combination of convex septal bowing and left ventricle hypertrophy. (*D*) Cine GRE left ventricular outflow tract plane showing supravalvular aortic stenosis, with poststenotic flow turbulence (*arrow*). The patient also had stenosis involving the branches of the abdominal aorta on MR angiography.

major surgery owing to the presence of widespread brain abnormalities, reflecting abnormal brain development in utero[10,11] In addition, new lesions are detected in more than half of the patients in the early postoperative period, mainly in the form of mild ischemic changes. These findings have potential implications for functional and cognitive outcome. The availability of MR imaging–compatible incubators with dedicated neonatal head and cardiac phased-array coils has opened up the possibility for these sick patients of combined cardiac and neurologic evaluation in a safe and efficient manner.

Pulmonary Veins

The most common indication for MR imaging is TAPVR, in which echo is unable to determine the course of the anomalous vein(s) and the site of insertion, or reliably exclude associated obstruction (see **Fig. 1**B). Screening for recurrent pulmonary venous obstruction after TAPVR repair is also a relatively common indication, and can be quite difficult to accomplish by echo in the postoperative setting. A less frequent indication

is neonatal scimitar syndrome, in which MR imaging is used to screen for anomalous pulmonary vein obstruction, aortopulmonary collaterals, lung morphology, and degree of left-right shunting (Qp:Qs). The protocol for pulmonary venous evaluation comprises an axial cine GRE sequence with overlapping thin slices across the pulmonary veins and pulmonary arteries, followed by 3D-CEMRA.

Pulmonary Arteries

Indications for MR imaging evaluation of the pulmonary artery in the neonatal period arise in the setting of pulmonary stenosis or atresia with ventricular septal defect (VSD). If the echo windows are suboptimal, MR imaging is indicated to screen for the source of pulmonary blood flow, confluence of the branch pulmonary arteries (**Fig. 5**), and branch pulmonary artery stenosis before BT shunt placement. The distinction between ductal dependent pulmonary blood flow and/or major aortopulmonary collaterals (MAPCAS) is critical to planning initial palliation in the setting of pulmonary artery/VSD. High-resolution 3D-CEMRA performed with breath-holding is important for optimal evaluation of

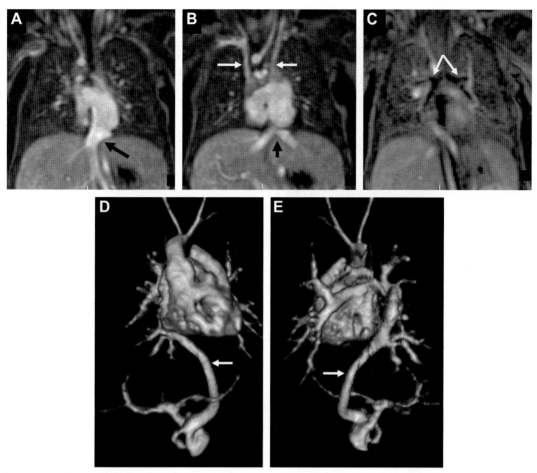

Fig. 4. A newborn with heterotaxy. (*A–C*) Maximum-intensity projections of a 3D contrast-enhanced MR angiography (3D-CEMRA) in a patient with heterotaxy and asplenia showing the inferior vena cava entering the left-sided atrium (*A*), separate insertion of the hepatic veins into the left-sided atrium (*black arrows* in *B*), bilateral superior vena cava without a connecting vein (*white arrows* in *B*), and bilateral eparterial bronchi (*white arrows* in *C*). (*D, E*) Anterior and posterior views of a volume-rendered 3D-CEMRA in the same patient showing infradiaphragmatic total anomalous pulmonary venous return to the portal vein (*white arrow*).

MAPCAS, with relevant findings including the size, number, and location of the collaterals, the presence of any associated stenosis of the collaterals, evidence of dual supply to the pulmonary segments, and any associated lung parenchymal abnormalities. Screening for aortopulmonary collaterals is challenging, and represents a limitation of MR imaging in the neonatal period, with CT angiography being favored in this setting.[1] MR imaging has also been used to diagnose and grade branch pulmonary artery stenosis in the setting of right ventricular outflow tract obstruction, as in Tetralogy of Fallot or single ventricle, before placement of a modified BT shunt to augment pulmonary blood flow. MR imaging can confirm a diagnosis of pulmonary sling, although evaluation of the serious airway abnormalities associated with pulmonary sling is more

reliably performed by CT (**Fig. 6**). An axial cine GRE sequence with overlapping thin slices, and contrast-enhanced MR angiography are usually adequate for morphologic evaluation of pulmonary blood flow, with phase-contrast sequences of the aorta, pulmonary arteries, and pulmonary veins being used if volumetric evaluation of pulmonary flow is desired.

Aorta

Indications for MR imaging of the aorta (**Fig. 7**) are usually in the setting of suspected coarctation, whereby echo is unable to reliably answer questions regarding severity (especially when echo evaluation is limited by the presence of a large patent ductus arteriosus), extent (discrete coarctation vs diffuse hypoplasia of the transverse

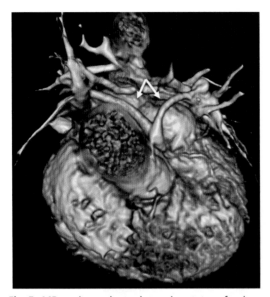

Fig. 5. MR angiography to determine status of pulmonary blood flow. Superior view of a volume-rendered 3D-CEMRA showing severely hypoplastic, but confluent branch pulmonary arteries in a neonate with pulmonary atresia (*white arrows*). The patient had multiple aortopulmonary collaterals as the source of pulmonary blood flow (not shown).

arch), or associated involvement of the head and neck arteries. Other indications include interrupted aortic arch, vascular rings, and rare aortopathies such as infantile Marfan syndrome and Loeys-Dietz syndrome.[12] The protocol comprises high-resolution black-blood, cine GRE and phase-contrast sequences performed in the oblique sagittal plane, aligned along the aortic arch. MR angiography is the best sequence for the aortic arch, providing information on the location, extent, and severity of stenosis, as well as on the presence of collaterals.

THE USE OF GADOLINIUM-BASED CONTRAST AGENTS IN NEONATES

Gadolinium is a toxic metal that binds to membranes, transport proteins, enzymes, lung, liver, spleen and bone. Gadolinium is complexed in a chelate, which allows it to interact with water in the body and provide increased relaxation while preventing free gadolinium from being exposed to body tissues. It is rapidly cleared from the body via glomerular filtration. Gadolinium-containing contrast agents have recently been associated with the development of nephrogenic systemic fibrosis (NSF) in patients with acute or chronic severe renal insufficiency (glomerular filtration rate [GFR] <30 mL/min/1.73 m^2), or acute renal

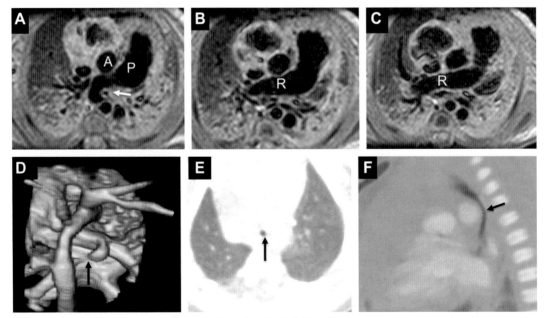

Fig. 6. A 10-day-old male with pulmonary sling. (*A–C*) Black-blood echoplanar T1 images showing anomalous origin of the left pulmonary artery (LPA) from the right pulmonary artery with course between the trachea (*white arrow*) and the esophagus. P is the main pulmonary artery. (*D*) Posterior volume-rendered projection of a 3D-CEMRA showing associated high-grade stenosis of the mid LPA (*black arrow*). (*E, F*) Axial and sagittal images from a computed tomographic angiogram revealing a rounded configuration of the trachea and long-segment tracheal stenosis (*black arrow*), consistent with complete cartilaginous tracheal rings.

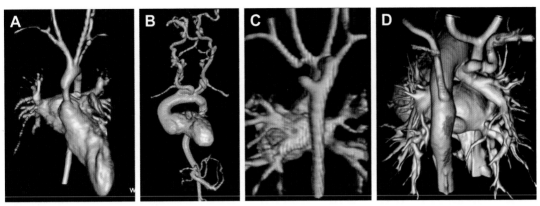

Fig. 7. Applications of MR imaging/MR angiography in the evaluation of aortic pathology in the newborn. 3D volume-rendered images of CEMRA in the following neonatal conditions: (*A*) supravalvular aortic stenosis; (*B*) infantile Marfan syndrome; (*C*) double aortic arch with posterior atresia of the left arch, constituting a vascular ring (posterior view); (*D*) type B interrupted aortic arch, with isolation of the right subclavian artery from the right pulmonary artery, large patent ductus arteriosus, and origin of the left subclavian artery from the proximal descending aorta (posterior view).

insufficiency of any severity due to the hepatorenal syndrome or in the perioperative liver transplantation period.[13]

Neonatal renal function is immature.[14] In normal infants aged 1 week, the mean GFR is 40 mL/min/1.73 m^2; at age 2 to 8 weeks, the GFR is 65 mL/min/1.73 m^2; and over the age of 8 weeks, the GFR is 95 mL/min/1.73 m^2. There is a theoretical possibility that neonates may be more susceptible to NSF because of functional renal immaturity. Therefore, it is recommended that gadolinium be used with caution after careful consideration in children younger than 1 year.[15] Contrast-enhanced MR angiography is performed routinely in children of all age groups on an off-label basis, often with double-dose gadolinium.[4,5,16–18] The pharmacokinetics of gadolinium in children, and follow-up studies specifically screening for NSF, are just starting to be evaluated in rigorous fashion.[19,20] Although there is a dearth of reports on the safety of gadolinium-based contrast agents in neonates and young patients, the existing reports suggest that doses of gadopentetate and gadodiamide of 0.1 to 0.2 mmol/kg are considered to be well tolerated in infants younger than 6 months.[18,19] A few cases of NSF have been reported in older children.[21] Macrocyclic agents such as gadoteridol, gadobutrol, and gadoterate meglumine may offer added protection against NSF, due to their enhanced stability relative to linear agents such as gadodiamide and gadopentetic acid. There is a school of thought that favors use of macrocyclic agents in neonates with functional renal immaturity. Only gadoteridol and gadobutrol are currently available in the United States, and there is no published report of their use in children younger than 2 years. This topic requires further study.

SUMMARY

MR imaging plays an important complementary role to echocardiography in the setting of neonatal CHD. Questions regarding systemic and pulmonary venous return, the status of the aortic arch, and branch pulmonary arteries constitute the bulk of indications for MR imaging. Familiarity with the anatomy before planning the study, achieving adequate sedation to reduce motion artifact, choosing the optimal coil to provide the required anatomic coverage, choosing the appropriate sequences and planes, and adapting the technique to suit the unique morphologic and functional needs in this age group are important prerequisites for a successful neonatal cardiac MR study.

REFERENCES

1. Krishnamurthy R. Neonatal cardiac imaging. Pediatr Radiol 2010;40(4):518–27.
2. Kellenberger CJ, Yoo SJ, Büchel ER. Cardiovascular MR imaging in neonates and infants with congenital heart disease. Radiographics 2007;27(1):5–18.
3. Blüml S, Friedlich P, Erberich S, et al. MR imaging of newborns by using an MR-compatible incubator with integrated radiofrequency coils: initial experience. Radiology 2004;231(2):594–601.
4. Prakash A, Torres AJ, Printz BF, et al. Usefulness of magnetic resonance angiography in the evaluation of complex congenital heart disease in newborns and infants. Am J Cardiol 2007;100(4):715–21.
5. Krishnamurthy R, Slesnick TC, Browne L, et al. Free breathing high temporal resolution time resolved

contrast enhanced MRA (4D MRA) at high rates using keyhole SENSE CENTRA in congenital heart disease. J Cardiovasc Magn Reson 2010; 12(Suppl 1):O31.

6. Geva T, Vick GW 3rd, Wendt RE, et al. Role of spin echo and cine magnetic resonance imaging in presurgical planning of heterotaxy syndrome. Comparison with echocardiography and catheterization. Circulation 1994;90(1):348–56.

7. Grosse-Wortmann L, Yun TJ, Al-Radi OK, et al. Borderline hypoplasia of the left ventricle in neonates: insights for decision-making from functional assessment with magnetic resonance imaging. J Thorac Cardiovasc Surg 2008;136:1429–36.

8. Browne LP, Kearney D, Taylor MD, et al. ALCAPA: the role of myocardial viability studies in determining prognosis. Pediatr Radiol 2010;40(2):163–7.

9. Krishnamurthy R, Chung T. Other complex congenital heart disease—heterotaxy, complex spatial relationships, conjoined twins and ectopia cordis. In: Fogel MA, editor. 'Principles and practice of cardiac magnetic resonance in congenital heart disease: form, function, and flow'. 1st edition. Oxford (United Kingdom): Wiley-Blackwell; 2010. p. 265.

10. Andropoulos DB, Brady KM, Easley RB, et al. Neuroprotection in pediatric cardiac surgery: what is on the horizon? Prog Pediatr Cardiol 2010;29(2):113–22.

11. McQuillen PS. Magnetic resonance imaging in congenital heart disease: what to do with what we see and don't see? [editorial]. Circulation 2009; 119:660–2.

12. Krishnamurthy R, Chung T. Pediatric cardiac MRI. In: Lucaya J, Strife JL, editors. 'Pediatric chest radiology', medical radiology diagnostic imaging. 2nd edition. Berlin: Springer-Verlag; 2007. p. 337.

13. Leiner T, Kucharczyk W. NSF prevention in clinical practice: summary of recommendations and guidelines in the United States, Canada, and Europe. J Magn Reson Imaging 2009;30(6):1357–63.

14. National Kidney Foundation. K/DOQ1 clinical practice guidelines for chronic kidney disease: evaluation, classification and stratification. Am J Kidney Dis 2002;39(Suppl 1):S1–266.

15. Riccabona M, Dacher JN, Olsen OE, et al. Gadolinium and nephrogenic systemic fibrosis—what to consider for pediatric MR imaging. Pediatric NSF Statement 2007. In: Fotter R, editor. Pediatric Uroradiology. 2nd revised edition. Berlin: Springer; 2008. p. 516–7.

16. El-Koussy M, Lövblad KO, Steinlin M, et al. Perfusion MRI abnormalities in the absence of diffusion changes in a case of moyamoya-like syndrome in neurofibromatosis type 1. Neuroradiology 2002; 44(11):938–41.

17. Evans AL, Widjaja E, Connolly DJ, et al. Cerebral perfusion abnormalities in children with Sturge-Weber syndrome shown by dynamic contrast bolus magnetic resonance perfusion imaging. Pediatrics 2006;117(6):2119–25.

18. Tsai-Goodman B, Geva T, Odegard KC, et al. Clinical role, accuracy, and technical aspects of cardiovascular magnetic resonance imaging in infants. Am J Cardiol 2004;94(1):69–74.

19. Martí-Bonmatí L, Vega T, Benito C, et al. Safety and efficacy of Omniscan (gadodiamide injection) at 0.1 mmol/kg for MRI in infants younger than 6 months of age: phase III open multicenter study. Invest Radiol 2000;35(2):141–7.

20. Hahn G, Sorge I, Gruhn B, et al. Pharmacokinetics and safety of gadobutrol-enhanced magnetic resonance imaging in pediatric patients. Invest Radiol 2009;44:776–83.

21. Jain SM, Wesson S, Hassanein A, et al. Nephrogenic fibrosing dermopathy in pediatric patients. Pediatr Nephrol 2004;19(4):467–70.

Congenital Cardiac Defects and MR-Guided Planning of Surgery

Emanuela R. Valsangiacomo Buechel, MD[a],*,
Mark A. Fogel, MD[b,c]

KEYWORDS

- Neonate • Congenital heart disease • Cardiac imaging
- MRI • Cardiac surgery

In neonates and infants with congenital heart disease (CHD), cardiovascular magnetic resonance (CMR) is an established imaging modality in all patients in whom echocardiography does not provide sufficient information and definitive diagnosis.

CMR is nowadays a well-used alternative to angiocardiography because of its noninvasiveness, and the noninvolvement of vascular catheterization or ionizing radiation. Therefore the use of CMR obviates the potential risks of cardiac catheterization in critically ill infants[1]; cardiac catheterization in newborns is limited to catheter-guided interventions, such as atrial septectomy or ductal stenting.

This article discusses the use of CMR in newborns with CHD before cardiac surgery. As imaging of the extracardiac vasculature is discussed in another article in this issue, the authors focus here on conotruncal anomalies, pulmonary venous anomalies, complex CHD in visceroatrial heterotaxy, and borderline hypoplastic left heart syndrome. One separate section is dedicated to the use of contrast medium in newborns.

CONOTRUNCAL ANOMALIES

Conotruncal anomalies are the result of an embryologic septation defect of the conotruncus and include interrupted aortic arch, truncus arteriosus communis, tetralogy of Fallot, pulmonary atresia, double-outlet right ventricle, transposition of the great arteries and ventricular septal defect associated with septal malalignment and/or aortic arch anomalies. Conotruncal anomalies represent the most frequent indication for performing preoperative CMR in newborns.[2] Interruption of the aortic arch and pulmonary blood supply in pulmonary atresia are presented by Krishnamurthy and Lee in another article in this issue.

In general, in conotruncal anomalies axial images acquired at the level of the cardiac basis can provide a first pictorial orientation showing the position of the great arteries within the heart and to each other, and provide an initial clue to the diagnosis of these defects (**Fig. 1**).

TRUNCUS ARTERIOSUS COMMUNIS
Background

Truncus arteriosus communis results from the failure of the conotruncus to divide into a separate aorta and pulmonary artery. Thus characteristic of this anomaly is a single large vessel (truncus) that arises from the midline base of the heart (see **Fig. 1**) and divides into the systemic, pulmonary, and coronary circulations.[3] A ventricular septal

[a] Division of Cardiology, Department of Pediatrics, University Children's Hospital Zurich, Steinwiesstrasse 75, CH-8032 Zurich, Switzerland
[b] Division of Cardiology, Department of Pediatrics, The Children's Hospital of Philadelphia, 34th Street and Civic Center Boulevard, Philadelphia, PA 19104, USA
[c] Department of Radiology, The Children's Hospital of Philadelphia, 34th Street and Civic Center Boulevard, Philadelphia, PA 19104, USA
* Corresponding author.
E-mail address: Emanuela.valsangiacomo@kispi.uzh.ch

Magn Reson Imaging Clin N Am 19 (2011) 823–840
doi:10.1016/j.mric.2011.08.005

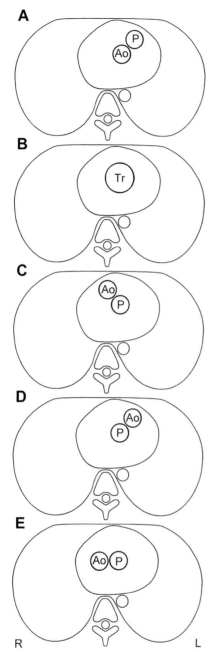

A

B

C

D

E

R   L

Fig. 1. Position of the great arteries in conotruncal anomalies, as seen in axial images at the level of the cardiac base. (A) Normal; (B) truncus arteriosus communis; (C) complete transposition of the great arteries; (D) corrected transposition of the great arteries; (E) double-outlet right ventricle. Ao, aorta; P, main pulmonary artery; Tr, arterial trunk.

defect located below the truncus always occurs. The classification of the different types (I–IV) of the disease is based on the description of the anatomy of the pulmonary arteries, as shown in

Fig. 2.[4] The truncal valve can be thickened or dysplastic and present tricuspid in 40% – 60%, quadricuspid in 25% – 30% and bicuspid in 10% – 30% of the patients.[4,5] Stenosis or regurgitation of the truncal valve is not uncommon. Anomalies of the pulmonary arteries occur rarely; however, isolated origin of a pulmonary artery from a duct or from an aortopulmonary collateral, absence of one pulmonary artery, stenosis or hypoplasia, and crossed or malpositioned pulmonary arteries have been described.[6] The aortic arch is right-sided in about one-third of the patients. Aortic coarctation or interrupted aortic arch is found in 15% to 20% of the cases. Finally, anomalies of the coronary arteries may present with variable patterns of origin that are independent from the number of truncal leaflets.[3]

Surgical correction for truncus arteriosus communis consists of ventricular septal defect (VSD) closure and insertion of a valved conduit between the right ventricle and the pulmonary arteries. Depending on the type of truncus arteriosus, the conduit can be sutured directly to the pulmonary trunk, or the complete pulmonary bifurcation can be reconstructed. In addition, reconstruction of the truncal valve may be required.

Preoperative Imaging

The following structures need to be carefully assessed by cardiac imaging before surgery:

- Pulmonary arteries
- VSD
- Truncal valve
- Ascending aorta and the aortic arch
- Coronary arteries.

Even if the primary anatomy can usually be defined by neonatal echocardiography, demonstration or exclusion of all potentially associated anomalies may require additional imaging.[5] A stack of axial images, acquired with the spin echo (SE) or the steady-state free precession (SSFP) sequence, demonstrate a single large vessel arising from the midline base of the heart,[7] and the pulmonary arteries, with or without a main stem, originating directly from the common trunk (**Fig. 3**). If several thin slices are acquired parallel to the plane of the truncal valve, the cusps of the truncus valve may be visualized.[8] Contrast-enhanced MR angiography (CEMRA) accurately defines the exact anatomy of the pulmonary arteries and of the aortic arch and its branches (**Fig. 4**). Velocity-encoded phase-contrast imaging (PC cine) can be used for exact quantification of the regurgitant volume and fraction of an insufficient truncal valve.

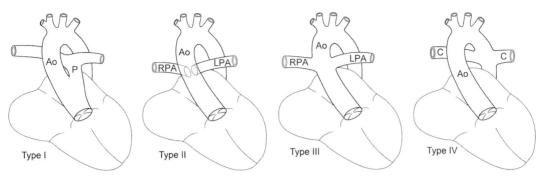

Fig. 2. Collett and Edwards classification of common arterial trunk on the basis of the pulmonary arterial origin. Ao, aorta; C, aortopulmonary collaterals; P, main pulmonary artery; LPA, left pulmonary artery; RPA, right pulmonary artery.

TETRALOGY OF FALLOT

Newborns with uncomplicated native tetralogy of Fallot (TOF) can be usually completely assessed by echocardiography. However, in severe forms with extremely diminutive pulmonary arteries, advanced anatomic imaging is essential for correct planning of a tailored treatment strategy, which usually begins with a palliative intervention and eventually ends with surgical repair. CMR, and particularly CEMRA, can be performed before palliation for visualization of the right ventricular outflow tract, main pulmonary artery, and the side branches.[9] The anatomic findings described will determine the choice of the appropriate palliation procedure, such as surgical Blalock-Taussig shunt or a catheter-guided stenting of the ductus arteriosus, or stenting of the right ventricular outflow tract.[10,11] In the presence of a dual lung supply, when lung perfusion is warranted by both the native pulmonary arteries and aortopulmonary collateral arteries, catheter-guided coiling of

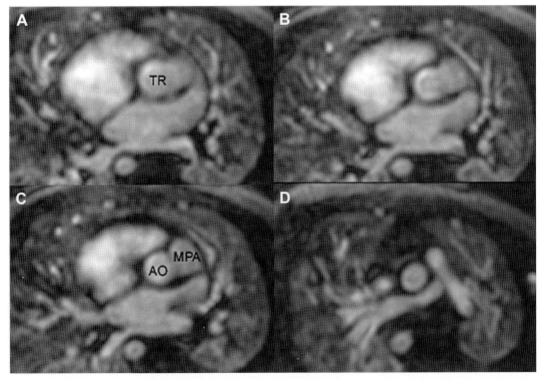

Fig. 3. A stack of steady-state free precession (SSFP) axial images showing (A) a single common trunk (Tr) at the base of the heart, (B, C) the main pulmonary artery (MPA) arising on the left side of the trunk, and (D) more cranially the bifurcation of the side branches. AO, aorta.

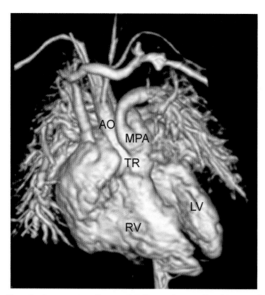

Fig. 4. Contrast-enhanced MR angiography (CEMRA) with 3D reconstruction of a truncus arteriosus communis. AO, Aorta ascendens; LV, left ventricle; MPA, main pulmonary artery; RV, right ventricle; TR, truncus arteriosus.

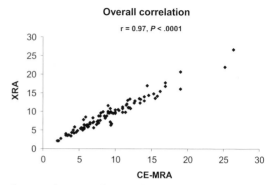

Fig. 5. The correlation between vascular measurements performed on CEMRA images and on conventional angiography (XRA) images. (*From* Valsangiacomo Büchel ER, DiBernardo S, Bauersfeld U, et al. Contrast-enhanced magnetic resonance angiography of the great arteries in patients with congenital heart disease: an accurate tool for planning catheter-guided interventions. Int J Cardiovasc Imaging 2005;21(2):313–22; with permission.)

selected aortopulmonary collaterals at the time of palliation increases flow into the native pulmonary arteries and therefore their growth.

During follow-up, CMR is the ideal tool for documenting growth of the pulmonary arteries and for planning surgical repair or other interventions. The accuracy of measurements of the vessel size on CEMRA images has been previously demonstrated even for vessels as small as 2 mm (**Fig. 5**).[12]

Such individually tailored management with a staged treatment approach, supported by repeated imaging of the pulmonary arteries, may eventually result in a successful surgical repair.[13]

DOUBLE-OUTLET RIGHT VENTRICLE
Background

Double-outlet right ventricle (DORV) is defined by a ventriculoarterial connection in which both great arteries arise completely or predominantly from the morphologically right ventricle (see **Fig. 1**). The spatial relationship of the great arteries to each other shows a wide spectrum, ranging from a normal position, to a side-by-side position, to a transposed position.[14] In DORV the ejected stroke volume of the left ventricle passes though a VSD, which is an integral part of the anomaly.[15] On the basis of its spatial relationship to the great arteries, the VSD is classified as subaortal, subpulmonal, doubly committed, or remote. Additional anatomic findings

potentially complicating management include total atrioventricular septal defect (particularly in right atrial isomerism), straddling of the atrioventricular valves, restrictive VSD, multiple VSD, some degree of ventricular hypoplasia, and obstructive anomalies of the aortic arch.[16] DORV has been frequently observed in hearts with right atrial isomerism.[17]

Preoperative Imaging

The diagnosis of DORV is usually done by echocardiography.[15] Initially the defect may be "naturally" palliated, if a pulmonary stenosis is present, or require palliation with a banding of the pulmonary artery or an aortopulmonary shunt. Surgical repair is then performed some months later. The primary aim of surgical correction is to direct blood flow from the left ventricle through the VSD into the aorta.[16] Accurate definition of the size and position of the VSD within the heart and of its relation to the aorta is crucial for planning surgical repair. Beekmana and colleagues[14] and Yoo and colleagues[18] demonstrated the usefulness of cross-sectional CMR for describing the pertinent features of VSD in DORV. By using transverse planes they found that the site of fusion of the outlet septum with the VSD margin was the most important diagnostic feature for differentiating subaortic from subpulmonal VSD; fusion was absent in doubly committed VSD. Similarly, Beekmana and colleagues[14] showed that CMR can accurately assess the spatial relationship between the semilunar valves and the VSD as well as the morphology of both outflow tracts

(**Fig. 6**). In 30% of the cases CMR provided additional information compared with conventional imaging. By contrast, CMR was not reliable in visualizing aberrant chordae tendinae, or straddling of the atrioventricular valves. In addition to intracardiac imaging, CEMRA and its 3-dimensional (3D) reconstructed images complete the anatomic information by showing the extracardiac venous and arterial anatomy in all its possible variances.

TRANSPOSITION OF THE GREAT ARTERIES
Complete Transposition of the Great Arteries

Transposition of the great arteries (TGA) can be entirely diagnosed by echocardiography. The most common associated anomalies include a VSD, left ventricular outflow tract obstruction, atrial septal defect, patent ductus arteriosus, and anomalies of the aortic arch such as right aortic arch, aortic coarctation, and double aortic arch. The origins of the coronary arteries are widely variable and need to be exactly described preoperatively, as during the arterial switch operation the surgeon will transfer the coronary arteries into the neo-aorta.

Advanced imaging is rarely required preoperatively, and occurrence of TGA in more complex CHD is the main indication for performing CMR in these patients (**Fig. 7**).

Congenitally Corrected Transposition of the Great Arteries

Congenitally corrected TGA (cTGA) is an entity characterized by atrioventricular and ventriculoarterial discordance. The right atrium is connected to the left ventricle and the left atrium is connected to the right ventricle. The aorta arises from the right ventricle and the pulmonary artery from the left ventricle (see **Fig. 1**). The aorta is located anteriorly and to the left of the pulmonary artery (**Fig. 8**). This defect is called corrected transposition of the great arteries as, unlike in TGA, which is a cyanotic CHD, in cTGA the normal hemodynamic pathways are maintained.

Recognition of cTGA at echocardiography can be challenging. Indeed cross-sectional imaging may facilitate the segmental approach to cardiac anatomy. SSFP axial images show the situs, the position of the heart, the systemic and pulmonary venous drainage, the morphology of both atria and both ventricles, and the origin of the great arteries; the connections among the cardiac segments can be accurately analyzed and defined (**Fig. 9**). If needed, subsequent oblique images can be helpful in further delineating the segmental connections. Finally, CEMRA enables recognition of additional cardiac and extracardiac findings.

Additional malformations in cTGA are common[19]:

- VSD (70%)
- Pulmonary valve stenosis (30%–50%)
- Dysplasia of the tricuspid valve (with Ebstein)
- Dextrocardia (20%)
- Situs inversus (5%–8%)
- Anomalies of the conduction system with high risk for complete heart block.

More rarely associated anomalies include superior/inferior position of the ventricles, aortic coarctation, interruption of the aortic arch, hypoplasia of one ventricle, common arterial trunk, and straddling or overriding of the left atrioventricular valve.

ANOMALIES OF THE PULMONARY VEINS
Background

Anomalous pulmonary venous connection is characterized by one or more pulmonary veins connecting to either the right atrium or a systemic vein, or to both. If all 4 pulmonary veins connect anomalously, they usually form a confluence behind the left atrium. This additional vascular structure behind the left atrium can be seen prenatally by fetal echocardiography, and represents one of the clues to the diagnosis of anomalous pulmonary venous connection in the fetus.[20] Total anomalous pulmonary venous connection (TAPVC) is classified as cardiac (27% of cases), supracardiac (51%), or infracardiac (15%) type, depending on the site of drainage (**Fig. 10**). A mixed type of TAPVC (7%) is present if part of the pulmonary

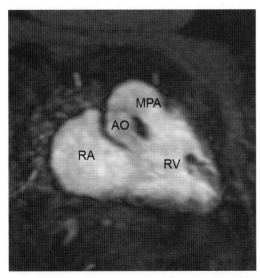

Fig. 6. CEMRA multi-intensity projection (mip) images of a newborn with double-outlet right ventricle. AO, aorta; MPA, main pulmonary artery; RA, right atrium; RV, right ventricle.

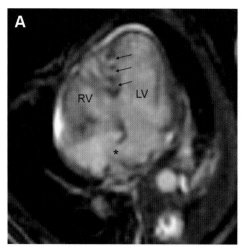
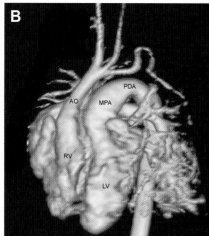

Fig. 7. (A) Complex transposition of the great arteries in a 3-day-old girl with transposition of the great arteries, atrial septal defect (*asterisk*), multiple ventricular septal defects (*arrows*), and suspected aortic coarctation. (B) CEMRA revealed an interrupted aortic arch. AO, aorta; LV, left ventricle; MPA, main pulmonary artery; PDA, patent ductus arteriosus; RV, right ventricle.

veins connects at one level and part to another.[21] In supracardiac or infracardiac type, a pulmonary venous channel, the so-called vertical vein, runs cranially, to drain into the superior systemic vein system, or caudally, crossing the diaphragm to drain into the infradiaphragmatic venous system (**Fig. 11**). Obstruction may occur at different levels within the course of the venous pathway (**Box 1**). Cardiac type and mixed type are often associated with more complex CHD, particularly visceroatrial heterotaxy.

Preoperative Imaging

Newborns with TAPVC present with cyanosis, lung congestion, and pulmonary hypertension, if the

pulmonary venous pathway is obstructed. Thus cardiac surgery is often required on an emergency basis. In these cases a quick and accurate diagnosis is required. Complete evaluation of TAPVC before surgical repair includes:

- Identification of venous confluence
- Identification of individual pulmonary veins joining the confluence

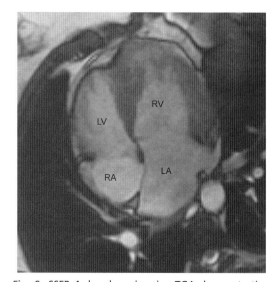

Fig. 9. SSFP 4-chamber view in cTGA demonstrating atrioventricular discordance. Right and left atrium can be distinguished by the morphology of the atrial appendages; right and left ventricle can be distinguished on the basis of characteristic trabeculation and moderator band of the right ventricle. LA, left atrium; LV, left ventricle; RA, right atrium; RV, right ventricle.

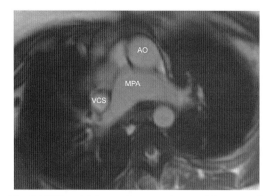

Fig. 8. SSFP axial image in a newborn with congenitally corrected transposition of the great arteries (cTGA). The ascending aorta is located anteriorly to the left of the main pulmonary artery. AO, aorta; MPA, main pulmonary artery; VCS, superior vena cava.

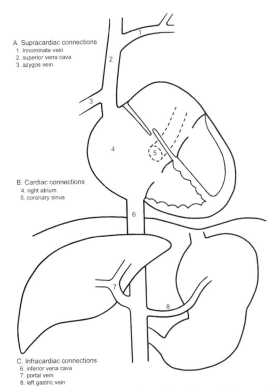

A. Supracardiac connections
1. Innominate vein
2. superior vena cava
3. azygos vein

B. Cardiac connections
4. right atrium
5. coronary sinus

C. Infracardiac connections
6. inferior vena cava
7. portal vein
8. left gastric vein

Fig. 10. Classification and possible sites of abnormal connection in total anomalous pulmonary venous connection.

- Identification of the site or sites of drainage
- Evaluation of any obstruction to the pulmonary venous blood flow
- Evaluation of the intracardiac anatomy
- Evaluation of associated cardiac lesions.

TAPVC can usually be adequately assessed by echocardiography[22]; however, in cases with complex pulmonary venous drainage advanced imaging with angiography is recommended. CMR is an equal alternative to conventional angiography, with some striking advantages in critically ill patients.[23]

Using SE, Masui and colleagues[24] demonstrated better detection rate (95%) for pulmonary venous anomalies, compared with echocardiography (38%) and conventional angiography (69%). Nowadays the SSFP sequence is preferred to SE, owing to the optimum natural contrast between the flowing blood and the surrounding structures, and to the short acquisition times.[25,26]

The introduction of CEMRA dramatically improved the diagnostic performance of CMR. In a group of 30 pediatric patients with pulmonary venous anomalies, the ability to visualize the pulmonary veins was 99% for CEMRA compared with 89% for transthoracic echocardiography. CEMRA provided a new diagnosis in one-third of the cases and clarified uncertain findings in another third.[27] Because the pulmonary veins are located close to other cardiac structures that may superimpose on overview images, the authors recommend reconstruction of the angiographic data, with the multi-intensity projection (mip) technique, as it allows visualization of each vein in two planes perpendicular to each other (double-oblique technique) and definition of their relationship to the adjacent structures in different views.

In patients for whom gadolinium has to be avoided, a stack of SSFP images in all 3 planes (axial, coronal, and sagittal) should be acquired. Similarly to fetal echocardiography, the venous confluence behind the left atrium can be visualized on the axial images[20]; the vertical vein can be recognized on the coronal and/or sagittal images. Further oblique planes can help visualize each single pulmonary vein and its site of drainage.

Blood flow measurements in the pulmonary arteries and pulmonary veins by PC cine sequence add hemodynamic information in the presence of

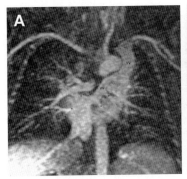
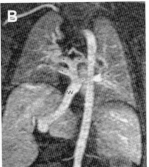

Fig. 11. CEMRA and mip reconstructed images in total anomalous pulmonary venous connection (TAPVC). (A) TAPVC of supracardial type with the vertical vein (VV) connecting to the innominate vein. Each single pulmonary vein is indicated by an asterisk. (B) TAPVC of infracardiac type. All 4 pulmonary veins (asterisks) merge in a vertical vein (VV) passing the diaphragm and connecting to the portal venous system in the liver.

pulmonary venous anomalies. Thus in the presence of partial anomalous pulmonary venous connection (PAPVC), the amount of intracardiac shunt can be quantified by measuring the flow in the aorta and in the pulmonary artery.

In suspected pulmonary venous obstruction, a feared complication postoperatively (**Fig. 12**),[28] changes in the pulmonary venous flow profile and/or in the pulmonary arterial flow distribution may occur.[29] The normal pulmonary venous flow pattern is characterized by one first peak of

forward flow during systole and a second peak during diastole, usually followed by a short reversed-flow wave, corresponding to atrial contraction (**Fig. 13**).[28] In the presence of obstruction, increased flow velocity is observed downstream of the obstruction, whereas flow velocity upstream of the obstruction is decreased and loses its typical biphasic pattern profile.[28,29] Therefore, flow ideally should be measured on both sides of a pulmonary venous obstruction.

In the presence of unilateral pulmonary venous obstruction, blood flow may redistribute within the lung, and flow measurement in the pulmonary arteries is strongly advisable.

The hypogenetic right lung complex, or scimitar syndrome,[30] is one of the rare indications for advanced cardiac Imaging of PAPVC in newborns. Some infants with scimitar syndrome may present with severe congestive heart failure and pulmonary hypertension, and require early surgical correction (**Fig. 14**).[31]

HETEROTAXY SYNDROME
Background

Visceral heterotaxy is a syndrome characterized by inconsistency of the situs of the thoracic and abdominal viscera. The abdominal and thoracic organs are incompletely or inappropriately lateralized,[32] resulting in a situs ambiguus. Heterotaxy syndrome is frequently associated with complex CHD, bronchial symmetry, and splenic anomalies, including asplenia or polysplenia. Atrial isomerism is another way to design this entity, based on the appearance of the atrial appendages, referring to right or left isomerism, depending on whether morphologically 2 left atria or 2 right atria are present.[33]

The most common characteristics of the associated cardiac defects are summarized in **Table 1**. Of note, hearts with left atrial isomerism tend to be biventricular and those with right atrial isomerism univentricular.[34] In addition, extracardiac anomalies may occur, including intestinal malrotation, hiatal hernia with partial thoracic stomach (particularly in right isomerism), and biliary atresia (left isomerism).[35,36]

Considering the complexity of the cardiac defects, a comprehensive and accurate delineation of cardiovascular anatomy and hemodynamics is essential for planning the correct surgical approach in each individual patient.

Preoperative Imaging

In heterotaxy syndrome, a well-structured and segmental approach is recommended during planning and reading of a diagnostic examination.

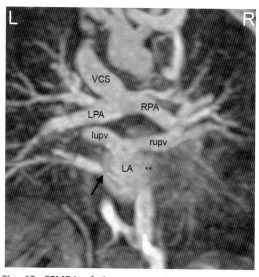

Fig. 12. CEMRA of the same patient as in **Fig. 11b** after TAPVC repair. The left upper (lupv) and right upper pulmonary veins (rupv) are widely patent; the left lower pulmonary vein presents a severe narrowing (*arrow*) at the junction to the left atrium (LA); the right lower pulmonary vein cannot be visualized as completely obstructed (*asterisks*). In addition, the patient underwent cavopulmonary connection; the superior vena cava (VCS) is now connected to the right (RPA) and left (LPA) pulmonary artery.

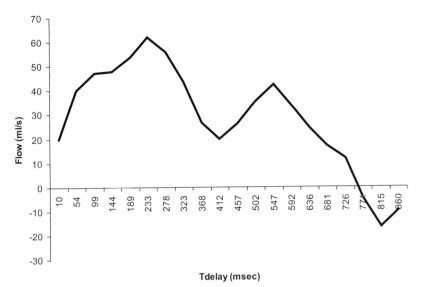

Fig. 13. Characteristic normal flow pattern in a pulmonary vein assessed by phase-contrast cine imaging.

Preoperative assessment of heterotaxy syndrome should include:

- Abdominal situs
- Spleen: asplenia, polysplenia
- Thoracic status: bronchi
- Morphology of the atrial appendages
- Cardiac position
- Cardiac segments
- Intracardiac anatomy (atrial defects, atrioventricular defects, ventricular defects, coronary sinus)

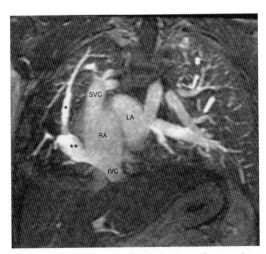

Fig. 14. Reconstructed CEMRA image of a newborn with scimitar syndrome. Most of the right lung is drained by a vertical pulmonary vein (*asterisk*), connecting to the right atrium at the junction (*double asterisk*) with the inferior vena cava. IVC, inferior vena cava; LA, left atrium; RA, right atrium; SVC, superior vena cava.

- Ventriculoarterial alignment
- Systemic venous anatomy
- Pulmonary venous anatomy and site of connection
- Pulmonary arteries
- Aortic arch.

CMR appears to be the ideal imaging technology to depict all of these characteristics in one single and noninvasive examination.[37] Geva and colleagues[38] demonstrated that the information obtained by CMR was more precise than that obtained by other imaging modalities and, not uncommonly, altered surgical planning. By combining echocardiography and CMR, the need for invasive cardiac catheterization is limited to patients in whom measurements of pulmonary vascular resistance are required or an interventional procedure has to be performed.

The SE or SSFP sequence can be used to define the thoracic and the abdominal situs. SE may be particular advantageous for demonstrating the anatomy of the main stem bronchi and their relations to the branch pulmonary arteries.[38] Symmetrical length of the bronchi or symmetric superior-inferior relation between the main bronchi and the proximal pulmonary arteries are indicative for a situs ambiguus (**Fig. 15**).[39] SSFP is particularly useful in defining the morphology of the atrial appendages (**Fig. 16**).

In the presence of unbalanced atrioventricular septal defect, measurements of the ventricular volumes by SSFP are essential for clinical decision as to performing biventricular repair or choosing univentricular palliation.[40] Anomalies of the pulmonary venous connection occur very frequently in

Table 1
Cardiac anatomy in heterotaxy syndromes

Defect	Right Isomerism	Left Isomerism
Bilateral superior venae cavae	45%	45%
Bilateral systemic venous drainage	70%	60%
Absence of coronary sinus	~100%	~60%
Interruption of inferior vena cava	<2.5%	80%
TAPVC extracardiac type	50% (obstruction in 50%)	Rare
Atrioventricular connection	Univentricular in 70%	Biventricular in ~75%
Ventriculoarterial connection	Concordant only in 4%	Concordant in ~70%
Pulmonary atresia or stenosis	80%	30%
Left sided obstructive lesion	<5%	~30%
Heart block/bradycardia	Rare	~70%

Abbreviation: TAPVC, total anomalous pulmonary venous connection.

heterotaxy syndrome and are major determinants of outcome. Pulmonary venous anomalies are accurately depicted by CEMRA,[30] as already discussed.

In conclusion, for the preoperative evaluation of heterotaxy syndrome CMR shows clear advantages over other imaging modalities; involvement of a pediatric cardiologist experienced in the imaging of complex CHD is recommended for a successful examination.[38]

MYOCARDIAL CONTRAST AGENTS

The use of gadolinium-based myocardial contrast agents has revolutionized the use of CMR and has enhanced its utility greatly, even in young children,

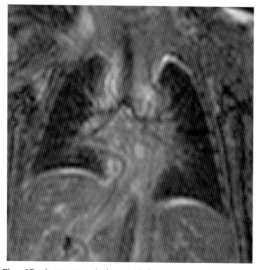

Fig. 15. A symmetric bronchial tree suggests heterotaxy syndrome. In this case a bilateral right bronchus morphology can be recognized.

as described earlier. In broad terms, gadolinium improves the ability to detect and identify the extent of disease, differentiates normal from abnormal tissue by defining and characterizing tissue, and can demonstrate pathologic activity. This agent dramatically reduces the spin lattice relaxation time of tissue (T1), and this reduction in T1 is used to visualize the vascular space. Three-dimensional imaging techniques, taking advantage of the increased T1 relaxation properties of the element, enables highly accurate assessment of 3D anatomy (**Fig. 17**) with submillimeter spatial resolution. This resolution is especially useful in the evaluation of the great vessels (aorta and pulmonary arteries), pulmonary veins, collaterals, and so forth. Using dynamic time-resolved sequences, even more exquisite delineation of anatomy can be attained along with temporal information as well. Gadolinium is also used in assessing myocardial perfusion both at rest and with adenosine administration, important for disease states such as pulmonary atresia with intact ventricular septum, in which the coronary circulation may be compromised. One of the most common uses today is in delineating myocardial scarring using the "delayed enhancement" approach (**Fig. 18**) along with identifying foreign material in the heart such as patches and baffles. This method exploits the kinetics of the contrast agent, whereby the volume of distribution of gadolinium is greater in necrotic myocardium than normal myocardium (gadolinium also gets "washed out" in normally perfused myocardium whereas this does not occur in scarred tissue). Finally, gadolinium can be used to characterize tissue such as in defining tumors, and to diagnose diseases such as myocarditis and arrhythmogenic right ventricular dysplasia (ARVD). In neonatal

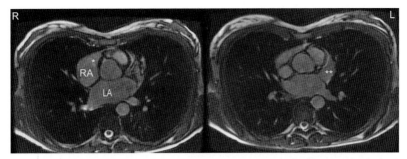

Fig. 16. Characterization of the atrial morphology on axial SSFP images. (*Left*) The morphologically right atrial appendage (*asterisk*) has an external triangular shape with a broad base and the apex pointed upward; internally the prominent crista terminalis and the pectinate muscles can be recognized. (*Right*) The left atrial appendage (*double asterisk*) has a tubular fingerlike shape with a narrow base, pointed anteriorly and downward. LA, left atrium; RA, right atrium.

CMR, its most important and common use is in defining 3D anatomy—everything from pulmonary artery architecture and aortic arch anatomy (see **Fig. 17**) to finding aortic to pulmonary collaterals in TOF with pulmonary atresia. Much less commonly, it has been used in tissue characterization (as in tumor identification), perfusion (eg, pulmonary atresia with intact ventricular septum and right ventricle–dependent coronary circulation), and viability (eg, neonatal insult causing myocardial infarction).

With such a diverse and important role, it is fair to assess the risk-benefit profile of the agent in children. Gadolinium traditionally has been deemed a relatively safe contrast agent, and literally tens of millions of patients have been exposed. All forms of the gadolinium are eliminated by the kidneys to a certain extent, many of them exclusively eliminated by the renal system such as gadodiamide. With the immature kidneys of infants, gadolinium may remain in the circulatory system longer and possibly exhibit increased toxicity. Some formulations such as gadoxetic acid are excreted by bile as well, and other toxic effects may be associated with infants in that regard.

It must be noted that not all gadolinium contrast agents are approved for use in all countries by agencies responsible for monitoring safety. For example, gadoversetamide is only approved in the United States by the Food and Drug Administration (FDA), whereas gadoterat is only approved for use in Europe by the European Agency for the Evaluation of Medicinal Products (EMEA). An agent such as gadodiamide, however, is approved

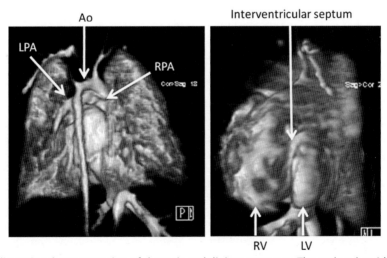

Fig. 17. Three-dimensional reconstruction of dynamic gadolinium sequence. The patient is a 4-kg neonate with a malaligned atrioventricular canal and a diffusely hypoplastic aorta. The reconstruction on the left is a posterior view demonstrating the aorta (Ao) and branch pulmonary arteries. The reconstruction on the right is a lateral view demonstrating the disparity in right ventricular (RV) and left ventricular (LV) sizes. LPA, left pulmonary artery; RPA, right pulmonary artery.

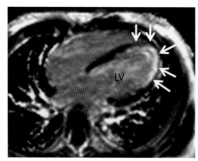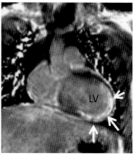

Fig. 18. Phase-sensitive delayed-enhancement imaging in a 2-week-old infant after arrest and neonatal insult. The 4-chamber (*left*) and left ventricular (LV) long axis views demonstrate apical and mid-short axis scarring (*arrows*).

for use by the FDA as well as the EMEA. Since 1988, at least 7 gadolinium-based contrast agents (GBCA) with different structural, physicochemical, and pharmacokinetic properties have been approved by the FDA. In the United States, gadolinium is not approved for use in the heart and its uses are considered "off-label."

Gadolinium Safety

In general, there are very few toxicities associated with gadolinium administration, with the exception of nephrogenic systemic sclerosis (NSF), discussed below. Adverse events are low, generally less than 5% in most adult studies, and are minor; idiosyncratic reactions are rare. Adverse events reported in all populations include reactions such as transient headache, nausea, vomiting, local "burning" or "coolness," hives, and temporary increase in serum bilirubin and iron. Anaphylactic reactions range from 1 in 200,000 to 1 in 400,000. There are only a few reported fatalities.

Focusing on children, much of what is known about the safety of gadolinium comes from applications other than its use in the heart.

Since 2006, a relatively rare but potentially fatal disease termed NSF has been linked to gadolinium exposure in patients with advanced renal disease. This disease most commonly involves the skin from the ankle to the mid-thigh and from the wrist to the mid-upper arm, with the face typically spared. There can be fever and general malaise. Papules, subcutaneous nodules, erythema, and plaques,[41] with some patients complaining of pruritus, can be present. Musculoskeletal involvement includes muscle and limb pain with possible contractures and reduction in mobility. The disease can extend to the lungs, myocardium, esophagus, and dura mater,[42] with hypercoagulopathy and thrombotic events possible. The onset of NSF can vary greatly, ranging from days to 6 months; the diagnosis is confirmed on biopsy

with spindle cells positive for CD34 immunostaining, fibroblast proliferation in the dermis, thickened collagen bundles, and increased macrophages and dendritic cells positive for CD68 and Factor XIIIA.

In 2000, Cowpers and colleagues[43] reported that patients undergoing hemodialysis presented with skin lesions termed "scleromyxedema-like," eventually coining the term "nephrogenic fibrosing dermopathy."[43] Eventually it was found that the disease involved other organ systems and the term NSF was then adopted,[44] followed in 2006 by the first reports suggesting the association with gadolinium chelates.[45] Since that time, regulatory agencies have provided guidance regarding NSF and the administration of GBCAs, with the current recommendation of the FDA[46] to avoid GBCAs in patients whose glomerular filtration rate is less than 30 mL/min/1.73 m^2.

It should be noted that pediatric cases of NSF are rare. There are few reports of patients 8 years of age or older contracting NSF,[47] and there are no reports of neonates or infants contracting the disease despite their immature renal function and low glomerular filtration rates.

THE BORDERLINE VENTRICLE

In the vast spectrum of CHD, there are several lesions that may contain either right or left ventricles with varying degrees of hypoplasia (**Figs. 19** and **20**). This hypoplasia may be very mild, such as the left ventricle in the case of TAPVC, or severe, such as in hypoplastic left heart syndrome. There are multiple reasons why these ventricles may be on the small side, such as hemodynamic (diversion of blood away from the ventricle, such as in the case of deviation of septum primum in hypoplastic left heart syndrome), anatomic with valve hypoplasia or atresia (eg, mitral or tricuspid atresia), or genetic. At either end of the range, surgery to create a single-ventricle circulation

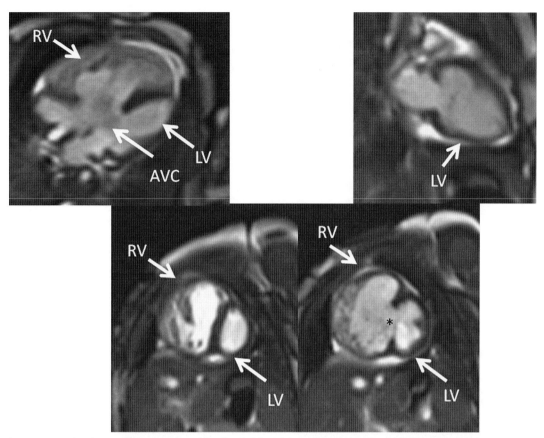

Fig. 19. SSFP cine images from a 5-day-old, 3-kg child with a malaligned atrioventricular canal and a borderline left ventricular size. The 4-chamber (*upper left*) and left ventricular (LV) long-axis view (*upper right*) demonstrate the malaligned atrioventricular canal (AVC), the atrial and ventricular septal defects, and the disparity in size between the two pumping chambers. The lower two images are short-axis views at different levels, again demonstrating the disparity in size between the two pumping chambers, including the large atrioventricular canal type ventricular septal defect (*asterisk*).

leading to the Fontan procedure or a two-ventricle repair is clear. However, because of this wide spectrum, there is obviously a "gray zone" where the ventricle may be large enough to support the circulation but it is unclear preoperatively that a two-ventricle repair would be successful. Indeed, the repair itself may make one ventricle larger but the other smaller (eg, in double-outlet right ventricle, the baffle from the left ventricle to the aorta will, by definition, remove cavity from the right ventricle making it smaller); the smaller ventricle itself may not be viable. It is in this region that physicians spend hours in the decision-making process and where imaging may make a difference.

Background

In the neonatal period, a patent ductus arteriosus (PDA) is nearly always present in the vast majority

of lesions, which allows for shunting between the systemic and pulmonary circulations. Similarly, a VSD performs the same function but at a different level. In the case of the borderline small left ventricle in the newborn, the PDA is the conduit that allows for the right ventricle to support the circulation and shunt blood from the pulmonary to systemic circulation. Similarly, in certain lesions where there is little left ventricular outflow tract obstruction, a VSD can also allow for the right ventricle to support the systemic circulation. As advantageous as this communication is, it presents a diagnostic dilemma because it is difficult to determine how much the left ventricle contributes to supporting the systemic circulation in this arrangement, which is important in understanding whether the left ventricle can be used as the systemic ventricle.

The clinician needs to decide whether the patient can undergo a two-ventricle repair or requires a single-ventricle approach (generally in

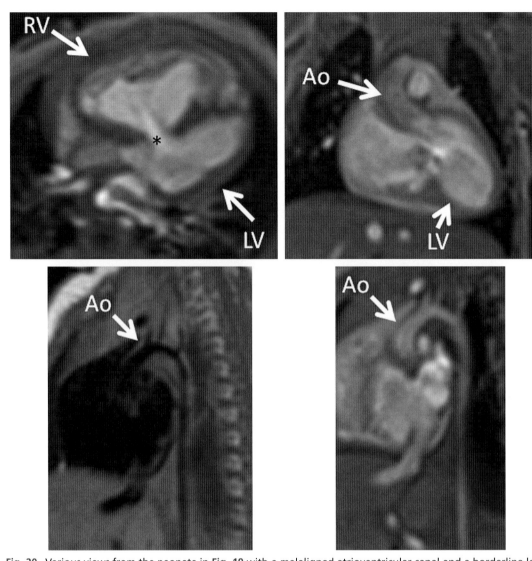

Fig. 20. Various views from the neonate in **Fig. 19** with a malaligned atrioventricular canal and a borderline left ventricular size. The upper left panel demonstrates a ventricular outflow tract view using gradient echo cine imaging, showing the ventricular septal defect (*asterisk*) and the disparity in size between the right (RV) and left ventricles (LV). Upper right is the orthogonal view of the upper left panel, also demonstrating a ventricular outflow tract view using gradient echo cine imaging. The lower images are the candy cane view of the aorta (Ao) using double-inversion dark blood imaging (*left*) and gradient echo cine imaging (*right*) showing the hypoplasia of the arch.

the newborn period), and each surgical pathway is different with unique problems and dissimilar outcomes. A two-ventricle repair will obviously be closer to the "normal" physiologic state and will have the left ventricle supporting the systemic circulation, whereas a single-ventricle repair will require staged surgical reconstruction, will not have a second ventricle to augment function, and will have the right ventricle, to varying degrees, supporting the systemic circulation with passive flow into the pulmonary bed via the "Fontan"

circuit; the clinician would be committing the patient to a Fontan reconstruction with the attendant morbidities (thrombosis, protein-losing enteropathy, congestive heart failure, and arrhythmia, to name a few). A two-ventricle repair also has the advantage of using the right ventricle as a pulmonary pumping chamber, which may aid in exercise tolerance. In addition, as many single-ventricle repairs in the neonatal period involve placement of systemic to pulmonary artery shunt, there is the risk of shunt occlusion.

It would seem from this discussion that a two-ventricle repair is always preferable; however, it is not that simple. In general, an operation to create a dual-chambered circulation is usually very complex and requires extensive surgery, with long cardiopulmonary bypass and deep hypothermic circulatory arrest times. Surgery can involve a right ventricle to pulmonary artery or other types of conduits, which usually will require revisions as the patient grows. There may be atrioventricular valve tissue in the pathway being created, putting the patient at risk for atrioventricular valve regurgitation by disruption of the suspension apparatus. A Ross-Kono procedure may be required, with possible semilunar valve insufficiency and aortic root dilation. Repair, therefore, may leave hemodynamic residua, and the treatment may be trading off one disease for another (eg, mitral or aortic insufficiency). As already mentioned, the baffling of blood from one ventricle to a great artery may make the other ventricle (the one being baffled through) smaller, which may make it nonviable. It is also far from clear that the two-ventricle repair will actually work, and a takedown of the reconstruction to a Norwood procedure carries a high risk (the opposite sequence of events appears to have a better result).[48–50]

There are other considerations when deciding whether a single-ventricle or two-ventricle repair is the optimal approach. Distal stenoses, whether it be at the aortic valve or great vessel level (eg, coarctation), will cause a pressure overload and must be repaired. Assessment of left ventricular performance must be taken into consideration, and the left ventricle itself may have varying degrees of endocardial fibroelastosis (EFE), which may affect ventricular function (**Fig. 21**). The architecture of the mitral valve also plays an important role; a parachute valve, a mitral arcade, a double-orifice mitral valve, and a broad spectrum of mitral hypoplasia may preclude a successful recruitment of the left ventricle. Shunt lesions may cause a volume load on the left ventricle, and these need to be addressed at surgery.

Two important questions arise when trying to make this decision. Is a poor two-ventricle repair better or worse than a good single-ventricle repair? If the decision is made to go down the single-ventricle route, would a two-ventricle repair have worked? The dilemma is clear.

Imaging in the Decision-Making Process of the Borderline Left Ventricle

Echocardiography has been the mainstay of imaging for patients with CHD, and this is no different in the borderline ventricle in the newborn period. Numerous studies abound in the literature,[51–55] but all are retrospective and small. In addition, institutional biases within each study preclude combining them to generalize about this methodology. Finally, the same criteria cannot be applied to every lesion (eg, critical aortic stenosis vs unbalanced atrioventricular canal[56]), making unified approaches much more difficult. Indeed the popularized Rhodes score[48] was used for aortic stenosis, and is not applicable to hypoplastic left heart complexes or malaligned atrioventricular canal defects.

CMR is the gold standard in determining ventricular volumes (see **Figs. 19** and **21**); this is an obvious advantage when deciding if a ventricle is too small to be used as a systemic pumping chamber. After a 4-chamber view is performed using SSFP cine images, a contiguous stack of short-axis cine images are performed from atrioventricular valve level to apex. By contouring the endocardial and epicardial borders of both ventricles at end-diastole and end-systole, ventricular volumes, cardiac index, ejection fraction, and

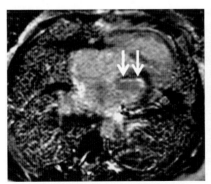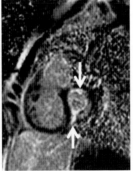

Fig. 21. A 4-chamber (*left*) and short-axis view (*right*) of a patient with hypoplastic left heart syndrome (aortic stenosis/mitral stenosis), which demonstrates endocardial fibroelastosis of the left ventricle (*arrows*) via delayed enhancement.

mass can be determined accurately. Flows through the semilunar valves can be used to assess systemic (Qs) and pulmonary blood flow (Qp) and to determine Qp/Qs. A "virtual baffle" can be created and traced during the postprocessing to estimate what the ventricular volumes, cardiac index, and ejection fraction might be if a baffle was placed in that position; of course this is just an estimate, as loading conditions will change after surgery. Similarly, atrioventricular valve apparatus, conal muscle, or other intracardiac structures can be visualized to determine whether they present an issue to baffle creation. A stack of contiguous "off-axis" images across the ventricle and great vessels in the outflow tract view spanning the ventricles may also be used to determine baffle geometry and placement, with subsequent volume and functional measurements. CMR is also useful in outlining EFE (see **Fig. 21**), which will enter into the decision regarding a two-ventricle repair.

There are some data in the literature supporting the use of CMR in this context; it has not been as widely used as echocardiography, due to unavailability and having to sedate the critical neonate before and during the study. Grosse-Wortmann and colleagues,[40] for example, published data in 2008 on 20 consecutive newborns with a mean age of 10 days who underwent CMR and echocardiography to assess the borderline small left ventricle. In their study, left ventricular volumes by echocardiography were approximately 50% of those determined by CMR (16.0 ± 7.0 mL/m^2 vs 33.5 ± 15.5 mL/m^2, respectively), consistently underestimating the value. Mitral valve z-score appeared to be the best predictor of left ventricular end-diastolic volume by CMR ($r = 0.77$, $P = .02$). By using the geometry of the ventricle by CMR, this study also suggested average potential volume increases for the left ventricle, which was a function of the major disease process (8.8% for aortic stenosis, 35.0% for endocardial cushion defects, and 23.0% for hypoplastic left heart complex). Surgical outcomes were also examined; 16 of 20 patients underwent biventricular repair, with only 5 (31.3%) having a preoperative left ventricular end-diastolic volume of greater than 20 mL/m^2 by echocardiography; none of the neonates with a CMR volume greater than 20 mL/m^2 sustained a perioperative death. The group used a left ventricular end-diastolic volume of greater than 20 mL/m^2 by CMR and calculating the potential left ventricular size increase along with the "left ventricular outflow tract" as being able to handle greater than 1 L/min/m^2 as important considerations of whether a biventricular repair was possible.

Left ventricular size is not the only thing that matters, and CMR can contribute to this determination. EFE can occur in patients with small left ventricles under pressure, such as with hypoplastic left heart syndrome, as already noted; CMR using delayed enhancement (see **Figs. 18** and **21**) can identify the presence and extent of EFE to guide the physician in deciding on prognosis regarding single-ventricle versus two-ventricle repair and possible therapeutic intervention. Indeed the presence of EFE has been linked to the viability of the left ventricle as a systemic pumping chamber,[54,57] and the surgical therapy for removal of the EFE has been attempted successfully, improving ventricular performance.[58] The use of CMR to identify these patients is an obvious advantage (see **Fig. 21**).

Similar to echocardiography, CMR can evaluate semilunar and atrioventricular valve anatomy and competency, and measure annular sizes, again important considerations in the decision-making process. Analogous to the recent article by Szwast and colleagues,[59] in which inflows into both ventricles were determined by color Doppler in patients with malaligned atrioventricular canal and was able to predict outcome, CMR, using phase-encoded velocity mapping, can apportion flow to both ventricles in these types of patients; a study, however, has yet to be performed. In addition, CMR can assess the great vessel anatomy and geometry, whether coarctation is present, and the relationships to other structures in the chest.

REFERENCES

1. Vitiello RMB, Nykanen D, Freedom RM, et al. Complications associated with pediatric cardiac catheterization. J Am Coll Cardiol 1998;32:1433–40.
2. Kellenberger CJ, Yoo SJ, Buechel ER. Cardiovascular MR imaging in neonates and infants with congenital heart disease. Radiographics 2007; 27(1):5–18.
3. Calder L, Van Praagh R, Van Praagh S. Truncus arteriosus communis. Am Heart J 1976;92:23–38.
4. Collett RW, Edwards JE. Persistent truncus arteriosus: a classification according to anatomic types. Surg Clin North Am 1949;29:1245–70.
5. Butto F, Lucas RV Jr, Edwards JE. Persistent truncus arteriosus: pathologic anatomy in 54 cases. Pediatr Cardiol 1986;7:95–101.
6. Rossiter SJ, Silverman JF, Shumway NE. Patterns of pulmonary arterial supply in patients with truncus arteriosus. J Thorac Cardiovasc Surg 1978;75:73–9.
7. Donnelly LF, Higgins CB. MR imaging of conotruncal abnormalities. Am J Roentgenol 1996;166(4):925–8.
8. Naehle CP, Schild H, Thomas D. Erstdiagnose einer quadrikuspiden Aortenklappe mittels MRT. Fortschröntgenstr 2009;181(05):487–90 [in German].

9. Dorfman AL, Geva T. Magnetic resonance imaging evaluation of congenital heart disease: conotruncal anomalies. J Cardiovasc Magn Reson 2006;8:645–59.

10. Okubo M, Benson LN. Intravascular and intracardiac stents used in congenital heart disease. Curr Opin Cardiol 2001;16(2):84–91.

11. Santoro G, Gaio G, Palladino MT, et al. Stenting of the arterial duct in newborns with duct-dependent pulmonary circulation. Heart 2008;94(7):925–9.

12. Valsangiacomo Büchel ER, DiBernardo S, Bauersfeld U, et al. Contrast-enhanced magnetic resonance angiography of the great arteries in patients with congenital heart disease: an accurate tool for planning catheter-guided interventions. Int J Cardiovasc Imaging 2005; 21(2):313–22.

13. Farouk A, Zahka K, Siwik E, et al. Individualized approach to the surgical treatment of tetralogy of Fallot with pulmonary atresia. Cardiol Young 2009; 19(1):76–85.

14. Beekmana RP, Roest AA, Helbing WA, et al. Spin echo MRI in the evaluation of hearts with a double outlet right ventricle: usefulness and limitations. Magn Reson Imaging 2000;18(3):245–53.

15. Mahle WT, Martinez R, Silverman N, et al. Anatomy, echocardiography, and surgical approach to double outlet right ventricle. Cardiol Young 2008;18(Suppl 3): 39–51.

16. Kleinert S, Sano T, Weintraub RG, et al. Anatomic features and surgical strategies in double-outlet right ventricle. Circulation 1997;96(4):1233–9.

17. Hashmi A, Abu-Sulaiman R, McCrindle BW, et al. Management and outcomes of right atrial isomerism: a 26-year experience. J Am Coll Cardiol 1998;31(5): 1120–6.

18. Yoo SJ, Lim TH, Park IS, et al. MR anatomy of ventricular septal defect in double-outlet right ventricle with situs solitus and atrioventricular concordance. Radiology 1991;181(2):501–5.

19. Losekoot TG. discordant atrioventricular connection and congenitally corrected transposition. In: Anderson RH, Shinebourne EA, Tynan M, editors. Pediatric cardiology. Edinburgh (United Kingdom): Churchill Livingstone; 1987. p. 867–88.

20. Valsangiacomo ER, Hornberger LK, Barrea C, et al. Partial and total anomalous pulmonary venous connection in the fetus: two-dimensional and Doppler echocardiographic findings. Pediatr Radiol 2003;22(3):257–63.

21. Musewe NN, Yoo SJ, Freedom RM. Anomalies of pulmonary venous connections including cor triatratum and stenosis of individual pulmonary veins. In: Freedom RM, Smallhorn JF, editors. Neonatal herat disease. London: Springer Verlag; 1992. p. 310–31.

22. Smallhorn JF FR. Pulsed Doppler echocardiograph in the preoperative evaluation of total anomalous pulmonary venous connection. J Am Coll Cardiol 1986;8(6):1413–20.

23. Reddy SC, Chopra PS, Rao PS. Mixed-type total anomalous pulmonary venous connection: echocardiographic limitations and angiographic advantages. Am Heart J 1995;129:1034–8.

24. Masui T, Seelos KC, Kersting-Sommerhoff BA, et al. Abnormalities of the pulmonary veins: evaluation with MR imaging and comparison with cardiac angiography and echocardiography. Radiology 1991; 181(3):645–9.

25. Beerbaum P, Korperich H, Barth P, et al. Noninvasive quantification of left-to-right shunt in pediatric patients: phase-contrast cine magnetic resonance imaging compared with invasive oximetry. Circulation 2001;103(20):2476–82.

26. Grosse-Wortmann L, Al-Otay A, Woo Goo H, et al. Anatomical and functional evaluation of pulmonary veins in children by magnetic resonance imaging. J Am Coll Cardiol 2007;49(9):993–1002.

27. Valsangiacomo E, Levasseur S, McCrindle B, et al. Contrast-enhanced MR angiography of pulmonary venous abnormalities in children. Pediatr Radiol 2003;33(2):92–8.

28. Valsangiacomo ER, Barrea C, Macgowan CK, et al. Phase-contrast MR assessment of pulmonary venous blood flow in children with surgically repaired pulmonary veins. Pediatr Radiol 2003;33(9):607–13.

29. Videlefsky N, Parks WJ, Oshinski J, et al. Magnetic resonance phase-shift velocity mapping in pediatric patients with pulmonary venous obstruction. J Am Coll Cardiol 2001;38(1):262–7.

30. Neill CA, Sabiston DC, Sheldon H. The familial occurrence of hypoplastic right lung with systemic arterial supply and venous drainage "scimitar syndrome". Bull Johns Hopkins Hosp 1960;107: 1–20.

31. Dupuis C, Breviere GM, Abou P. "Infantile" form of the scimitar syndrome with pulmonary hypertension. Am J Cardiol 1993;71:1326–30.

32. Van Praagh S, Sanders SP. Cardiac malpositions with special emphasis on visceral heterotaxy (asplenia and polysplenia syndromes). In: Nadas AS, editor. "Nadas" pediatric cardiology. Philadelphia: Hanley&Belfus; 1992. p. 589–608.

33. Anderson RH. Atrial structure in the presence of visceral heterotaxy. Cardiol Young 2000;10:299–302.

34. Gilljam T, McCrindle BW, Smallhorn JF, et al. Outcomes of left atrial isomerism over a 28-year period at a single institution. J Am Coll Cardiol 2000;36(3):908–16.

35. Ticho BS, Goldstein AM, Van Praagh R. Extracardiac anomalies in the heterotaxy syndromes with focus on anomalies of midline-associated structures. Am J Cardiol 2000;85(6):729–34.

36. Phoon CK, Neill CA. Asplenia syndrome: insight into embryology through an analysis of cardiac and

extracardiac anomalies. Am J Cardiol 1994;73(8):581–7.

37. Yoo SJ, Kim YM, Choe YH. Magnetic resonance imaging of complex congenital heart disease. Int J Cardiovasc Imaging 1999;15:151–60.

38. Geva T, Vick GW 3rd, Wendt RE, et al. Role of spin echo and cine magnetic resonance imaging in pre-surgical planning of heterotaxy syndrome. Comparison with echocardiography and catheterization. Circulation 1994;90(1):348–56.

39. Hong YK, Park YW, Ryu SJ, et al. Efficacy of MRI in complicated congenital heart disease with visceral heterotaxy syndrome. J Comput Assist Tomogr 2000;24:671–82.

40. Grosse-Wortmann L, Yun T-J, Al-Radi O, et al. Borderline hypoplasia of the left ventricle in neonates: insights for decision-making from functional assessment with magnetic resonance imaging. J Thorac Cardiovasc Surg 2008;136(6):1429–36.

41. Cowpers SE, Su LD, Bhawan J, et al. Nephrogenic fibrosing dermopathy. Am J Dermatopathol 2001;23:383–93.

42. Gibson SE, Farver CF, Prayson RA. Multiorgan involvement in nephrogenic fibrosing dermopathy: an autopsy case and review of the literature. Arch Pathol Lab Med 2006;130;209–12.

43. Cowpers SE, Robin HS, Steinberg SM, et al. Scleromyxoedema-like cutaneous disease in renal dialysis patients. Lancet 2000;356(9234):1000–1.

44. Daram SR, Cortese CM, Bastani B. Nephrogenic fibrosing dermopathy/nephrogenic systemic fibrosis: report of a new case with literature review. Am J Kidney Dis 2005;46:754–9.

45. Marckmann P, Skov L, Rossen K, et al. Nephrogenic systemic fibrosis: suspected causative role of gadodiamide used for contrast enhanced magnetic resonance imaging. J Am Soc Nephrol 2006;17:2359–62.

46. Available at: http://www.fda.gov/Drugs/DrugSafety/PostmarketDrugSafetyInformationforPatientsandProviders/ucm142884.htm. Accessed on April 11, 2011.

47. Penfield J. Nephrogenic systemic fibrosis and the use of gadolinium-based contrast agents. Pediatr Nephrol 2008;23:2121–9.

48. Rhodes LA, Colan SD, Perry SB, et al. Predictors of survival in neonates with critical aortic stenosis. Circulation 1991;84:2325–35.

49. Hickey EJ, Caldarone CA, Blackstone EH, et al. Critical left ventricular outflow tract obstruction: the disproportionate impact of biventricular repair in borderline cases. J Thorac Cardiovasc Surg 2007;134:1429–36.

50. Pearl JM, Cripe LW, Manning PB. Biventricular repair after Norwood palliation. Ann Thorac Surg 2003;75:132–6.

51. Parsons MK, Moreau GA, Graham TP, et al. Echocardiographic estimation of critical left ventricular size in infants with isolated aortic valve stenosis. J Am Coll Cardiol 1991;18:1049–55.

52. Leung MP, McKay R, Smith A, et al. Critical aortic stenosis in early infancy: anatomic and echocardiographic substrates of successful open valvotomy. J Thorac Cardiovasc Surg 1991;101:526–35.

53. Latson LA, Cheatham JP, Gutgesell HP. Relation of the echocardiographic estimate of left ventricular size to mortality in infants with severe left ventricular outflow obstruction. Am J Cardiol 1981;48:887–91.

54. Gundry SR, Behrendt DM. Prognostic factors in valvotomy for critical aortic stenosis in infancy. J Thorac Cardiovasc Surg 1986;92:747–54.

55. Pelech AN, Dyck JD, Trusler GA, et al. Critical aortic stenosis. Survival and management. J Thorac Cardiovasc Surg 1987;94:510–7.

56. Cohen MS, Jacobs ML, Weinberg PM, et al. Morphometric analysis of unbalanced common atrioventricular canal using two-dimensional echocardiography. J Am Coll Cardiol 1996;28:1017–23.

57. Mocellin R, Sauer U, Simon B, et al. Reduced left ventricular size and endocardial fibroelastosis as correlates of mortality in newborns and young infants with severe aortic valve stenosis. Pediatric Cardiology 1983;4:265–72.

58. Emani SM, Bacha EA, McElhinney DB, et al. Primary left ventricular rehabilitation is effective in maintaining two-ventricle physiology in the borderline left heart. J Thorac Cardiovasc Surg 2009;138:1276–82.

59. Szwast AL, Marino BS, Rychik J, et al. Usefulness of left ventricular inflow index to predict successful biventricular repair in right-dominant unbalanced atrioventricular canal. Am J Cardiol 2011;107:103–9.

MR Imaging of the Neonatal Musculoskeletal System

Charlotte Gilbert, MBChB, RANZCR[a],*,
Paul Babyn, MDCM, FRCP(C)[b]

KEYWORDS

- Magnetic resonance imaging • Neonates
- Musculoskeletal system • Radiography

Evaluation of the neonatal musculoskeletal system with magnetic resonance (MR) imaging is not commonly needed. Radiography and ultrasound remain the initial imaging modalities for most common and uncommon musculoskeletal conditions encountered in this age group. However, because of the exquisite tissue contrast provided by MR imaging, its use is expanding, especially for evaluation of complex malformations, infections, and tumors of the neonatal musculoskeletal system. The ability of MR to image the abundant cartilage present within the neonate makes MR imaging invaluable in the assessment of the neonatal musculoskeletal system.

MR imaging of the neonate poses several unique challenges that may arise either before or during scanning. Considerations include patient transport, the need for sedation and monitoring, as well as safe patient positioning. When imaging, careful consideration of coil selection, scan parameters, and sequences is vital. The interpretation of images may also be challenging because the appearance of the neonatal musculoskeletal system and type of underlying disorder often differ from those encountered in older children.

This article discusses some practical aspects of MR imaging of the neonatal musculoskeletal system. It reviews the normal neonatal appearance of the musculoskeletal system and focuses on some common and uncommon musculoskeletal disorders for which MR imaging has been shown to be of benefit in the neonate.

EXAMINATION TECHNIQUE
Patient Preparation

Close cooperation between the neonatal service and the radiology department is required for successful acquisition of a diagnostic neonatal MR study. We carry out MR examinations in the neonate as far as possible without the use of anesthesia, instead using a feed-wrap-and-snooze technique. This technique is described in a step-by-step approach by Mathur and colleagues.[1]

There are several principles to optimize success in pediatric musculoskeletal imaging.[2] When sedation or general anesthesia are needed, the MR compatibility of any necessary ventilatory or monitoring equipment must be considered. The number of intravenous solutions should be minimized as much as possible. The neonate is wrapped snugly and placed in a regular transfer incubator or, if available, a specialized neonatal MR-compatible incubator. The advantage of an MR-compatible incubator is that fewer patient transfers are required, which reduces the

[a] 9 Kelly Street, Auckland, New Zealand
[b] Department of Medical Imaging, University of Saskatchewan and Saskatoon Health Region, Royal University Hospital, Room 1566.1, 103 Hospital Drive, Saskatoon, Saskatchewan S7N 0W8, Canada
* Corresponding author.
E-mail address: lotgilbert@yahoo.com

Magn Reson Imaging Clin N Am 19 (2011) 841–858
doi:10.1016/j.mric.2011.08.001

likelihood of disturbing the neonate or dislodging monitoring leads and intravenous lines. The use of a dedicated nurse, familiar with neonatal procedures and associated specialized equipment, helps to smoothly transfer from nursery to MR scanner and back again. Clear and up-to-date communication with the ward about the anticipated study start is important to enable suitable scheduling of feeds, generally 30 to 40 minutes before scan initiation.

Field of View and Coil Selection

It is important to find an appropriate balance between the desired anatomic coverage, required spatial and matrix resolution, and signal/noise ratio. These factors, along with coil sensitivity and magnetic field strength, help determine the field of view (FOV) and slice thickness to be used. The use of small FOVs with similar matrix sizes to those used in adult studies decreases the signal/noise ratio greatly and may create excessive noise and uninterpretable images. However, if the FOV is too large for a given matrix size, then the spatial resolution may not be adequate for evaluation of neonatal anatomy. Generally, selection of a pixel size of just less than 1 mm by 1 mm with slice thicknesses of 3 to 5 mm is adequate.

The volumes to be imaged in the neonate for detailed evaluation may be small, requiring dedicated imaging coils able to acquire the required small FOVs in adequate detail. At present, in our institution, we primarily use either the head coil, and place the entire baby within the coil for larger anatomic coverage or, for smaller regions, use surface coils.

Choice of Scan Sequences and Parameters

As for all pediatric MR imaging, the order of sequence selection is important. The sequences with the highest anticipated yield should be performed first, so that, if the neonate rouses, enough of the study will hopefully have been completed to give diagnostic information. In general, MR imaging studies of the neonatal musculoskeletal system include a variety of standard fast spin-echo and gradient sequences with or without fat suppression, such as T1-weighted (T1-W), T2-weighted (T2-W), spoiled gradient echo or fast low angle shot, and short tau inversion recovery (STIR). Both two-dimensional and three-dimensional sequences are being used.

T1-W images

T1-W images are helpful in the interpretation of bone marrow involvement in patients with yellow marrow, with abnormalities typically appearing as low signal on T1-W images. However, in the neonate, hematopoietic marrow predominates, which also appears low signal on T1-W images, obscuring recognition of focal or more diffuse marrow lesions. Use of in-phase and out-of-phase sequences may help.[3]

Water-sensitive images

STIR and fat-suppressed TSE T2-W imaging are the most commonly used water-sensitive images. Fat-suppressed T2-W imaging is the preferred method when magnetic field inhomogeneity is not a concern because it is more efficient than STIR imaging. Fat-suppressed T2-W imaging is also the method used when contrast enhancement is present because STIR suppresses any signal that has a short T1, including gadolinium.

Proton density

Proton density imaging has a high signal/noise ratio that can provide excellent spatial resolution for evaluation of musculoskeletal structures. It is one of the most commonly used sequences in musculoskeletal imaging in older children and adults and also works well in neonates, particularly with fat suppression.

Gradient echo sequences

Gradient echo (GRE) images are particularly useful for imaging cartilage and for looking for magnetic susceptibility artifacts, as seen in hemorrhage. Hyaline epiphyseal and physeal cartilage is of high or intermediate signal, whereas hemorrhage shows as blooming. This sequence is particularly useful in distinguishing between cartilage and adjacent joint fluid. With increasing T2 weighting, signal contrast is increased between cartilage (lower signal) and fluid (higher signal). Three-dimensional gradient sequences are often used for dedicated joint imaging and multiplanar reconstruction.

Use of 3 Tesla MR imaging

The experience with 3 Tesla (3T) MR imaging of the neonate is still in its infancy. With 3T, there is increased signal available, which is used to decrease overall examination time and/or increase image resolution. In practice, for neonatal imaging, a combination of these benefits is usually used to both reduce overall scan time and improve spatial resolution. Early experience with pediatric 3T MR imaging has shown that it can provide good image quality even at small FOVs, showing cartilage, ligaments, and nerves in good detail. In addition, the ability to decrease examination time helps to decrease motion artifact and the need for sedation, which can reduce potential patient complications and aid work flow. However, changes in imaging parameters are required when moving from 1.5T to 3T. The T2 relaxation times at 3T are slightly reduced, whereas the T1 relaxation times are more prolonged, making it difficult to achieve the same contrast resolution. Artifacts related to movement, flow, susceptibility, and chemical shift can cause a problem at higher magnet field strength. Although certain devices and implants may not be safe at 3T,[4] this is not a significant problem in this age group, given the rarity of implants in this patient population. The increased acoustic noise of the 3T scanner may also be problematic, especially for the sleeping neonate.

Use of Contrast

At present, contrast product guidelines warn that the safety and efficacy of gadolinium-based contrast agents have not been established in patients less than the 2 years of age. The pharmacokinetics of the neonatal population has not been well studied; however, it is known that the glomerular filtration rate of neonates and young infants is lower than that of adults, and that the pharmacokinetic volume of distribution is also different. It is also unclear whether 1 type of MR contrast agent is better than another in this patient population.

Despite this caveat, contrast is used because it can add useful information when performing MR imaging of the neonatal musculoskeletal system, similarly to studies in older children. We generally use a similar dosages to those for infants when contrast is needed.

Following contrast agent injection, there is prominent enhancement of the normal cartilaginous physis, the juxtaphyseal tissues, and the subperiosteal fibrovascular tissues. After 30 to 60 minutes, sufficient contrast extravasates into the joint space to act as an indirect arthrogram.[2] In inflammatory conditions such as infection and arthritis, the epiphyseal vascular channels may become even more prominent. In the case of infection or concern for avascularity, contrast administration can be helpful in showing areas that may need drainage or debridement. Tumors and vascular malformations can become more conspicuous following contrast administration, and may be better characterized by their enhancement characteristics or show areas of internal necrosis.

NORMAL MR IMAGING APPEARANCE OF THE NEONATAL MUSCULOSKELETAL SYSTEM

Intramembranous ossification is responsible for the development of the facial bones and cranium, whereas the skull base, long and tubular bones, clavicles, and vertebral column develop by endochondral ossification from cartilaginous models. Thus, hyaline cartilage is more abundant within the neonate than in the older child, particularly within the epiphyses and growth plates.

Epiphyseal hyaline cartilage, also known as the chondroepiphysis, is the precursor to the ossified end of long bones. In the neonate, the epiphyses are predominantly all cartilaginous, converting to bone later with subsequent development and growth of the secondary ossification center. The chondroepiphyses are of homogeneous intermediate signal intensity (SI) on T1-W images and are low SI on water-sensitive images. The cartilaginous ends of bones are supplied by a unique vascular arrangement coursing through the cartilage embedded within tubular structures called epiphyseal vascular canals. These vascular canals contain arterioles, venules, capillaries, and loose connective tissues. Articular cartilage is also hyaline but it has a more organized structure than epiphyseal cartilage and appears as a thin, hyperintense rim surrounding the developing epiphysis on water-sensitive images.

In neonates and young children, the physis is flatter and less undulating than in older children. Two distinct regions of the physis are seen on MR imaging. The first is the cartilaginous zone, which is of intermediate to high SI on water-sensitive images. This zone is easy to separate from epiphyseal cartilage, which is of lower SI. On T1-W images, the physis is difficult to visualize separately from the adjacent unossified epiphysis.[2] The second zone of the physis is that of provisional calcification. This zone is of low SI on all sequences because it contains a more mineralized matrix.[5]

The epiphyseal vasculature courses through the cartilaginous ends of the long bones within the cartilage canals. The vasculature extends across the physis from the metaphysis into the epiphysis until approximately 12 to 18 months of age when the physis acts as a barrier between the epiphyseal vascularity and the metaphyseal vascularity.[5] This anatomic fact is of clinical importance because of the rapid spread of infection within bone and cartilage within the neonate. The cartilage canals have a linear parallel appearance before development of the ossification centers and converge around the ossification center.[6]

Fibrocartilage appears similar to that seen in older children and adults, with low signal on all standard sequences. Khanna and Thapa[7] recently reviewed the MR appearances of developing cartilage.

Bone

Long bones

In the third-trimester fetus, and in the newborn, the diaphyseal cortex is thick, with only a small central medullary cavity that eventually enlarges to form the mature marrow cavity. During this time, the SI of cortical bone is low on all sequences. Bones typically appear low signal on T1-W images because of both the presence of hematopoietic marrow and increased trabeculation. The marrow space starts enlarging within the first week of life. It is initially entirely hematopoietic and vascular with low T1-W SI, and high SI on water-sensitive images.[5] Marrow conversion to fatty marrow begins during the first year of life but is not well advanced in the neonatal period. On MR imaging, the characteristics of normal marrow depend on the relative amounts of the marrow constituents, including hematopoietic elements and marrow fat. Normal neonatal hematopoietic marrow is lower than or equal to muscle SI on T1-W imaging and of increased signal on T2-W imaging and following contrast enhancement.

The bony envelope

The periosteum is a thin, low-SI structure that parallels the bone cortex. It is loosely attached along the shaft of the bone, but tightly held at the level of the physis where it is termed the perichondrium. The perichondrium surrounds the physeal cartilage and allows for circumferential growth. It is most prominent in newborns.[5]

There is a layer of fibrovascular tissue that separates the periosteum from the cortex. This layer is most easily seen at the metaphysis where it appears as a metaphyseal stripe on longitudinal images, and a cuff on transverse images. It has a high SI on water-sensitive images and enhances vividly after contrast administration. In areas of loose attachment of the periosteum, subperiosteal collections of blood, pus, or tumor can form.

Spine

The various structures of the spine also undergo marked changes during infancy. These structures have 3 distinct stages of evolution. The description in this article compares the T1-W SI of the bone and cartilage with that of skeletal muscle. Stage 1, from birth to approximately 1 month of age, shows prominent hyperintense cartilage at the superior and inferior margins of the vertebral body, and hypointense ossification centers. A central band of higher SI is occasionally seen corresponding with the radiolucent band seen on radiographs. At this stage, the vertebral body is ovoid in shape. Stage 2 is from approximately 1 to 6 months, and shows increasing SI in the ossification centers, from the endplates inwards, with decreasing prominence of the cartilage. Stage 3, from approximately 7 months, shows increasingly rectangular vertebral bodies that are centrally intense, with a further decrease in the amount of cartilage.[8] The neonatal spinal marrow signal is lower than that of the adjacent disc.

NEONATAL MUSCULOSKELETAL DISORDERS AND THE USE OF MR IMAGING

Abnormalities of the spine, pelvis, and extremities are common in neonates. In many cases, the abnormality is evident on clinical examination, as in the absence of all or part of a limb, and no imaging is required. Other conditions, such as developmental dysplasia of the hip, are more difficult to diagnose and may require imaging. Imaging is useful in confirming the diagnosis or assessing for potential complications. Imaging can also provide information for preoperative planning, or can be used in follow-up. Radiographs remain the first-line imaging modality for almost all conditions, giving an overview of skeletal density and ossification, alignment, and presence of calcification. Ultrasound is also widely used because it has several advantages: lower cost than MR imaging, can be performed portably, and seldom requires sedation. Despite the distinct role of ultrasound in certain conditions, its sensitivity remains operator dependant. The role of MR imaging in neonatal musculoskeletal conditions is expanding, with its greatest advantage being its multiplanar capability to visualize the nonossified elements of the musculoskeletal system.

Congenital and Developmental Conditions

Neonates with certain skeletal dysplasias with underlying cartilage abnormalities, such as achondrogenesis II and hypochondrogenesis, have been shown histologically to have increased size and number of cartilage canals. MR imaging can reveal these abnormalities in the number and distribution of the cartilage canals.

Congenital anomalies are those that occur early during the embryonic period, whereas developmental deformities occur later in fetal or neonatal life. Limb buds appear in the upper body by the 23rd gestational day and appear for the lower limbs a few days later. Development can be affected by genetic, vascular, nervous, and teratologic influences, the timing of which is reflected both in the specific musculoskeletal abnormality and any concurrent anomalies, such as the many associated findings commonly identified with abnormalities of the radius.[9]

Upper extremity

Congenital and developmental disorders of the upper limb occur less commonly than those of the lower limbs.[10,11] Of the disorders that present in the neonatal period, many do not require MR imaging at this time. For example, radiography provides all the information required in cases of polydactyly or congenital amputations. Other entities, such as radioulnar synostosis, may not present until later in life, and those abnormalities involving the radius that may be associated with syndromes are generally further worked up with ultrasound. However, MR imaging can be helpful in unique anomalies that are rarely encountered, such as intrathoracic development of a right upper limb.

Lower extremity

Depiction of the unossified skeletal structures of the lower limbs with MR imaging is more important in planning treatment of children with a broader variety of congenital deformities of the lower extremities.[12]

Developmental dysplasia of the hip

In infancy, the most common clinical concern of the lower limb is developmental dysplasia of the hip (DDH). Hip dysplasia in the neonate may also arise from multiple causes including neuromuscular conditions, such as cerebral palsy and arthrogryposis, as well as teratologic causes or ligament laxity.[13–15] In most cases, DDH is diagnosed clinically and with ultrasound. Radiography may be used once the femoral head ossification centers have appeared. In certain refractory cases of DDH, as well as in other causes of hip dysplasia, MR imaging has a role both in preoperative planning and postoperative care.

MR can show the cartilaginous parts of the pelvis and hip and analyze the relationship of the femoral head to the acetabulum and labrum without the radiation required with computed tomography (CT). An MR classification of DDH has been described, but this is not in common use, especially for the neonatal age group. With MR, the sequences used should be limited to 1 or 2 in total in the coronal and/or axial planes so that studies can be completed without need for sedation. Generally, cartilage-specific GRE or fat-suppressed T1-W sequences are used. Fat-saturated spin-echo T1-W images or gradient sequences with flip angles of 34° to 45°, show epiphyseal cartilage appearing bright, with ossified bone, and the labrum appearing dark.

MR imaging is helpful to confirm satisfactory concentric hip reduction in casts. With MR imaging, it is possible to see potential impediments to reduction, such as an inverted labrum or prominent pulvinar fat. Other causes of inability to concentrically reduce the hip include a redundant ligamentum teres, whereas the capsule, iliopsoas tendon, or transverse acetabular ligaments may all become interposed, also preventing hip relocation.[13] Routine MR imaging has been recommended by some investigators in all casted open or closed reduced dislocations to confirm reduction because up to 4% to 14% of patients may not have satisfactory reduction in casts. This recommendation has not yet been widely adopted. MR imaging has also been used to evaluate the degree of abduction and extent of femoral head perfusion. Relative increased abduction is associated with an increased risk of vascular compromise. Gadolinium enhancement may show abnormalities of the femoral head and physeal vascularity with reduced perfusion. Timely correction of potential ischemia of the femoral head may obviate the development of chondronecrosis.[16]

Proximal focal femoral deficiency

Proximal focal femoral deficiency (PFFD) is a congenital condition with unilateral hypoplasia or complete or partial absence of the proximal femur associated with proximal femoral varus deformity. Associated abnormalities include asymmetry in muscle size with decrease in ipsilateral musculature and vessels. Abnormalities of the more distal limb may also be present, including agenesis of the cruciate ligaments and fibular agenesis. Several classification schemes have been proposed based on radiographic appearance or proposed therapy with the most widely known being the Aitken classification. In this classification, class A is a shortened femur with coxa vara and a normal acetabulum. Class B shows no apparent connection between the femoral head and shaft. In class C, the acetabulum is abnormal with a small or absent femoral head, whereas, in class D, both the femoral head and acetabulum are missing. However, cartilaginous connections are not well identified on radiograph and radiographic classification may be unreliable and underestimate the extent of cartilage present.[17]

When radiographic assessment fails to show the femoral head or proximal femur, MR imaging can help to identify the presence or absence of a cartilaginous anlage for the femoral head. MR imaging is more accurate than radiographic evaluation and can delineate the presence of cartilage across a proximal femoral bony gap to enable earlier appropriate intervention.[17,18] Thin-section coronal and axial imaging is required if a small femoral head is not to be missed.[13]

Congenital pseudarthrosis of the tibia

Congenital pseudarthrosis is an uncommon entity that usually becomes evident within the first year of life with angulation seen within the calf. There is typically unilateral segmental osseous weakness of the tibia resulting in anterolateral angulation of the tibia. MR imaging depicts the morphology of the pseudarthrosis and adjacent soft tissue deformity better than radiography. MR imaging can clearly show the type of pseudarthrosis, its length and structure, and whether there is union or nonunion of the bone. This information is of prognostic significance because the pseudarthrosis and affected periosteum need to be surgically removed. Associated soft tissue abnormalities, such as neurofibroma, can also be shown, although these may be at a site distant from the pseudarthrosis.[19] On MR imaging, the pseudarthrosis appears hyperintense on fat-suppressed and T2-W images, whereas, on T1-W images, it is usually hypointense. Contrast may help to define the lesion.

Congenital patellar dislocation

The patella develops as a sesamoid bone anterior to the femur. Congenital anomalies of the patella include its absence, hypoplasia, or dislocation. Absence or hypoplasia occur as part of several syndromes including nail-patella syndrome and genitopatella syndrome. Congenital dislocation of the patella (CPD) is uncommon.

CPD is believed to arise from failure of internal rotation of the myotome that forms the femur, the quadriceps muscle, and the extensor mechanism of the knee, occurring during the 8th to 10th week of embryologic life.[19] CPD usually presents at birth with characteristic genu valgum, flexion contracture, and external rotation of the tibia. However, some cases with less distinctive features do not present until later in childhood. Casting or surgical intervention is required to realign the maldeveloped, laterally displaced extensor mechanism to reduce or avoid long-term sequelae of knee dysfunction and early knee degeneration.[20]

Radiographs are used to confirm the diagnosis in older infants and children in whom the patella has ossified. Changes are also seen in the appearance of the femur and joint space. However, in the neonate, diagnosis is more difficult. Sonography can be used to identify the presence of a congenital dislocated patella. However, MR imaging provides an overall detailed anatomic perspective and permits better understanding of mutual anatomic relationships of involved structures.[21] Assessment with MR imaging can be performed with a 3D gradient sequence to highlight the cartilaginous patella. MR evaluation should describe the size, shape, and orientation of the developing patella, the size and position of the quadriceps muscle and its tendon, the patellar tendon, and the medial and lateral patellar retinacula. Assessment of the bones, including the femoral sulcus, the menisci, and ligaments of the knee, should also be included.[22] Thin sections are needed to avoid missing a small, hypoplastic patella.

Ankle/foot

Distinct entities of the foot and ankle, other than those related to a more generalized condition, are uncommon in the neonate. The most common concern is clubfoot, which occurs in 1:1000 newborns in North America.[13] The 2 classifications are postural or positional, which can be manipulated back into the correct alignment, or fixed. Imaging is performed after 4 to 12 weeks of unsuccessful conservative treatment, routinely with radiography. MR imaging is rarely needed for clubfoot. Although rarely used, the theoretic advantage of MR imaging is in visualizing the relationships of the cartilage anlagen.

Spine and pelvis

Evaluation of the lumbar neonatal spine is possible with ultrasound caused because of the cartilaginous nature of most vertebral bodies at this stage. The most common clinical finding in an otherwise normal infant, prompting evaluation, is the presence of a sacral dimple. Skilled clinicians can obtain a great deal of detail and information with ultrasound, but MR imaging is the modality of choice for a more detailed evaluation of the spinal column and cord, and any abnormality found on ultrasound is usually followed up with MR imaging (**Fig. 1**).

Congenital spine abnormalities result from interruption of the normal spinal development and can occur at any developmental stage. The entities range from simple solitary conditions affecting the spinal cord, such as a conus cyst, to more complex lesions such as spinal dysraphisms. Vertebral anomalies can also be solitary or occur as part of complex associations such as VACTERL (vertebral abnormalities, anal atresia, cardiac abnormalities, tracheoesophageal fistula and/or esophageal atresia, renal agenesis and dysplasia, and limb defects). Vertebral anomalies can be associated with pelvic abnormalities such as in caudal regression syndrome and sacral agenesis.

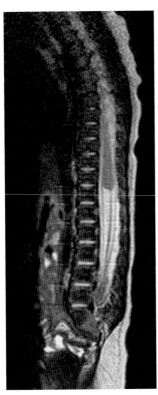

Fig. 1. One-week-old neonate with caudal regression syndrome and absence of the sacral segments. The cord ends at the level of T11, with a club-shaped distal cord.

A complete discussion of congenital spinal anomalies is beyond the scope of this review.

Conjoined Twins

Imaging is of paramount importance in the preoperative assessment of conjoined twins. MR imaging can be used prenatally, typically using single-shot fast spin-echo sequences. It has a larger FOV than sonography, which may be helpful in understanding the extent of fusion present. Commonly both CT and MR imaging are used after birth to give information regarding the bones, organs, vascular anatomy, and, when required, central nervous system. The classification of the twinning is according to the most prominent site of connection, with the most common site being the thorax (termed thoracopagus). Other connections include the abdomen (omphalopagus), sacrum (pygopagus), pelvis (ischiopagus), skull (craniopagus), face (cephalopagus), and back (rachipagus).[23] MR imaging can better show soft tissue anomalies, whereas CT better shows complex bony anatomy.

Musculoskeletal Infection

Although infection, including osteomyelitis, during the first month of life is uncommon, it is critical to consider this condition. Prompt treatment may avoid septic shock or devastating sequelae such as joint destruction. Infection of the neonatal musculoskeletal system differs from that seen in older children, often with a distinct presentation, patterns of bony involvement, and imaging appearance. Bones and joints of the lower limbs are most commonly affected but there can be involvement of the upper limbs, pelvis, and spine. Discitis is most commonly seen in the lumbar spine. The cartilaginous end plates are traversed by numerous canals through which small blood vessels pass. These vessels terminate adjacent to the intervertebral disc. There is a reduced rate of vertebral body infection because of the difference in neonatal blood supply. Sepsis may be multifocal in the neonate, including with neonatal septic arthritis, which can also be bilateral.

In the neonate, symptoms are often nonspecific, which may result in delayed diagnosis. In most cases, there is little or no evidence of infection, and presenting symptoms can be as vague as irritability or poor feeding. Clinical signs may include local swelling and erythema, or limitation or absence of spontaneous movement, termed pseudoparalysis of the affected limb.[24] The causal agent in the neonatal age group is most commonly *Staphylococcus aureus*, and the most frequent mode of transmission is hematogenous spread.[20] Other infectious agents include group B hemolytic streptococci and, less commonly, *Escherichia coli* and *Klebsiella*.[25] Neonates in intensive care are at increased risk of direct inoculation following procedures such as line placements. Delay in diagnosis and treatment, age of onset of infection, premature birth, and virulence of infecting organism influence the outcome. Delayed diagnosis can lead to marked deformity of any involved epiphysis and adjacent physis leading to an irregular ossification center, delayed appearance, or deformity after skeletal maturity.

As in older infants, it is the long bones, particularly of the lower extremities, that are most commonly affected. Infection begins in the dilated capillary loops of the metaphysis adjacent to the cartilaginous growth plate. In the neonate, persistent small vessels penetrate the cartilaginous epiphyseal plate and end in large venous lakes within the epiphysis.[26] Infection in the metaphysis may lead to invasion of the growth plate, spread through the transphyseal vessels into the epiphysis, or rupture through the cortex into the joint, subperiosteal space, or surrounding tissue.

By 12 to 18 months, the vascular connections between the metaphysis and epiphysis are significantly reduced and the cartilaginous growth plate acts as a relative barrier against the spread of infection.[26]

The diagnosis of osteomyelitis is based on the clinical response to antibiotics in conjunction with one or more of the following: positive blood cultures, growth from bone aspirates, positive cerebrospinal fluid culture, and typical radiographic changes that may be present initially or in follow-up.[27]

When clinical suspicion of osteomyelitis is raised in a neonate, the role of imaging is to identify all sites of bony abnormality, whether unifocal or multifocal, and whether there are any collections requiring drainage. Imaging evaluation begins with radiography. Soft tissue swelling and loss of soft tissue planes can be seen as early as 48 hours after the onset of symptoms; however, bony changes may not be seen until 7 to 10 days. Other findings can include joint space widening, subluxation, or frank dislocation. Radiographs may help differentiate other disorders clinically masquerading as osteomyelitis, including neonatal fractures and tumors.

The sensitivity of nuclear medicine studies in neonates is less than in older children, with a significant false-negative rate.[27] Sonography can detect soft tissue edema, subperiosteal collections, and joint effusions, but there is no consensus as to the role it should have in the work-up of suspected osteomyelitis. For experienced clinicians, it can be of use in the neonate for extremity osteomyelitis and septic arthritis, for which it can confirm joint effusions and guide needle aspirations.[28]

MR imaging has been shown to be of higher sensitivity and specificity in detecting osteomyelitis than skeletal scintigraphy. MR is excellent in depicting the presence of osteomyelitis and its complications, which include soft tissue and bone abscesses, physeal involvement, and septic arthritis, or, in the spine, the epidural space.[29] Discitis is more common in infants, whereas vertebral body infection is more common in adults.

Marrow edema is the earliest finding of acute osteomyelitis. On MR imaging, there is low SI on T1-W images, and increased SI on water-sensitive images. This condition occurs within 1 to 2 days after the onset of symptoms.[30] Early in the course of infection, the interface between normal and abnormal marrow is poorly defined, becoming better defined with increasing marrow signal as the infection progresses. Surrounding soft tissue inflammation is seen as ill-defined, high T2-W SI. Cortical bone may also show high T2-W SI, reflecting areas of destruction or infiltration, whereas periosteal reaction is seen as layered high SI on T2-W images. Subperiosteal collections are usually low SI on T1-W and high SI on T2-W images. The use of gadolinium intravenous contrast does not significantly improve the sensitivity or specificity of the diagnosis of osteomyelitis.[31] However, it is useful in distinguishing between edema and an abscess collection, and also in improving the confidence of physeal involvement or septic arthritis (**Fig. 2**). MR can be helpful in showing paraspinal abscesses along with spinal cord compression. Gadolinium administration is not needed if the unenhanced sequences do not show any evidence of inflammation.

Primary pyomyositis is a purulent, mostly staphylococcal infection occurring in skeletal muscle. Neonatal pyomyositis is less common than septic arthritis or osteomyelitis. MR imaging is helpful to differentiate between the early stage of diffuse muscle inflammation and subsequent abscess formation. MR is warranted if patients have clinical features of septic hip without ultrasound showing hip effusion or periosteal thickening.[32]

Trauma and Fractures

Neonatal brachial plexus injury
Neonatal brachial plexus palsy occurs in 1.5/1000 live births. Risk factors include shoulder dystocia, macrosomia, and breech delivery. Presentation of decreased spontaneous movements can be confused with other entities such as a fracture of the clavicle or humerus, or infection with septic arthritis and osteomyelitis.[9] Neonatal brachial plexus injury spontaneously recovers in 60% to 90%,[10] but, in those who do not resolve, there is weakness of the external rotators of the shoulder: the infraspinatus and teres minor.[11] MR can show the muscle asymmetry. Early nerve grafting within 3 months may improve functional outcome.[33] The decision as to whether surgery will be performed is based on the clinical severity of internal rotation contracture and external rotation weakness. Preoperative MR imaging of the glenohumeral deformity is helpful in surgical planning because the humeral head and glenoid are predominately cartilaginous.[11] However, this is not generally undertaken in the neonatal period.

Accidental or birth trauma versus nonaccidental injury
Fractures seldom occur during the birthing process. However, their incidence has decreased in recent years, presumably because of the increased number of caesarian sections for complicated pregnancies such as breech position and macrosomia.

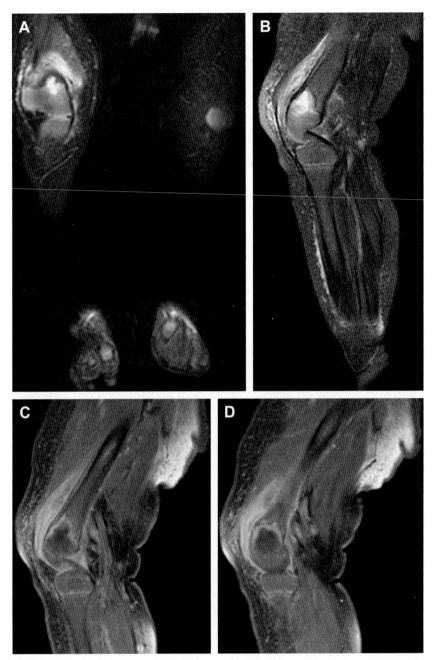

Fig. 2. Newborn with neonatal lupus, right foot swelling, and fever. Complicated osteomyelitis is present with an intraosseous abscess collection in the distal right femur well shown on the coronal and sagittal T2-W images (*A* and *B*) and postcontrast T1-W fat-suppressed images (*C* and *D*). The osteomyelitis involves the cartilaginous epiphysis, physis, and metaphysis. Adjacent soft tissue increased signal in keeping with inflammation is present along with periosteal reaction.

Commonly encountered birth fractures are seen in the clavicle and humerus. A delayed presentation of a neonatal fracture may raise the suspicion of nonaccidental injury.[34–36] The diagnosis of a neonatal fracture is usually made with plain film. In rare cases involving a physeal separation, ultrasound and MR imaging may be used to provide further delineation because radiography may not identify the displaced epiphysis because of its lack of ossification.[34]

Physeal separations are rare in newborns. There may be proximal or distal humeral, femoral, or even tibial involvement. Traumatic separation of the distal humeral epiphysis is usually the result of rotatory shear forces, typically seen following a difficult birth or child abuse. The injury can be overlooked in the newborn and not present until 9 to 30 days after birth. Clinical examination shows swollen elbow, pseudoparalysis, and muffled crepitus on movement. Radiographs show an altered relationship between distal humerus and proximal forearm, which is displaced posteromedially. MR imaging can show the fracture separation. Concomitant physeal fracture and infection can be seen as a rare complication of neonatal osteomyelitis or septic arthritis.[37] The hip is the joint most commonly affected with sepsis in such a fashion.

Neonatal compartment syndrome

Neonatal compartment syndrome is rare, of unknown cause, and is present at birth.[38] It produces skin lesions that involve 1 upper limb from elbow to wrist with variable severity. It is often mistaken for other entities such as amniotic band syndrome, neonatal gangrene, and necrotizing fasciitis. Early diagnosis is important but often difficult. Neonatal compartment syndrome differs from compartment syndrome in older children in that the length of ischemic insult is often unknown. On physical examination, areas of ischemia or necrosis are seen. It may require fasciotomy, surgical debridement, or skin grafting. MR imaging can identify the extent of ischemia and necrosis present and help guide surgical debridement of underlying muscle groups.

Benign Soft Tissue Tumors

Soft tissue tumors account for approximately 25% of all neonatal tumors. More than two-thirds are benign.[39] Imaging is often requested to help establish a diagnosis, and to evaluate lesion extent. MR imaging is the best modality to evaluate soft tissue masses and, in some cases, imaging features are diagnostic, such as in lipomas, hematomas, and subcutaneous fat necrosis.[9] However, histology is still often required to establish a definitive diagnosis.[40] The most common soft tissue masses in childhood are the vascular abnormalities. The classification system most widely used is that by Mulliken and Glowacki,[41] established in 1982. This system classifies lesions by clinical findings, histology, and cellular kinetics. Hemangiomas are neoplastic vascular lesions. They appear after birth and involute for a few years after a rapid growth phase. Vascular malformations are errors in vascular development that are always present at birth. They are classified by the main vascular channel within the lesion.[40]

Hemangiomas

The diagnosis of hemangiomas of infancy is most commonly made on clinical grounds alone, but imaging is required for atypical features such as lesions that are partly or totally subcutaneous. Most have a benign course, but there are some associated risks, such as with periocular or airway hemangiomas. The MR features reflect the biologic phase of the lesion. In the proliferative phase, the well-defined, lobulated lesion is isointense to muscle on T1-W images, and hyperintense on T2-W. Following contrast, there is homogeneously diffuse and persistent enhancement. Signal voids of the high-flow vessels are present on SE sequences. In the involuting phase, T1-W SI increases with time, reflecting its decreased vascularity and fatty replacement.[40]

Congenital hemangiomas are a separate group from hemangiomas of infancy. This group includes rapidly involuting congenital hemangiomas (RICH) and noninvoluting congenital hemangiomas (NICH).

Kaposiform hemangioendothelioma (KHE) is a rare vascular tumor that presents as a blue-red lesion within the first few months of life. It is associated with Kasabach-Merritt phenomenon, which is characterized by thrombocytopenia and hemorrhage in 50% of cases. This condition has a high mortality. On MR imaging, KHE can be differentiated from hemangiomas of infancy. There is involvement of multiple planes and thickening of the skin as well as subcutaneous stranding, edema, occasional hemosiderin deposits, and feeding vessels that are less prominent than in hemangioma of infancy. There can be changes to adjacent osseous structures caused by infiltration.[40]

Vascular malformations

The classification of vascular malformations is based on the main feeding vascular channel present.[42] They can be arteriovenous, venous, lymphatic, capillary, or mixed.

Arteriovenous malformations are high-flow lesions characterized by direct communication between the arterial and venous systems, with no capillary bed. Forty percent of cases are present at birth, and grow with the child. MR imaging shows enlarged vascular channels with dilated feeding and draining vessels. There is no associated mass. Perilesional edema may be present. The high-flow vessels appear as signal void foci on SE sequences, or high SI on enhanced images. Skin thickening and fat deposition may also be present.

Venous malformations have anomalous venous channels present. They may be small, or extensive, and may occur as part of syndromes such as Klippel-Trenaunay or Maffucci syndromes. On MR imaging, they show dilated tortuous veins, or lobulated masses made of multiple locules. The locules represent the dilated venous spaces separated by thin interstitial septa. They are isointense to hypointense to muscle on T1-W images, hyperintense on T2-W, and show patchy enhancement after gadolinium. Phleboliths may be present and appear as small, rounded signal void foci, and should be confirmed with radiography. Fluid-fluid levels may also be seen.

Localized lymphatic malformations (lymphangiomas) are divided into macrocystic (previously cystic hygromas) and microcystic types. Combined forms can also be seen. They are more frequent in the head and neck and usually visible at birth. On MR imaging, macrocystic lesions are clearly defined cysts, usually of low signal on T1-W images and high signal on T2-W images (**Fig. 3**). There are often fluid-fluid levels. The signal from within the cyst can vary based on the contents of the cyst, and whether hemorrhage

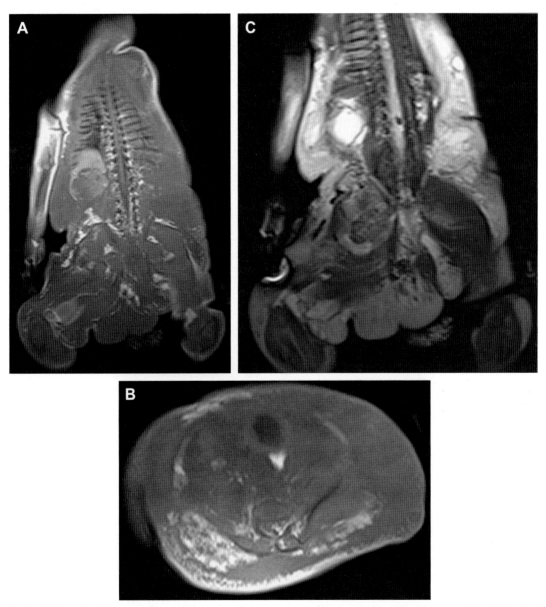

Fig. 3. A 27-week-old infant with hemihypertrophy and extensive lower trunk lymphangioma examined on day 1 of life primarily for central nervous concerns. Coronal and axial T1-W images (*A* and *B*) show extensive asymmetry of the chest and abdominopelvic wall, with predominantly low signal. High signal is present on coronal fat-suppressed turbo spin-echo T2-W imaging (*C*).

has occurred. With gadolinium, there is only enhancement of the septa, not the cyst itself, distinguishing this lesion from venous malformations. The tiny cysts of the microcystic type are not distinguishable on MR imaging. Instead, the lesions appear as diffuse areas of low signal on T1-W images and high signal on T2-W images. Following gadolinium, there may be mild or no enhancement.

Fibrous tumors

Fibrous tumors are uncommon in infancy. The most common is infantile myofibromatosis, which can involve skin, muscle, bone, and viscera. It is classified according to whether it is unicentric or multicentric (more common in girls) and whether there is visceral involvement. The typical appearance is of multiple soft tissue nodules in the subcutaneous tissues (usually affecting the head, neck, and trunk), or involving the skeleton, intestinal tract, heart, and lungs. If there is visceral involvement, the disease is lethal in 75% of cases, but otherwise recovery typically occurs.[43]

MR imaging SI can be variable, but is usually low on T1-W imaging and high or centrally low with high signal periphery on T2-W imaging. The center can be slightly high on T1-W imaging (**Fig. 4**). After gadolinium contrast, there can be peripheral enhancement, reflecting central necrosis or hemorrhage.[40,44,45]

Fibrous hamartoma of infancy

Fibrous hamartoma of infancy is a subcutaneous, freely mobile, painless tumor that is most common in the shoulder girdle of boys who are less than 2 years old. Histologically, the tumor comprises immature round to spindle cells arranged in an organized way with mucoid matrix admixed with mature fat.

On MR imaging, there are intermediate SI strands of fibrous tissue interspersed with fat. Lesions are usually 2.5 cm to 5 cm, but can be as large as 15 cm. The trabeculated appearance on MR imaging suggests fibrous hamartoma of infancy in the appropriate clinical setting.[40] The lesions are treated by excision.[43]

Fatty tumors

Lipoblastomas and lipoblastomatosis are benign neoplasms of immature or mature adipocytes. They are most common in the lower extremities, and most common in boys less than 3 years of age but can be present at birth. These tumors are usually bright on T2-W imaging and variable on T1-W imaging, depending on the maturity of the fat cells and the amount of myxoid material present. There is minimal enhancement when the tumor is predominately composed of fat.

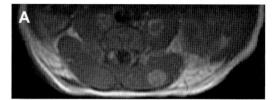
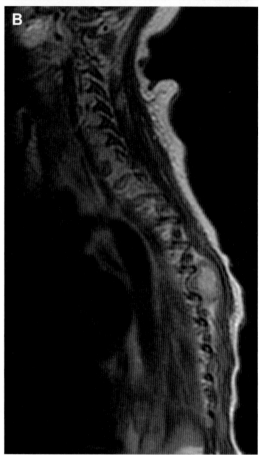

Fig. 4. One-week-old girl with multiple soft tissue nodules subsequently proved to be infantile myofibromatosis. Multiple small nodular lesions were noted within the retroperitoneal and paraspinal musculature. The lesions were isointense or increased in signal on axial (*A*) and sagittal (*B*) T1-W imaging compared with muscle and low signal on T2-W imaging.

Lipoblastoma is encapsulated, whereas lipoblastomatosis is not. Lipoblastomatosis can be infiltrative, and recur if resection is incomplete. Liposarcoma is rare in children, especially the very young. However, liposarcoma cannot be differentiated from lipoblastomatosis at MR imaging and tumor karyotyping is suggested.[41] MR imaging shows a mass that is isointense to muscle on T1-W images, and hyperintense on T2-W images with subtle and patchy linear areas of decreased SI.

Nerve sheath tumors

Neurofibromas are the result of proliferation of the connective tissue of the nerve sheaths. They occur commonly in patients with neurofibromatosis type 1. Plexiform neurofibromas have a more extensive extracellular matrix. There are 3 different types of growth pattern: superficial, displacing, and invasive. MR imaging features are typically of a beaded, undulating lesion isointense to muscle on T1-W imaging, and hyperintense on T2-W with avid enhancement. On cross section there is the typical target sign on T2-W images, which is the result of a central zone of tightly packed hypointense dense collagen surrounded by hyperintense myxomatous matrix. If the target is not present, this may be caused by hemorrhagic, cystic, or necrotic degeneration, and raises concern for malignant degeneration. This condition occurs in approx 10% of those with neurofibromatosis type 1, usually in a preexisting plexiform tumor.[43]

Fibromatosis colli

Fibromatosis colli usually presents in the first 2 to 3 weeks of life as a firm anterior neck mass that can lead to torticollis. The underlying disorder is a fusiform or eccentric expansion of the sternocleidomastoid muscle, which occurs in approximately 0.4% of infants. Its cause is unclear. The typical course of the mass is to increase in size for several weeks, and then spontaneously resolve in 90% in the next 8 months. Pathology examination shows myofibroblasts and fibroblasts in varying stages of differentiation. The younger the baby, the more immature the cells.[43]

Sonography is diagnostic in most cases, showing a well-defined, unilateral, fusiform expansion of the sternocleidomastoid muscle. On MR imaging, the mass is isointense to muscle on T1-W imaging, and hyperintense on T2-W images. There may be subtle patchy and linear areas of decreased SI. Alternative diagnoses of infection or tumor should be considered if there are any atypical features, such as extension beyond the sternocleidomastoid muscle or vascular encasement.

Subcutaneous fat necrosis of the newborn

Subcutaneous fat necrosis of the newborn is a rare, benign process in full-term infants. Trauma, hypoxia, and hypothermia may all play a role in the cause. Clinically, the lesions usually become apparent within the first month of life. The lesions are firm, well defined, nontender, and mobile. On imaging, there may be diffuse subcutaneous thickening to discrete nodules. They are usually found in the subcutaneous regions of the shoulders, back, buttocks and thighs, and cheeks. Fat necrosis is usually a self-limiting process with rare complications including hypercalcemia. The lack of a discrete mass in the imaging of fat necrosis is an important negative. Imaging characteristics of fat necrosis are linear abnormalities in SI (**Fig. 5**) (low on T1-W and T2-W images or high on T2-W images) and confinement to the subcutaneous tissue, often with lack of a discrete mass.[46]

Malignant Soft Tissue Tumors

Fibrosarcoma

Congenital or infantile fibrosarcoma is a separate entity from fibrosarcoma in older children and adults.[47] Occurring in children less than 1 year of age, it is most often found in the extremities. These tumors are large and bulky, and histologically are composed of anaplastic immature spindle cells arranged in a herringbone pattern. Metastases are rare, but there can be local invasion and recurrence following surgery.[43,48]

Fibrosarcomas can be cystic or solid. They are isointense to muscle on T1-W images, and of inhomogeneous high signal on T2-W images. Fibrosarcomas may also have inhomogeneous enhancement with gadolinium.[49]

Rhabdomyosarcoma

Rhabdomyosarcomas can present within the first month of life. In this age group, the location of this tumor differs, being more commonly found in the abdomen and pelvis or extremities, rather than the head and neck as in older patients. Prognosis is associated with the histologic type and tumor extent of the tumor, whether local or distant.[20,48]

MR imaging helps suggest the site of origin of the tumor, and identifies local and nodal spread. Following surgery, it is used for evaluation of recurrence. The tumor appears isointense on T1-W imaging, intermediate to high on T2-W imaging, and there is usually intense enhancement following contrast administration (**Fig. 6**). Vessels within the tumor may have high flow leading to signal voids.[43]

Liposarcoma

Liposarcomas are exceedingly rare in the neonate, but remain in the differential of soft tissue masses that contain fat. Histologically, they can be difficult to distinguish from lipoblastomas. Liposarcoma has metastatic potential, but metastases are rare. With surgical excision, prognosis is good. Of the different histologic types, myxoid tends to occur in infants.[48] At MR imaging, it is not possible

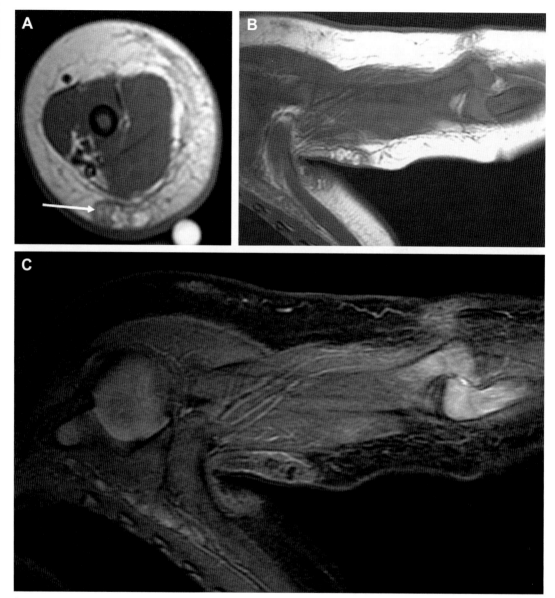

Fig. 5. A 3-month-old girl with induration and swelling adjacent to the left shoulder noted shortly after birth, consistent with subcutaneous fat necrosis. Axial and coronal (*A* and *B*) T1-W views of left arm show uniform hypodense hematopoietic bone marrow. Low signal irregularity of the periaxillary subcutaneous fat is present (*arrow*). Fast spin-echo inversion recovery (*C*) showing increased signal on coronal fast-spin echo inversion recovery view.

to reliably distinguish liposarcoma from lipoblasto-matosis, and genetic testing is required.[43]

Synovial sarcoma

Synovial sarcomas originate from mesenchymal cells that differentiate to look like synovium, rather than being derived from synovium itself. They are more commonly seen in adults, but can occur in children and infants. The lesions are usually found in the lower extremities, classically around a joint, and more rarely in the abdominal and thoracic walls. The prognosis is excellent with complete resection.[28]

Radiographically, the findings are nonspecific. Usually, a soft tissue mass of water density is present and, in up to 30% of cases, calcification may be seen. Bone involvement may be present in up to 20% of cases. Spread is along myofascial planes, and the size of the tumor is often larger than is clinically suspected.[28]

Synovial sarcomas are usually large at diagnosis, with lobulated margins and the appearance

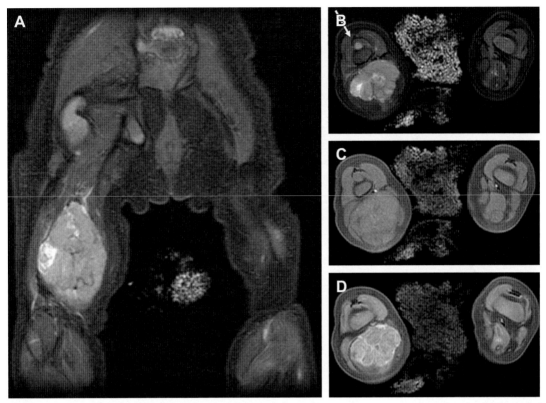

Fig. 6. A 3-week-old girl with metastatic posterior right thigh rhabdomyosarcoma. Coronal and axial (A and B) fast spin-echo (FSE) T2-W images show large, high-signal, posterior thigh mass. Axial fat-suppressed T1-W images before and after intravenous administration of contrast (C and D) show intense enhancement. Numerous other, smaller lesions were present in the pelvic thigh musculature (arrow).

of a capsule. On T1-W imaging, they are isointense to muscle, whereas on T2-W imaging it is heterogeneous but hyperintense. There may be hemorrhage and fluid-fluid levels, or the tumor may be entirely cystic. In 25%, mineralization may be present.[43]

Sacrococcygeal teratomas

Sacrococcygeal teratomas most commonly present at antenatal imaging or in the newborn as a mass in the sacrum or buttocks. They range from benign well-differentiated cystic lesions to malignant solid masses. In general, teratomas are derived from pluripotent stem cells with the ability to differentiate into any of the 3 germ cell layers. The location of sacrococcygeal teratomas is usually postsacral, but they can be presacral and there is often an association with vertebral anomalies. In general, there is a good outcome, but malignancy can be present.[20] MR findings depend on the specific underlying disorder, typically with large solid and cystic tumor components **(Fig. 7)**.

Bone Tumors

MR imaging may further characterize a lesion following radiography, and be used for staging and treatment planning as well as in posttherapy follow-up. MR imaging is nonspecific in histology characterization, and radiography remains the basis for generating a differential diagnosis. MR imaging has the ability to show both intraosseous and extraosseous components of aggressive tumors.[50] Estimation of the intramedullary extent, cortical involvement, and epiphyseal and joint space invasion are all possible, as well as evaluation for same bone and skip lesions. MR imaging is also useful for the assessment of ligamentous, tendinous, and neurovascular involvement. It provides important information for surgical planning, and assessment of response to therapy through signal characteristics and tumor size.

MR imaging should include conventional T1-W and T2-W sequences with and without fat saturation; STIR and T1-W images after contrast administration are acquired in at least 2

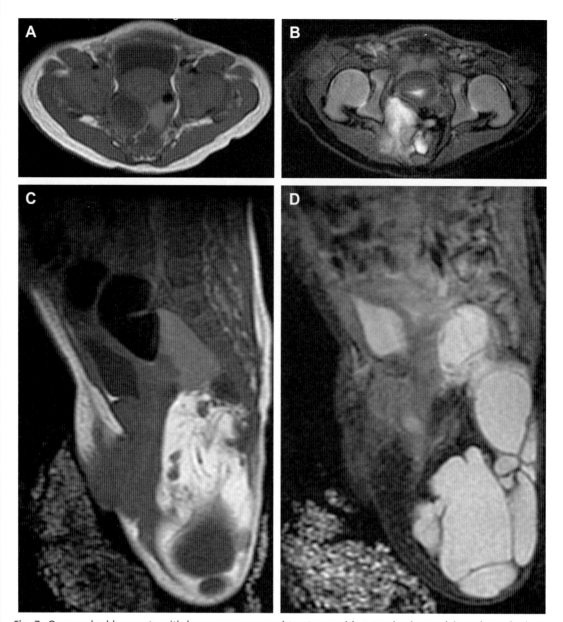

Fig. 7. One-week-old neonate with large sacrococcygeal teratoma with extensive intrapelvic and exophytic ex-trapelvic components (*A–D*). Complex cystic and solid components are present with extensive fat, well shown on the axial T1-W (*A*) and FSE fat-suppressed T2-W (*B*) images of the pelvis and the sagittal T1-W and fat-suppressed T2-W images (*C* and *D*) of the lower spine and pelvis.

planes. Pathologic tissues generally appear as low SI on T1 images and high on T2-W and STIR images.[51]

Bone tumors, both benign and malignant, are rare in the neonate. Ewing sarcoma has been re-ported in neonates, and is predominantly of the axial skeleton,[52] with a rare case of an infant with MR findings of a neoplastic process in the humerus ultimately also shown to be Ewing sarcoma.[53]

Metastases to Bone and Soft Tissue

Neuroblastoma

Neuroblastoma is the second most common solid malignancy of infancy and childhood, and the most common malignancy of the newborn. Nearly 60% have metastatic disease at diagnosis, most commonly to the liver (65%), subcutaneous nodules (32%), and bone (3%). A case was pre-sented with metastasis to the heart and skeletal muscle, for which MR imaging was the superior imaging modality, showing the skeletal muscle metastasis that CT had not shown. MR imaging shows low T1-W and high T2-W SI with prominent gadolinium enhancement.[54]

Miscellaneous: postmortem imaging

As the number of autopsies has been declining worldwide, increased interest in other methods of obtaining postmortem information has developed. Postmortem radiology, or virtual autopsy, may be a more acceptable alternative to relatives of the deceased than an formal invasive autopsy. Conventional radiography remains the main form of postmortem imaging. Gestational age and the presence of underlying anomalies such as skeletal dysplasias can be assessed. MR imaging has been used mostly for assessment of the central nervous system, body, and extremity.[55]

SUMMARY

Experience in MR imaging of the neonatal musculoskeletal system is rapidly increasing. The exquisite ability of MR imaging to image the soft tissues, especially cartilage, without radiation is its key strength. Although it is not practical or sensible to undertake MR imaging in conditions in which radiography and ultrasound provide adequate information, MR is proving to be a useful adjunct and problem-solving tool in many neonatal musculoskeletal conditions.

REFERENCES

1. Mathur AM, Neil JJ, McKinstry RC, et al. Transport, monitoring, and successful brain MR imaging in unsedated neonates. Pediatr Radiol 2008;38:260–4.

2. Jaramillo D, Laor T. Pediatric musculoskeletal MRI: basic principles to optimize success. Pediatr Radiol 2008;38:379–91.

3. Burdiles A, Babyn PS. Pediatric bone marrow MR imaging. Magn Reson Imaging Clin N Am 2009;17:391–409, v.

4. Chavhan GB, Babyn PS. Pediatric musculoskeletal imaging at 3 Tesla. Semin Musculoskelet Radiol 2009;13:181–95.

5. Laor T, Jaramillo D. MR imaging insights into skeletal maturation: what is normal? Radiology 2009;250:28–38.

6. Barnewolt C, Shapiro F, Jaramillo D. Normal gadolinium-enhanced MR imaging of the developing appendicular skeleton. Part 1. Cartilaginous epiphysis and physis. AJR Am J Roentgenol 1997;169:183–9.

7. Khanna P, Thapa M. The growing skeleton: MR imaging appearances of developing cartilage. Magn Reson Imaging Clin N Am 2009;17(3):411–21.

8. Sze G, Baierl P, Bravo S. Evolution of the infant spinal column: evaluation with MR imaging. Radiology 1991;181:819–27.

9. Herring JA. Tachdjian's pediatric orthopedics. Philadelphia: Saunders Elsevier; 2007.

10. Greenwald AG, Schute PC, Shiveley JL. Brachial plexus birth palsy: a 10-year report on the incidence and prognosis. J Pediatr Orthop 1984;4:689–92.

11. Emery KH. MR imaging in congenital and acquired disorders of the pediatric upper extremity. Magn Reson Imaging Clin N Am 2009;17:549–70, vii.

12. Laor T, Jaramillo D, Hoffer FA, et al. MR imaging in congenital lower limb deformities. Pediatr Radiol 1996;26:381–7.

13. Dwek JR. The hip: MR imaging of uniquely pediatric disorders. Magn Reson Imaging Clin N Am 2009;17:509–20, vi.

14. Westhoff B, Wild A, Seller K, et al. Magnetic resonance imaging after reduction for congenital dislocation of the hip. Arch Orthop Trauma Surg 2003;123:289–92.

15. Jaramillo D, Villegas-Medina O, Laor T, et al. Gadolinium-enhanced MR imaging of pediatric patients after reduction of dysplastic hips: assessment of femoral head position, factors impeding reduction, and femoral head ischemia. AJR Am J Roentgenol 1998;170:1633–7.

16. Tiderius C, Jaramillo D, Connolly S, et al. Post-closed reduction perfusion magnetic resonance imaging as a predictor of avascular necrosis in developmental hip dysplasia: a preliminary report. J Pediatr Orthop 2009;29(1):14–20.

17. Maldjian C, Patel TY, Klein RM, et al. Efficacy of MRI in classifying proximal focal femoral deficiency. Skeletal Radiol 2007;36:215–20.

18. Carpineta L, Faingold R, Albuquerque PA, et al. Magnetic resonance imaging of pelvis and hips in infants, children, and adolescents: a pictorial review. Curr Probl Diagn Radiol 2007;36:143–52.

19. Mahnken AH, Staatz G, Hermanns B, et al. Congenital pseudarthrosis of the tibia in pediatric patients: MR imaging. AJR Am J Roentgenol 2001;177:1025–9.

20. Martin R, Fanaroff A, Walsh M. Fanaroff and Martin's Neonatal perinatal medicine: disease of the fetus and infant. 8th edition. St Louis: Mosby; 2005.

21. Borowski A, Grissom L, Littleton AG, et al. Diagnostic imaging of the knee in children with arthrogryposis and knee extension or hyperextension contracture. J Pediatr Orthop 2008;28:466–70.

22. Koplewitz BZ, Babyn PS, Cole WG. Congenital dislocation of the patella. AJR Am J Roentgenol 2005;184:1640–6.

23. Kingston CA, McHugh K, Kumaradevan J, et al. Imaging in the preoperative assessment of conjoined twins. Radiographics 2001;21:1187–208.

24. Korakaki E, Aligizakis A, Manoura A, et al. Methicillin-resistant *Staphylococcus aureus* osteomyelitis

and septic arthritis in neonates: diagnosis and management. Jpn J Infect Dis 2007;60:129–31.

25. Trobs R, Moritz R, Buhligen U, et al. Changing pattern of osteomyelitis in infants and children. Pediatr Surg Int 1999;15:363–72.

26. Asmar BI. Osteomyelitis in the neonate. Infect Dis Clin North Am 1992;6:117–32.

27. Ash JM, Gilday DL. The futility of bone scanning in neonatal osteomyelitis: concise communication. J Nucl Med 1980;21:417–20.

28. Israels SJ, Chan HS, Daneman A, et al. Synovial sarcoma in childhood. AJR Am J Roentgenol 1984; 142:803–6.

29. Jaramillo D, Treves ST, Kasser JR, et al. Osteomyelitis and septic arthritis in children: appropriate use of imaging to guide treatment. AJR Am J Roentgenol 1995;165:399–403.

30. Ranson M. Imaging of pediatric musculoskeletal infection. Semin Musculoskelet Radiol 2009;13: 277–99.

31. Averill LW, Hernandez A, Gonzalez L, et al. Diagnosis of osteomyelitis in children utility of fat-suppressed contrast-enhanced MRI. AJR Am J Roentgenol 2009;192:1232–8.

32. Falesi M, Regazoni BM, Wytlenbach M, et al. Primary pelvic pyomyositis in a neonate. J Perinatol 2009;29(12):830–1.

33. Chuang DC, Mardini S, Ma HS. Surgical strategy for infant obstetrical brachial plexus palsy: experiences at Chang Gung Memorial Hospital. Plast Reconstr Surg 2005;116:132–42 [discussion: 143–4].

34. Brown J, Eustace S. Neonatal transphyseal supracondylar fracture detected by ultrasound. Pediatr Emerg Care 1997;13:410–2.

35. Stranzinger E, Kellenberger CJ, Braunschweig S, et al. Whole-body STIR MR imaging in suspected child abuse: an alternative to skeletal survey radiography? Eur J Radiol Extra 2007;63:43–7.

36. Campbell AN, Chan HS, O'Brien A, et al. Malignant tumours in the neonate. Arch Dis Child 1987;62: 19–23.

37. Schiavon R, Borgo A, Micaghio A. Septic physeal separation of proximal femur in a newborn. J Orthop Traumatol 2009;10:105–10.

38. Allen LM, Benacci JC, Trane RN. Neonatal compartment syndrome. Am J Perinatol 2010;27:103–6.

39. Minard-Colin V, Orbach D, Martelli H, et al. Soft tissue tumors in neonates. Arch Pediatr 2009;16: 1039–48 [in French].

40. Navarro OM. Imaging of benign pediatric soft tissue tumors. Semin Musculoskelet Radiol 2009; 13:196–209.

41. Mulliken JB, Glowacki J. Hemangiomas and vascular malformations in infants and children: a classification based on endothelial characteristics. Plast Reconstr Surg 1982;69:412–22.

42. Moukaddam H, Pollak J, Haims AH. MRI characteristics and classification of peripheral vascular malformations and tumors. Skeletal Radiol 2009;38:535–47.

43. Stein-Wexler R. MR imaging of soft tissue masses in children. Magn Reson Imaging Clin N Am 2009;17: 489–507, vi.

44. Koujok K, Ruiz RE, Hernandez RJ. Myofibromatosis: imaging characteristics. Pediatr Radiol 2005;35: 374–80.

45. Teo HE, Peh WC, Chan MY, et al. Infantile lipofibromatosis of the upper limb. Skeletal Radiol 2005;34: 799–802.

46. Anderson DR, Narla LD, Dunn NL. Subcutaneous fat necrosis of the newborn. Pediatr Radiol 1999;29: 794–6.

47. Gulhan B, Kupeli S, Yalcin B, et al. An unusual presentation of infantile fibrosarcoma in a male newborn. Am J Perinatol 2009;26:331–3.

48. Palumbo JS, Zwerdling T. Soft tissue sarcomas of infancy. Semin Perinatol 1999;23:299–309.

49. Jimenez RM, Jaramillo D, Connolly SA. Imaging of the pediatric hand: soft tissue abnormalities. Eur J Radiol 2005;56:344–57.

50. Moore SG, Bisset GS 3rd, Siegel MJ, et al. Pediatric musculoskeletal MR imaging. Radiology 1991;179: 345–60.

51. Balassy C, Hormann M. Role of MRI in paediatric musculoskeletal conditions. Eur J Radiol 2008;68: 245–58.

52. van den Berg H, Dirksen U, Ranft A, et al. Ewing tumors in infants. Pediatr Blood Cancer 2008;50: 761–4.

53. Hsieh HY, Hsiao CC, Chen WS, et al. Congenital Ewing's sarcoma of the humerus. Br J Radiol 1998; 71:1313–6.

54. Faingold R, Babyn PS, Yoo SJ, et al. Neuroblastoma with atypical metastases to cardiac and skeletal muscles: MRI features. Pediatr Radiol 2003;33:584–6.

55. Sieswerda-Hoogendoorn T, van Rijn RR. Current techniques in postmortem imaging with specific attention to paediatric applications. Pediatr Radiol 2010;40:141–52 [quiz: 259].

Index

Note: Page numbers of article titles are in **boldface** type.

Magn Reson Imaging Clin N Am 19 (2011) 859–861
doi:10.1016/S1064-9689(11)00111-5

United States Postal Service

Statement of Ownership, Management, and Circulation
(All Periodicals Publications Except Requestor Publications)

1. Publication Title	2. Publication Number	3. Filing Date
Magnetic Resonance Imaging Clinics of North America	0 1 1 1 - 9 0 0 9	9/16/11

4. Issue Frequency	5. Number of Issues Published Annually	6. Annual Subscription Price
Feb, May, Aug, Nov	4	$309.00

7. Complete Mailing Address of Known Office of Publication (Not printer) (Street, city, county, state, and ZIP+4®)

Elsevier Inc.
360 Park Avenue South
New York, NY 10010-1710

Contact Person
Stephen Bushing
Telephone (Include area code)
215-239-3688

8. Complete Mailing Address of Headquarters or General Business Office of Publisher (Not printer)

Elsevier Inc., 360 Park Avenue South, New York, NY 10010-1710

9. Full Names and Complete Mailing Addresses of Publisher, Editor, and Managing Editor (Do not leave blank)

Publisher (Name and complete mailing address)

Kim Murphy, Elsevier, Inc., 1600 John F. Kennedy Blvd. Suite 1800, Philadelphia, PA 19103-2899

Editor (Name and complete mailing address)

Barton Dudlick, Elsevier, Inc., 1600 John F. Kennedy Blvd. Suite 1800, Philadelphia, PA 19103-2899

Managing Editor (Name and complete mailing address)

Barton Dudlick, Elsevier, Inc., 1600 John F. Kennedy Blvd. Suite 1800, Philadelphia, PA 19103-2899

10. Owner (Do not leave blank. If the publication is owned by a corporation, give the name and address of the corporation immediately followed by the names and addresses of all stockholders owning or holding 1 percent or more of the total amount of stock. If not owned by a corporation, give the names and addresses of the individual owners. If owned by a partnership or other unincorporated firm, give its name and address as well as those of each individual owner. If the publication is published by a nonprofit organization, give its name and address.)

Full Name	Complete Mailing Address
Wholly owned subsidiary of	4520 East-West Highway
Reed/Elsevier, US holdings	Bethesda, MD 20814

11. Known Bondholders, Mortgagees, and Other Security Holders Owning or Holding 1 Percent or More of Total Amount of Bonds, Mortgages, or Other Securities. If none, check box. ☐ None

Full Name	Complete Mailing Address
N/A	

12. Tax Status (For completion by nonprofit organizations authorized to mail at nonprofit rates) (Check one)
The purpose, function, and nonprofit status of this organization and the exempt status for federal income tax purposes:
☐ Has Not Changed During Preceding 12 Months
☐ Has Changed During Preceding 12 Months (Publisher must submit explanation of change with this statement)

PS Form 3526, September 2007 (Page 1 of 3 (Instructions Page 3)) PSN 7530-01-000-9931 PRIVACY NOTICE: See our Privacy policy in www.usps.com

---

13. Publication Title	14. Issue Date for Circulation Data Below
Magnetic Resonance Imaging Clinics of North America	August 2011

15. Extent and Nature of Circulation		Average No. Copies Each Issue During Preceding 12 Months	No. Copies of Single Issue Published Nearest to Filing Date
a. Total Number of Copies (Net press run)		2710	1766
b. Paid Circulation (By Mail and Outside the Mail)	(1) Mailed Outside-County Paid Subscriptions Stated on PS Form 3541 (Include paid distribution above nominal rate, advertiser's proof copies, and exchange copies)	1151	1232
	(2) Mailed In-County Paid Subscriptions Stated on PS Form 3541 (Include paid distribution above nominal rate, advertiser's proof copies, and exchange copies)		
	(3) Paid Distribution Outside the Mails Including Sales Through Dealers and Carriers, Street Vendors, Counter Sales, and Other Paid Distribution Outside USPS®	325	345
	(4) Paid Distribution by Other Classes Mailed Through the USPS (e.g. First-Class Mail®)		
c. Total Paid Distribution (Sum of 15b (1), (2), (3), and (4))	▶	1476	1577
d. Free or Nominal Rate Distribution (By Mail and Outside the Mail)	(1) Free or Nominal Rate Outside-County Copies Included on PS Form 3541	72	55
	(2) Free or Nominal Rate In-County Copies Included on PS Form 3541		
	(3) Free or Nominal Rate Copies Mailed at Other Classes Through the USPS (e.g. First-Class Mail)		
	(4) Free or Nominal Rate Distribution Outside the Mail (Carriers or other means)		
e. Total Free or Nominal Rate Distribution (Sum of 15d (1), (2), (3) and (4))	▶	72	55
f. Total Distribution (Sum of 15c and 15e)	▶	1548	1632
g. Copies not Distributed (See instructions to publishers #4 (page #3))	▶	1162	134
h. Total (Sum of 15f and g)	▶	2710	1766
i. Percent Paid (15c divided by 15f times 100)		95.35%	96.63%

16. Publication of Statement of Ownership

☐ If the publication is a general publication, publication of this statement is required. Will be printed in the November 2011 issue of this publication.   ☐ Publication not required

17. Signature and Title of Editor, Publisher, Business Manager, or Owner	Date
[signature] Stephen R. Bushing –Inventory Distribution Coordinator	September 16, 2011

I certify that all information furnished on this form is true and complete. I understand that anyone who furnishes false or misleading information on this form or who omits material or information requested on the form may be subject to criminal sanctions (including fines and imprisonment) and/or civil sanctions (including civil penalties).

PS Form 3526, September 2007 (Page 2 of 3)

Moving?

Make sure your subscription moves with you!

To notify us of your new address, find your **Clinics Account Number** (located on your mailing label above your name), and contact customer service at:

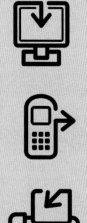

Email: journalscustomerservice-usa@elsevier.com

800-654-2452 (subscribers in the U.S. & Canada)
314-447-8871 (subscribers outside of the U.S. & Canada)

Fax number: 314-447-8029

Elsevier Health Sciences Division
Subscription Customer Service
3251 Riverport Lane
Maryland Heights, MO 63043

ELSEVIER